Study Guide for

Fundamentals of Nursing

Ninth Edition

Study Guide for

Fundamentals of Nursing

Ninth Edition

Geralyn Ochs, RN, AGACNP-BC, ACNP-BC, ANP-BC
Associate Professor of Nursing
Coordinator of the Adult Gerontological Acute Care Nurse Practitioner Program
St. Louis University School of Nursing
St. Louis, Missouri

ELSEVIER

ELSEVIER

3251 Riverport Lane
St. Louis, Missouri 63043

Notices

Knowledge and best practice in this field are constantly changing. As new research and experience broaden our understanding, changes in research methods, professional practices, or medical treatment may become necessary.

Practitioners and researchers must always rely on their own experience and knowledge in evaluating and using any information, methods, compounds, or experiments described herein. In using such information or methods they should be mindful of their own safety and the safety of others, including parties for whom they have a professional responsibility.

With respect to any drug or pharmaceutical products identified, readers are advised to check the most current information provided (i) on procedures featured or (ii) by the manufacturer of each product to be administered, to verify the recommended dose or formula, the method and duration of administration, and contraindications. It is the responsibility of practitioners, relying on their own experience and knowledge of their patients, to make diagnoses, to determine dosages and the best treatment for each individual patient, and to take all appropriate safety precautions.

To the fullest extent of the law, neither the Publisher nor the authors, contributors, or editors, assume any liability for any injury and/or damage to persons or property as a matter of products liability, negligence or otherwise, or from any use or operation of any methods, products, instructions, or ideas contained in the material herein.

Executive Content Strategist: Tamara Myers
Content Development Manager: Jean Sims Fornango
Senior Content Development Specialist: Tina Kaemmerer
Publishing Services Manager: Hemamalini Rajendrababu
Project Manager: Minerva Irene Viloria

Printed in the United States of America

Last digit is the print number: 9 8 7 6 5 4 3 2

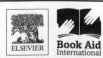

Working together
to grow libraries in
developing countries

www.elsevier.com • www.bookaid.org

Introduction

The *Study Guide for Fundamentals of Nursing*, Ninth Edition, has been developed to encourage independent learning for beginning nursing students. As a beginning nursing student, you may be wondering, "How will I possibly learn all of the material in this chapter?" The essential objective of this study guide is to assist you in this endeavor by helping you learn *what* you need to know and then testing what you have learned with hundreds of review questions.

This study guide follows the textbook layout chapter for chapter. For each chapter your instructor assigns, you will use the same chapter number in this study guide. The outline format was designed to help you learn to read nursing content more effectively and with greater understanding. Each chapter of this study guide has several sections to assist you to comprehend and recall.

The *Preliminary Reading* section is designed to teach prereading strategies. You will become familiar with the chapter by first reading the chapter title, key terms, objectives, key points (found at the end of each chapter), as well as all main headings. Also pay close attention to all illustrations, tables, and boxes. This can be done rather quickly and will give you an overall idea of the content of the chapter.

Next you will find the *Comprehensive Understanding* section, which is in outline format. This will prove to be a very valuable tool not only as you first read the chapter but also as you review for exams. This outline identifies both topics and main ideas for each chapter as an aid to concentration, comprehension, and retaining textbook information. By completing this outline, you will learn to "pull out" key information in the chapter. As you write the answers in the study guide, you will be reinforcing that content. Once completed, this outline will serve as a review tool for exams.

The review questions in each chapter provide a valuable means of testing and reinforcing your knowledge of the material. All questions are multiple choice. As a further means for independent learning, each answer requires a rationale (the reason *why* the option you selected is correct). After you have completed the review questions, you can check the answers in the back of the study guide.

Chapters 27 and 34–50 include exercises based on the care plans and concept maps found in the text. These exercises provide practice in synthesizing nursing process and critical thinking as you, the nurse, care for patients. Taking one aspect of the nursing process, you will be asked to imagine you are the nurse in the case study and write your answers in the appropriate boxes. You will have to think about what knowledge, experiences, standards, and attitudes might be used in caring for the patient.

When you finish answering the review questions and exercises, take a few minutes for self-evaluation using the Answer Key. If you answered a question incorrectly, begin to analyze the thoughts that led you to the wrong answer:

- Did you miss the key word or phrase?
- Did you read into something that wasn't stated?
- Did you not understand the subject matter?
- Did you use an incorrect rationale for selecting your response?

Each incorrect response is an opportunity to learn. Go back to the text and reread any content that is still unclear. In the long run, it will be a time-saving activity.

The learning activities presented in this study guide will assist you in completing the semester with a firm understanding of nursing concepts and process that you can rely on for your entire professional career.

Contents

UNIT VII PHYSIOLOGICAL BASIS FOR NURSING PRACTICE

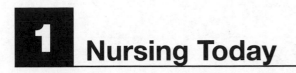

Nursing Today

PRELIMINARY READING

Chapter 1, pp. 1-13

COMPREHENSIVE UNDERSTANDING

Nursing as a Profession

1. According to Benner, an expert nurse goes through five levels of proficiency. Identify them.

    a. _____

    b. _____

    c. _____

    d. _____

    e. _____

2. What are the ANA Standards of Practice?

    a. _____

    b. _____

    c. _____

    d. _____

    e. _____

    f. _____

3. Define *nursing* (according to the American Nursing Association [ANA]).

    _____

    _____

    _____

4. Identify the ANA Standards of Professional Performance.

    a. _____

    b. _____

    c. _____

    d. _____

    e. _____

    f. _____

g. _____

h. _____

i. _____

j. _____

5. Describe nursing's code of ethics.

_____

_____

_____

Professional Responsibilities and Roles

Match the following.

6. _____ Autonomy
7. _____ Caregiver
8. _____ Advocate
9. _____ Educator
10. _____ Communicator
11. _____ Manager
12. _____ Advanced Practice Registered Nurse (APRN)
13. _____ Clinical Nurse Specialist (CNS)
14. _____ Nurse Practitioner
15. _____ Certified Nurse-Midwife (CNM)
16. _____ Certified Registered Nurse Anesthetist (CRNA)
17. _____ Nurse educator
18. _____ Nursing administrator
19. _____ Nurse researcher

a. Investigates problems to improve nursing care and to expand the scope of nursing practice
b. Independent nursing interventions that the nurse initiates without medical orders
c. Is central to the nurse–patient relationship
d. Helps the patient maintain and regain health, manage disease and symptoms, and attain a maximal level of function and independence
e. Manages patient care and the delivery of specific nursing services within a health care agency
f. Has personnel, policy, and budgetary responsibility for a specific nursing unit
g. Explains, demonstrates, reinforces, and evaluates the patient's progress in learning
h. Works primarily in schools of nursing and staff development
i. Expert clinician in a specialized area of practice
j. Involves the independent care for women in normal pregnancy, labor, and delivery and care of newborns
k. Detects and manages self-limiting acute and chronic stable medical conditions
l. Provides surgical anesthesia
m. Four core roles: certified nurse-midwife, certified nurse practitioner, clinical nurse specialist, and certified registered nurse anesthetist
n. Protects patients' human and legal rights and provides assistance in asserting these rights

Historical Highlights

20. How did Florence Nightingale see the role of the nurse in the early 1800s?

_____

_____

_____

Match the following.

21. _____ Clara Barton
22. _____ Lillian Wald and Mary Brewster
23. _____ Mary Adelaide Nutting
24. _____ Mary Mahoney

a. First professionally trained African-American nurse
b. Instrumental in moving nursing education into universities
c. Opened the Henry Street Settlement, focusing on the health needs of the poor
d. Founder of the American Red Cross

Contemporary Influences

25. What are the external forces that have affected nursing practice in the twenty-first century?

    a. _____

    b. _____

    c. _____

    d. _____

    e. _____

26. Explain *compassion fatigue*:

    _____

    _____

    _____

Trends in Nursing

27. Identify the competencies of the QSEN initiative.

    a. _____

    b. _____

    c. _____

    d. _____

    e. _____

28. Define the term *genomics*.

    _____

    _____

    _____

Professional Registered Nurse Education

Match the following.

29. _____ Associate's degree
30. _____ Baccalaureate degree
31. _____ Master's degree
32. _____ Doctor of Philosophy
33. _____ Doctor of Nursing Practice
34. _____ In-service education
35. _____ Continuing education

a. A practice-focused doctorate
b. Emphasizes research-based clinical practice
c. Emphasizes advanced knowledge in basic sciences and research-based clinical courses
d. A 4-year program that includes social sciences, arts, and humanities
e. Rigorous research and theory development
f. Formal, organized educational programs offered by various institutions
g. Instruction or training provided by health care agencies

Nursing Practice

36. What is the purpose of Nurse Practice Acts?

    _____

    _____

    _____

37. The examination for RN *licensure* provides:

    _____

    _____

    _____

38. The value of *certification* is:

_____

_____

_____

Professional Nursing Organizations

39. The goals of any professional nursing organization is to:

_____

_____

_____

REVIEW QUESTIONS

Select the appropriate answer and cite the rationale for choosing that particular answer.

40. The factor that best advanced the practice of nursing in the twenty-first century was:
    1. Growth of cities
    2. Teachings of Christianity
    3. Better education of nurses
    4. Improved conditions for women

    Answer: _____ Rationale: _____

    _____

    _____

41. Graduate nurses must pass a licensure examination administered by the:
    1. State Boards of Nursing
    2. National League for Nursing
    3. Accredited school of nursing
    4. American Nurses Association

    Answer: _____ Rationale: _____

    _____

    _____

42. A group that lobbies at the state and federal levels for advancement of nurses' role, economic interests, and health care is the:
    1. State Boards of Nursing
    2. American Nurses Association
    3. American Hospital Association
    4. National Student Nurses Association

    Answer: _____ Rationale: _____

    _____

    _____

2 The Health Care Delivery System

PRELIMINARY READING

Chapter 2, pp. 14-30

COMPREHENSIVE UNDERSTANDING

1. The Institute of Medicine (2011) vision to transform health care delivery states that nurses need:

   a. _____

   b. _____

   c. _____

   d. _____

Health Care Regulation and Reform

Match the following.

2. _____ Professional standards review organizations (PSROs)
3. _____ Utilization review (UR) committees
4. _____ Prospective payment system (PPS)
5. _____ Diagnosis-related groups (DRGs)
6. _____ Capitation
7. _____ Resource utilization groups (RUGs)
8. _____ Managed care

a. Review the admissions and identify and eliminate overuse of diagnostic and treatment services
b. Eliminated cost-based reimbursement
c. Review the quality, quantity, and cost of hospital care
d. Used in long-term care
e. Hospitals receive a set dollar amount based on an assigned group
f. Providers receive a fixed amount per patient
g. Provider or health care system receives a predetermined capitated payment for each patient

Emphasis on Population Wellness

9. The emphasis of the health care industry today is shifting from managing _____ to managing _____.

Health Care Settings and Services

10. Explain what integrated delivery networks (IDNs) are.

    _____

    _____

    _____

11. Give examples of each of the levels of health care services available in the US health care system.

    a. Primary care (health promotion): _____

    b. Preventive care: _____

    c. Secondary acute care: _____

    d. Tertiary care: _____

    e. Restorative care: _____

    f. Continuing care: _____

Preventive and Primary Health Care Services

12. Explain the difference between:

    a. Primary health care: _____

    b. Preventive care: _____

Secondary and Tertiary Care (Acute Care)

13. Disease management is: _____

14. Give some examples of acute care facilities.

    a. _____

    b. _____

    c. _____

    d. _____

15. Because of _____, more services are available on nursing units, thus minimizing the need to transfer and transport patients across multiple areas.

16. *Discharge planning* begins: _____

17. _____ is a centralized, coordinated, multidisciplinary process that ensures that the patient has a plan for continuing care after leaving the health care agency.

18. List the tips on making a referral process.

    a. _____

    b. _____

    c. _____

    d. _____

19. Identify the instructions needed before patients leave health care facilities.

    a. _____

    b. _____

    c. _____

    d. _____

    e. _____

    f. _____

    g. _____

20. Identify the two reasons why an *intensive care unit* (ICU) is the most expensive health care delivery site.

    a. _____

    b. _____

21. The goal of *restorative care* is:

    _____

    _____

    _____

22. *Home care* services include:

    a. _____

    b. _____

    c. _____

    d. _____

23. Give some examples of home nursing care.

    a. _____

    b. _____

    c. _____

    d. _____

    e. _____

24. _____ restores a person to the fullest physical, mental, social, vocational, and economic potential possible.

Match the following.

25. _____ Extended care facility   a. 24-hour intermediate and custodial care
26. _____ Continuing care   b. Include immediate care and skilled nursing facilities
27. _____ Nursing center   c. Services are for people who are disabled, not functionally independent or
28. _____ Assisted living   who suffer a terminal disease
29. _____ Respite care   d. Long-term care setting with greater resident autonomy
30. _____ Adult day care center   e. Provides short-term relief to the family members who care for the patient
31. _____ Hospice   f. Allows patients to retain more independence by living at home
                                             g. Focus of care is palliative, not curative, treatment

32. Health care reform has stimulated the development of two systems focused on coordinating medical care. Briefly explain each model.

    a. Accountable Care Organizations (ACO): _____

    b. Patient-centered medical home (PCMH): _____

Issues in Health Care Delivery

33. List some of the factors that are contributing to a nursing shortage.

    _____

    _____

    _____

34. The Institute of Medicine (IOM) identified five interrelated competencies that are essential in the twenty-first century. Briefly explain.

    a. Provide patient-centered care: _____

    b. Work in interdisciplinary teams: _____

    c. Use evidence-based practice: _____

    d. Apply quality improvement: _____

    e. Use informatics: _____

35. List the 10 rules of performance in a redesigned health care system.

    a. _____

    b. _____

    c. _____

    d. _____

    e. _____

    f. _____

g. _____

h. _____

i. _____

j. _____

36. Quality health care is: _____

37. The goal of pay for performance programs is: _____

38. Hospital Consumer of Assessment of Healthcare Providers and Systems (HCAHPS) is: _____
_____

39. Concepts of *patient-centered care* include:

a. _____

b. _____

c. _____

d. _____

40. Health care organizations that apply for Magnet status must demonstrate:

a. _____

b. _____

c. _____

41. The revised Magnet model has five components affected by global issues; please identify.

a. _____

b. _____

c. _____

d. _____

e. _____

42. Explain nurse-sensitive outcomes and give some examples.

_____

_____

_____

43. _____ uses information and technology to communicate, manage knowledge, mitigate error, and support decision making.

44. Define globalization.

_____

_____

_____

45. *Vulnerable populations* are identified as:

a. _____

b. _____

c. _____

Quality and Performance Improvement

46. Quality data are the outcome of both of the following; please explain.

a. Quality improvement (QI): _____

_____

_____

b. Performance improvement (PI): _____

_____

_____

REVIEW QUESTIONS

Select the appropriate answer and cite the rationale for choosing that particular answer.

47. Health promotion programs are designed to help patients:
    1. Reduce the incidence of disease
    2. Maintain maximal function
    3. Reduce the need to use more expensive health care services
    4. All of the above

Answer: _____   Rationale: _____

_____

_____

48. Rehabilitation services begin:
    1. When the patient enters the health care system
    2. After the patient's physical condition stabilizes
    3. After the patient requests rehabilitation services
    4. When the patient is discharged from the hospital

Answer: _____ Rationale: _____

_____

_____

49. An example of an extended care facility is a:
    1. Home care agency
    2. Skilled nursing facility
    3. Suicide prevention center
    4. State-owned psychiatric hospital

Answer: _____ Rationale: _____

_____

_____

50. A patient and his or her family facing the end stages of a terminal illness might best be served by a:
    1. Hospice
    2. Rehabilitation center
    3. Extended care facility
    4. Crisis intervention center

Answer: _____ Rationale: _____

_____

_____

3 Community-Based Nursing Practice

PRELIMINARY READING

Chapter 3, pp. 31-40

COMPREHENSIVE UNDERSTANDING

Community-Based Care

1. Community-based care focuses on: _____

2. Community-based health care focuses on: _____

3. Identify some of the challenges in community-based health care.

   _____

   _____

4. Give some examples of a comprehensive community assessment.

   _____

   _____

5. Identify five social determinants of health.

   _____

   _____

6. Define health disparities.

   _____

   _____

Community Health Nursing

7. Briefly describe the differences between:

   a. Public health nursing focus: _____

   b. Community health nursing focus: _____

Community-Based Nursing

8. Community-based nursing care takes place in: _____

9. Vulnerable populations are those patients who:

   a. _____

   b. _____

   c. _____

Identify the risk factors for the following vulnerable groups.

10. Immigrant population: _____

11. Poverty and homelessness: _____

12. Abused patients: _____

13. Mental illness: _____

14. Older adults: _____

A nurse in a community-based practice must have a variety of skills and talents in assisting patients within the community. Briefly explain the competencies the nurse needs in the following roles.

15. Caregiver: _____

16. Case manager: _____

17. Change agent: _____

18. Patient advocate: _____

19. Collaborator: _____

20. Counselor: _____

21. Educator: _____

22. Epidemiologist: _____

Community Assessment

23. There are three components of a community that need to be assessed. Identify them and give an example of each.

    a. _____

    b. _____

    c. _____

REVIEW QUESTIONS

Select the appropriate answer and cite the rationale for choosing that particular answer.

24. Which of the following is an example of an intrinsic risk factor for homelessness?
    1. Severe anxiety disorders
    2. Psychotic mental disorders
    3. Living below the poverty line
    4. Progressive chronic alcoholism

Answer: _____   Rationale: _____

_____

_____

25. When the community health nurse refers patients to appropriate resources and monitors and coordinates the extent and adequacy of services to meet family health care needs, the nurse is functioning in the role of:
    1. Advocate
    2. Counselor
    3. Collaborator
    4. Case manager

Answer: _____   Rationale: _____

_____

_____

26. The first step in community assessment is determining the community's:
    1. Goals
    2. Set factors
    3. Boundaries
    4. Throughputs

Answer: _____   Rationale: _____

_____

_____

4 Theoretical Foundations of Nursing Practice

PRELIMINARY READING

Chapter 4, pp. 41–51

COMPREHENSIVE UNDERSTANDING

Theory

Match the following concepts that relate to theories.

1. _____ Nursing theories
2. _____ Theory
3. _____ Phenomenon
4. _____ Concepts
5. _____ Definitions
6. _____ Assumptions
7. _____ Grand theories
8. _____ Middle-range theories
9. _____ Descriptive theories
10. _____ Prescriptive theories

a. Label given to describe an idea about an event or group of situations
b. Address nursing interventions for a phenomenon, guide practice change, and predict consequences
c. More limited in scope and less abstract
d. Ideas and mental images
e. A conceptualization of some aspect of nursing communicated for the purpose of describing, explaining, predicting, or prescribing nursing care
f. Concepts, definitions, and assumptions or propositions
g. Describe phenomena and identify circumstances in which the phenomena occur
h. Define a particular concept based on the theorist's perspective
i. "Taken for granted" statements
j. Structural framework for broad, abstract ideas about nursing

Domain of Nursing

Match the following.

11. _____ Domain
12. _____ Paradigm
13. _____ Conceptual framework
14. _____ Nursing metaparadigm
15. _____ Person
16. _____ Environment
17. _____ Nursing

a. All possible conditions affecting the patient and the setting of health care delivery
b. The diagnosis and treatment of human responses to actual or potential health problems
c. Perspective of a profession
d. Links science, philosophy, and theories accepted and applied by the discipline
e. Provides a way to organize major concepts and visualize the relationship
f. Is the recipient of nursing care
g. What nursing is, what it does, and what we do

Shared Theories

18. Shared theory explains: _____

19. Explain the following components of the nursing process as it pertains to systems.

   a. Input: _____

   b. Output: _____

   c. Feedback: _____

   d. Content: _____

Selected Nursing Theories

Match the following nursing theories.

20. _____ Nightingale's
21. _____ Peplau's
22. _____ Henderson's
23. _____ Benner
24. _____ Orem's
25. _____ Leininger's
26. _____ Roy's
27. _____ Watson's

a. Five stages of skill acquisition of nurses
b. Culturally specific nursing care
c. Patient's self-care needs
d. The patient's environment was the focus of nursing care
e. Nurse–patient relationship
f. The goal is to help the patient adapt to various domains
g. Help patient perform 14 basic needs through physiological, psychological, sociocultural, spiritual, and developmental domains
h. Philosophy of transpersonal caring

Link Between Theory and Knowledge Development in Nursing

28. Research refines the knowledge base of nursing. Briefly explain each one.

a. Theory generating: _____

b. Theory testing: _____

REVIEW QUESTIONS

Select the appropriate answer and cite the rationale for choosing that particular answer.

29. Which of the following models is based on the physiological, sociocultural, and dependence–independence adaptive modes?
    1. Roy's adaptation model
    2. Orem's model of self-care
    3. King's model of personal, interpersonal, and social systems
    4. Rogers' life process interactive person–environmental model

Answer: _____ Rationale: _____

_____

_____

30. Nursing metaparadigm includes the following linkages:
    1. Person
    2. Health
    3. Environment or situation
    4. All of the above

Answer: _____ Rationale: _____

_____

_____

5 Evidence-Based Practice

PRELIMINARY READING

Chapter 5, pp. 52-64

COMPREHENSIVE UNDERSTANDING

The Need for Evidence-Based Practice

1. Define *evidence-based practice*.

   _____

   _____

2. Identify the steps of evidence-based practice.

   a. _____

   b. _____

   c. _____

   d. _____

   e. _____

   f. _____

   g. _____

3. Identify the five elements of a PICOT question.

   a. _____

   b. _____

   c. _____

   d. _____

   e. _____

4. Identify the sources where you can find the evidence.

   a. _____

   b. _____

   c. _____

   d. _____

5. A *peer-reviewed* article is: _____

6. What are clinical guidelines?

   _____

   _____

7. _____ are the gold standard for research.

Critiquing the Evidence

Briefly explain the following elements of evidence-based articles.

8. Abstract: _____

9. Introduction: _____

10. Literature review: _____

11. A clinical article describes: _____

12. Identify and define the four subsections that a research article contains in the manuscript narrative.

    a. _____

    b. _____

    c. _____

    d. _____

Nursing Research

13. Define *nursing research*. _____

14. Define *outcomes research*. _____

15. Define *scientific method*. _____

16. List the five characteristics of scientific research.

    a. _____

    b. _____

    c. _____

    d. _____

    e. _____

Briefly describe the following quantitative methods.

17. Experimental: _____

18. Nonexperimental: _____

19. Surveys: _____

20. Evaluation: _____

21. Qualitative nursing research is: _____

Research Process

22. Identify the nursing process step that corresponds to each step in the research process.

    a. Identify the area of interest or clinical problem: _____

    b. Develop research hypotheses: _____

    c. Determine how the study will be conducted: _____

    d. Conduct the study: _____

    e. Evaluation: _____

23. Briefly explain informed consent in relation to conducting a study.

_____

_____

REVIEW QUESTIONS

Select the appropriate answer and cite the rationale for choosing that particular answer.

24. Research studies can most easily be identified by:
    1. Examining the contents of the report
    2. Looking for the study only in research journals
    3. Reading the abstract and introduction of the report
    4. Looking for the word *research* in the title of the report

    Answer: _____ Rationale: _____

    _____

    _____

25. A research report includes all of the following except:
    1. The researcher's interpretation of the study results
    2. A description of methods used to conduct the study
    3. A summary of other research studies with the same results
    4. A summary of literature used to identify the research problem

    Answer: _____ Rationale: _____

    _____

    _____

26. Practice guidelines for the treatment of adults with low back pain is an example of:
    1. Clinical guidelines
    2. Quantitative nursing research
    3. Outcomes management research
    4. A randomized controlled trial (RCT)

    Answer: _____ Rationale: _____

    _____

    _____

6 Health and Wellness

PRELIMINARY READING

Chapter 6, pp. 65-78

COMPREHENSIVE UNDERSTANDING

Healthy People Documents

1. The four overarching goals of *Healthy People 2020* are:

    a. _____

    b. _____

    c. _____

    d. _____

Definition of Health

2. Define *health*. _____

    _____

Models of Health and Illness

3. Identify some practices of each health behavior.

    a. Positive health behavior: _____

    b. Negative health behavior: _____

4. Describe the three components of the health belief model.

    a. _____

    b. _____

    c. _____

5. The health promotion model focuses on three areas. They are:

    a. _____

    b. _____

    c. _____

6. Define the main concepts of the holistic health model.

    _____

    _____

    _____

Variables Influencing Health and Health Beliefs and Practices

7. Briefly describe the following internal variables.

   a. Developmental stage: _____

   _____

   b. Intellectual background: _____

   _____

   c. Perception of functioning: _____

   _____

   d. Emotional factors: _____

   _____

   e. Spiritual factors: _____

   _____

8. Briefly describe the following external variables.

   a. Family practices: _____

   b. Socioeconomic factors: _____

   c. Cultural background: _____

Health Promotion, Wellness, and Illness Prevention

9. Define *health promotion*.

   _____

   _____

10. Wellness education includes: _____

11. Define *illness prevention*.

   _____

   _____

12. Identify the differences between passive and active strategies for health promotion.

   _____

   _____

13. Define the following levels of preventive care.

   a. Primary: _____

   b. Secondary: _____

   c. Tertiary: _____

Risk Factors

14. Define *risk factor.*

   _____

   _____

15. Identify at least two risk factors for each of the following categories.

   a. Genetic and physiological factors: _____

   _____

   b. Age: _____

   _____

   c. Environment: _____

   _____

   d. Lifestyle: _____

   _____

Risk Factor Modification and Changing Health Behaviors

16. Briefly explain the five stages of health behavior change.

   a. Precontemplation: _____

   b. Contemplation: _____

   c. Preparation: _____

   d. Action: _____

   e. Maintenance: _____

Illness

17. Define *illness*.

   _____

   _____

18. Explain the two general classifications of illness.

   a. Acute illness: _____

   b. Chronic illness: _____

19. Illness behavior involves: _____

20. Give examples of the following variables that influence illness.

   a. Internal variables: _____

   b. External variables: _____

Impact of Illness on the Patient and Family

21. The patient and family commonly experience the following. Briefly explain each one.

   a. Behavioral and emotional changes: _____

   b. Impact on body image: _____

   c. Impact on self-concept: _____

   d. Impact on family roles: _____

   e. Impact on family dynamics: _____

REVIEW QUESTIONS

Select the appropriate answer and cite the rationale for choosing that particular answer.

22. Internal variables influencing health beliefs and practices include:
    1. Developmental stage
    2. Intellectual background
    3. Emotional and spiritual factors
    4. All of the above

    Answer: _____ Rationale: _____

    _____

    _____

23. Any variable increasing the vulnerability of an individual or a group to an illness or accident is a(an):
    1. Risk factor
    2. Illness behavior
    3. Lifestyle determinant
    4. Negative health behavior

    Answer: _____ Rationale: _____

    _____

    _____

24. Marsha states, "My chubby size runs in our family. It's a glandular condition. Exercise and diet won't change things much." The nurse determines that this is an example of Marsha's:
    1. Health beliefs
    2. Active strategy
    3. Acute situation
    4. Positive health behavior

    Answer: _____ Rationale: _____

    _____

    _____

7 Caring in Nursing Practice

PRELIMINARY READING

Chapter 7, pp. 79-89

COMPREHENSIVE UNDERSTANDING

Theoretical Views on Caring

1. Define *caring*.

   _____

   _____

2. Explain Leininger's concept of care from a transcultural perspective.

   _____

   _____

3. Summarize Watson's transpersonal caring.

   _____

   _____

4. What does Watson mean by "transformative model"?

   _____

   _____

5. Swanson's theory of caring consists of five categories. Explain each.
   a. Knowing:

   _____

   _____

   b. Being with:

   _____

   _____

   c. Doing for:

   _____

   _____

   d. Enabling:

   _____

   _____

   e. Maintaining belief:

   _____

   _____

6. List the common themes in nursing caring theories.

    a. _____

    b. _____

    c. _____

    d. _____

Ethics of Care

7. Identify the nurse's responsibilities in relation to the ethics of care.

    _____

    _____

Caring in Nursing Practice

8. Summarize the concept of presence.

    _____

    _____

9. The outcomes of nursing presence include:

    a. _____

    b. _____

    c. _____

10. The use of touch is one comforting approach. Explain the differences between the three categories of touch.

    a. Task oriented:

    _____

    _____

    b. Caring:

    _____

    _____

    c. Protective:

    _____

    _____

11. Describe what listening involves.

    _____

    _____

    _____

12. Two elements that facilitate knowing are:

    a. _____

    b. _____

13. Barriers to knowing the patient are:

    a. _____

    b. _____

14. List the 11 caring behaviors that are perceived by families.

a. _____

b. _____

c. _____

d. _____

e. _____

f. _____

g. _____

h. _____

i. _____

j. _____

k. _____

The Challenge of Caring

15. Summarize the challenges facing nursing in today's health care system.

_____

_____

REVIEW QUESTIONS

Select the appropriate answer and cite the rationale for choosing that particular answer.

16. Leininger's care theory states that the patient's caring values and behaviors are derived largely from:
1. Gender
2. Culture
3. Experience
4. Religious beliefs

Answer: _____   Rationale: _____

_____

17. The central common theme of the caring theories is:
1. Maintenance of patient homeostasis
2. Compensation for patient disabilities
3. Pathophysiology and self-care abilities
4. The nurse–patient relationship and psychosocial aspects of care

Answer: _____   Rationale: _____

_____

18. For the nurse to effectively listen to the patient, he or she needs to:
1. Lean back in the chair
2. Sit with the legs crossed
3. Maintain good eye contact
4. Respond quickly with appropriate answers to the patient

Answer: _____   Rationale: _____

_____

19. The nurse demonstrates caring by:
1. Maintaining professionalism at all costs
2. Doing all the necessary tasks for the patient
3. Following all of the health care provider's orders accurately
4. Helping family members become active participants in the care of the patient

Answer: _____   Rationale: _____

_____

8 Caring for the Cancer Survivor

PRELIMINARY READING

Chapter 8, pp. 90-100

COMPREHENSIVE UNDERSTANDING

The Effects of Cancer on Quality of Life

1. A cancer survivor is at risk for a wide range of treatment-related problems. Briefly explain the following.

   a. Second cancer: _____

   b. Late effects of chemotherapy: _____

   c. Chemotherapy-induced peripheral neuropathy: _____

   d. Cancer-related fatigue (CRF): _____

   e. Chemotherapy-related cognitive impairment: _____

2. Explain the following psychological effects of cancer.

   a. Fear of cancer recurrence: _____

   b. Posttraumatic stress disorder (PTSD): _____

   c. Disrupted interpersonal relationships: _____

3. Identify the social impact that cancer causes across the life span.

   a. Adolescents and young adults: _____

   b. Adults (30–59 years): _____

   c. Older adults: _____

Cancer and Families

4. Summarize the issues affecting families of patients with cancer.

   _____

   _____

Implications for Nursing

5. List the types of questions that you may use to assess the cancer survivor.

   _____

   _____

6. Explain the transactional model of cancer family caregiving skill as it relates to the following patterns of care.

   a. Self-caregiving pattern: _____

   b. Collaborative care pattern: _____

   c. Family caregiving pattern: _____

7. Identify at least three important patient education topics for cancer survivors and their families.

a. _____

b. _____

c. _____

Components of Survivorship Care

8. The four essential components of survivorship care are:

a. _____

b. _____

c. _____

d. _____

REVIEW QUESTIONS

Select the appropriate answer and cite the rationale for choosing that particular answer.

9. Many cancer survivors report attention problems, loss of memory, and difficulty recognizing and solving problems. This is an example of impaired:
   1. Social well-being
   2. Physical well-being
   3. Spiritual well-being
   4. Psychological well-being

Answer: _____ Rationale: _____

_____

_____

10. All of the following are the numerous social concerns that older adults are faced with as a result of cancer except:
    1. Retirement
    2. Fixed income
    3. Isolation from social supports
    4. Ample medical insurance coverage

Answer: _____ Rationale: _____

_____

_____

11. The essential components of survivorship are all of the following except:
    1. Surveillance for cancer spread
    2. Care for the patient by oncologists only
    3. Intervention for consequences of cancer
    4. Prevention and detection of new cancers and recurrent cancer

Answer: _____ Rationale: _____

_____

_____

9 Cultural Awareness

PRELIMINARY READING

Chapter 9, pp. 101-116

COMPREHENSIVE UNDERSTANDING

Health Disparities

1. Define *health disparity*.

   _____

   _____

2. Social determinants of health are:

   _____

   _____

3. Health care disparities are:

   _____

   _____

Culture

Match the following.

4. _____ Culture
5. _____ Intersectionality
6. _____ Oppression
7. _____ Transcultural nursing
8. _____ Culturally congruent care
9. _____ Cultural awareness
10. _____ Cultural knowledge
11. _____ Cultural skills
12. _____ Cultural encounters
13. _____ Cultural desire

a. A formal and informal system of advantages and disadvantages tied to a membership in social groups
b. Care that fits a person's life patterns, values, and system of meaning
c. Concept that applies to a group of people whose members share values and ways of thinking and acting that are different from those of people who are outside the group
d. Motivation and commitment to caring that moves an individual to learn from others
e. Self-examination of one's own background, recognizing bias and prejudices
f. Belong simultaneously to multiple social groups with changing social and political contexts
g. Ability to assess social, cultural, and biophysical factors that influence patient care
h. Comparative study of cultures in order to understand their similarities and differences
i. Sufficient comparative knowledge of diverse groups
j. Cross-cultural interactions that provide opportunities to learn about other cultures

Cultural Competency

14. Cultural competence refers to:

    _____

    _____

15. Linguistic competence is:

_____

_____

16. Identify the culturally oriented question types to use in a comprehensive cultural assessment.

a. _____

b. _____

c. _____

d. _____

e. _____

f. _____

g. _____

h. _____

i. _____

j. _____

17. List some helpful hints when trying the teach-back method.

a. _____

b. _____

c. _____

d. _____

18. State the requirements that all organizations are to follow for provision of language access services.

a. _____

b. _____

c. _____

d. _____

Core Measures

19. *Core measures* are: _____

_____

20. List the six steps to implement equity-focused quality improvement.

a. _____

b. _____

c. _____

d. _____

e. _____

f. _____

REVIEW QUESTIONS

Select the appropriate answer and cite the rationale for choosing that particular answer.

21. When providing care to patients with varied cultural backgrounds, it is imperative for the nurse to recognize that:
    1. Cultural considerations must be put aside if basic needs are in jeopardy.
    2. Generalizations about the behavior of a particular group may be inaccurate.
    3. Current health standards should determine the acceptability of cultural practices.
    4. Similar reactions to stress will occur when individuals have the same cultural background.

Answer: _____   Rationale: _____

_____

_____

22. To be effective in meeting various ethnic needs, the nurse should:
    1. Treat all patients alike
    2. Be aware of patients' cultural differences
    3. Act as if he or she is comfortable with the patient's behavior
    4. Avoid asking questions about the patient's cultural background

Answer: _____   Rationale: _____

_____

_____

23. The most important factor in providing nursing care to patients in a specific ethnic group is:
    1. Communication
    2. Time orientation
    3. Biological variation
    4. Environmental control

Answer: _____   Rationale: _____

_____

_____

10 Caring for Families

PRELIMINARY READING

Chapter 10, pp. 117-131

COMPREHENSIVE UNDERSTANDING

The Family

1. Define the three important attributes that characterize contemporary families.

   a. Durability: _____

   _____

   b. Resiliency: _____

   _____

   c. Diversity: _____

   _____

2. A family is defined as:

   _____

   _____

Family Forms and Current Trends

3. Summarize the various family forms.

   a. Nuclear family: _____

   _____

   b. Extended family: _____

   _____

   c. Single-parent family: _____

   _____

   d. Blended family: _____

   _____

   e. Alternative family: _____

   _____

4. Explain the following threats and concerns facing the family.

   a. Changing economic status: _____

   _____

   b. Homelessness: _____

   _____

c. Domestic violence: _____

_____

d. Acute and/or chronic illness: _____

_____

5. Explain how the following events might impact caring for the family.

a. Trauma: _____

_____

b. End of life: _____

_____

Approaches to Family Nursing: An Overview

Summarize the general perspectives when providing nursing care to the family as a whole and the patient.

6. Developmental stages: _____

_____

_____

7. Structure may enhance or detract from the family's ability to respond to stressors. Briefly explain each of the following.

a. Rigid structure: _____

_____

b. Open or flexible structure: _____

_____

8. Family functioning focuses on the processes used by the family to achieve its goals. Identify these processes.

_____

_____

_____

9. Describe the Family Health System approach to identifying the needs of families.

a. _____

b. _____

c. _____

d. _____

e. _____

10. Explain the following attributes of healthy families.

a. Hardiness:

_____

_____

b. Resiliency:

_____

_____

Family Nursing

Identify the three levels and focuses proposed for family nursing practice. Briefly explain each.

11. Family as context: _____

12. Family as patient: _____

13. Family as system: _____

Nursing Process for the Family

14. Three factors underlie the family approach to the nursing process. Name them.

   a. _____

   b. _____

   c. _____

15. Identify and define the five areas to include in a family assessment.

   a. _____

   b. _____

   c. _____

   d. _____

   e. _____

16. A comprehensive, culturally sensitive family assessment is critical in order to:

   a. _____

   b. _____

   c. _____

   d. _____

17. Summarize the challenges for family nursing in relation to each of the following.

   a. Discharge planning: _____

   b. Cultural diversity: _____

Implementing Family-Centered Care

18. When implementing family-centered care, the following need to be addressed. Briefly explain.

   a. Family caregiving: _____

   b. Health promotion: _____

   c. Acute care: _____

   d. Restorative and continuing care: _____

REVIEW QUESTIONS

Select the appropriate answer and cite the rationale for choosing that particular answer.

19. Family structure can best be described as:
    1. A complex set of relationships
    2. A basic pattern of predictable stages
    3. The pattern of relationships and ongoing membership
    4. Flexible patterns that contribute to adequate functioning

    Answer: _____ Rationale: _____

    _____

    _____

20. When planning care for a patient and using the concept of family as patient, the nurse:
    1. Includes only the patient and his or her significant other
    2. Considers the developmental stage of the patient and not the family
    3. Understands that the patient's family will always be a help to the patient's health goals
    4. Realizes that cultural background is an important variable when assessing the family

    Answer: _____ Rationale: _____

    _____

    _____

21. Interventions used by the nurse when providing care to a rigidly structured family include:
    1. Attempting to change the family structure
    2. Providing solutions for problems as they arise
    3. Exploring with the family the benefits of moving toward more flexible modes of action
    4. Administering nursing care in a manner that provides minimal opportunity for change

    Answer: _____ Rationale: _____

    _____

    _____

11 Developmental Theories

PRELIMINARY READING

Chapter 11, pp. 132-140

COMPREHENSIVE UNDERSTANDING

Developmental Theories

1. Briefly summarize Gesell's theory of development.

   _____

   _____

2. Briefly summarize theories of psychoanalytical/psychosocial theory.

   _____

   _____

3. Explain the five stages of Freud's psychoanalytic model of personal development.

   a. Stage 1: Oral: _____

   _____

   _____

   b. Stage 2: Anal: _____

   _____

   _____

   c. Stage 3: Phallic: _____

   _____

   _____

   d. Stage 4: Latency: _____

   _____

   _____

   e. Stage 5: Genital: _____

   _____

   _____

Match the following stages of Erickson (psychosocial development) with the appropriate years.

4. _____ Trust vs. mistrust   a. 3–6 years
5. _____ Autonomy vs. shame   b. Birth to 1 year
6. _____ Initiative vs. guilt   c. Puberty
7. _____ Industry vs. inferiority   d. 1–3 years
8. _____ Identity vs. role confusion   e. 6–11 years
9. _____ Intimacy vs. isolation   f. Middle age
10. _____ Generativity vs. self-absorption   g. Young adult
11. _____ Integrity vs. despair   h. Old age

12. Define *temperament.*

_____

_____

13. Identify the three basic classes of temperament and briefly explain each.

    a. _____

    b. _____

    c. _____

14. Havinghurst's stage: crisis theory incorporates three primary sources for developmental tasks, which are:

    a. _____

    b. _____

    c. _____

15. Contemporary life-span approach considers:

_____

_____

16. Identify the four periods of Piaget's theory of cognitive development.

    a. _____

    b. _____

    c. _____

    d. _____

Kohlberg identified six stages of moral development under three levels. Briefly describe each.

17. Level I: Preconventional level:

_____

_____

    a. Stage 1: _____

_____

_____

    b. Stage 2: _____

_____

_____

18. Level II: Conventional level:

_____

_____

    a. Stage 3: _____

_____

_____

b. Stage 4: _____

_____

_____

19. Level III: Postconventional level: _____

_____

_____

a. Stage 5: _____

_____

_____

b. Stage 6: _____

_____

_____

REVIEW QUESTIONS

Select the appropriate answer and cite the rationale for choosing that particular answer.

20. According to Piaget, the school-age child is in the third stage of cognitive development, which is characterized by:
    1. Concrete operations
    2. Conventional thought
    3. Postconventional thought
    4. Identity vs. role diffusion

    Answer: _____   Rationale: _____

    _____

    _____

21. According to Erikson, the developmental task of adolescence is:
    1. Industry vs. inferiority
    2. Identity vs. role confusion
    3. Autonomy vs. shame and doubt
    4. Role acceptance vs. role confusion

    Answer: _____   Rationale: _____

    _____

    _____

22. According to Erikson's developmental theory, the primary developmental task of the middle years is to:
    1. Achieve intimacy
    2. Achieve generativity
    3. Establish a set of personal values
    4. Establish a sense of personal identity

    Answer: _____   Rationale: _____

    _____

    _____

23. According to Kohlberg, children develop moral reasoning as they mature. Which of the following is most characteristic of a preschooler's stage of moral development?
    1. The rules of correct behavior are obeyed.
    2. Behavior that pleases others is considered good.
    3. Showing respect for authority is important behavior.
    4. Actions are determined as good or bad in terms of their consequences.

    Answer: _____   Rationale: _____

    _____

    _____

12 Conception Through Adolescence

PRELIMINARY READING

Chapter 12, pp. 141-158

COMPREHENSIVE UNDERSTANDING

Intrauterine Life

1. Identify the three trimesters of a full-term pregnancy, and state when each occurs.

   a. _____

   b. _____

   c. _____

2. Identify some of the common concerns that are verbalized by the expectant mother that are attributable to fetal growth and hormonal changes.

   _____

   _____

Transition from Intrauterine to Extrauterine Life

3. The assessment tool used to assess newborns is the Apgar score. Identify the components.

   a. _____

   b. _____

   c. _____

   d. _____

   e. _____

4. Direct nursing care at birth includes _____, _____, and _____

5. Give some examples of how to encourage parent–child attachment immediately after birth.

   _____

   _____

Newborn

Match the following terms that address the newborn.

6. _____ Neonatal period
7. _____ Molding
8. _____ Anterior fontanel
9. _____ Early cognitive development
10. _____ Infant positioning
11. _____ Posterior fontanel
12. _____ Normal behavior
13. _____ Health promotion of the infant

a. Screenings, car seats, and cribs
b. Closes at the end of the second to third month
c. Overlapping of the soft skull bones
d. First month of life
e. Innate behavior, reflexes, and sensory functions
f. Sleep on their back
g. Sucking, crying, sleeping, and activity
h. Closes at 12–18 months

Infant

14. Infancy is the period from _____ to _____

15. Summarize the changes in size, weight, and height that occur in the first 12 months.

    _____

    _____

16. Describe the cognitive changes that occur in infants.

    _____

    _____

17. Identify the language development in infants and how to help parents further develop infants' language.

    _____

    _____

18. Explain the following psychosocial changes that occur.

    a. Separation and individuation: _____

    _____

    b. Play: _____

    _____

19. Explain the following in relation to health risks of the infant.

    a. Injury prevention: _____

    _____

    b. Child maltreatment: _____

    _____

20. Give an example of health promotion activities for the following.

    a. Nutrition: _____

    _____

    b. Supplementation: _____

    _____

    c. Immunizations: _____

    _____

    d. Sleep: _____

    _____

Toddler

21. Toddlerhood ranges from _____ to _____

22. Summarize the fine motor capabilities that occur during this stage.

    _____

    _____

23. Summarize the cognitive changes that occur during this stage.

_____

_____

24. Describe language ability at this stage.

_____

_____

25. Describe the psychosocial changes of a toddler.

_____

_____

26. Describe the play of a toddler.

_____

_____

27. Identify the health risks of a toddler.

_____

_____

28. Identify the health promotion activities for this age group related to the following.

    a. Nutrition: _____

_____

    b. Toilet training: _____

_____

Preschoolers

29. The preschool period ranges from _____ to _____

30. Summarize the height and weight changes that occur in preschoolers.

_____

_____

31. Describe the more complex thinking processes a preschooler develops.

_____

_____

32. Explain the following.

    a. Psychosocial changes: _____

_____

    b. Language: _____

_____

33. Describe the concept of play for the preschooler.

_____

_____

34. Explain health promotion activities related to the following for this group.

   a. Nutrition: _____

   _____

   b. Sleep: _____

   _____

   c. Vision: _____

   _____

School-Age Children

35. The school-age years range from _____ to _____

36. Puberty signals _____

37. Summarize the physical changes that occur in school-age children.

   _____

   _____

38. Define the cognitive skills that develop in school-age children.

   _____

   _____

39. Summarize psychosocial development in relation to the following.

   a. Psychosocial changes: _____

   _____

   b. Peer relationships: _____

   _____

   c. Sexual identity: _____

   _____

   d. Stress: _____

   _____

40. Identify the health risks for school-age children.

   _____

   _____

41. Give an example of a health promotion intervention that is appropriate for school-age children.

   a. Perceptions: _____

   _____

   b. Health education: _____

   _____

   c. Health maintenance: _____

   _____

   d. Safety: _____

   _____

   e. Nutrition: _____

   _____

Adolescents

42. The adolescent period ranges from _____ to _____

43. List the four major physical changes that occur.

    a. _____

    b. _____

    c. _____

    d. _____

44. Menarche is:

    _____

    _____

45. Briefly explain the cognitive abilities of this group.

    _____

    _____

46. Identify some strategies for communicating with adolescents.

    _____

    _____

47. Explain the following components of personal total identity.

    a. Sexual identity: _____

    _____

    b. Group identity: _____

    _____

    c. Family identity: _____

    _____

    d. Health identity: _____

    _____

48. Identify the leading causes of death for adolescents.

    a. _____

    b. _____

    c. _____

49. List the six warning signs of suicide for adolescents.

    a. _____

    b. _____

    c. _____

    d. _____

    e. _____

    f. _____

50. Define the two eating disorders that follow.

   a. Anorexia nervosa: _____

   _____

   b. Bulimia nervosa: _____

   _____

51. Identify health promotion interventions for adolescents in regard to the following.

   a. Substance abuse: _____

   _____

   b. Sexually transmitted infections: _____

   _____

   c. Pregnancy: _____

   _____

52. Identify the concerns of minority adolescents.

   _____

   _____

53. Explain how a nurse could help a teen disclose his or her sexual orientation.

   _____

   _____

REVIEW QUESTIONS

Select the appropriate answer and cite the rationale for choosing that particular answer.

54. The mother of a 2-year-old expresses concern that her son's appetite has diminished and that he seems to prefer milk to other solid foods. Which response by the nurse reflects knowledge of principles of communication and nutrition?
   1. "Have you considered feeding him when he doesn't seem interested in feeding himself?"
   2. "Oh, I wouldn't be too worried; children tend to eat when they're hungry. I just wouldn't give him dessert unless he eats his meal."
   3. "That is not uncommon in toddlers. You might consider increasing his milk to two quarts per day to be sure he gets enough nutrients."
   4. "A toddler's rate of growth normally slows down. It's common to see a toddler's appetite diminish in response to decreased calorie needs."

   Answer: _____ Rationale: _____

   _____

   _____

55. To stimulate cognitive and psychosocial development of the toddler, it is important for parents to:
   1. Set firm and consistent limits
   2. Foster sharing of toys with playmates and siblings
   3. Provide clarification about what is right and wrong
   4. Limit confusion by restricting exploration of the environment

   Answer: _____ Rationale: _____

   _____

   _____

56. Which of the following is true of the developmental behaviors of school-age children?
   1. Fears center on the loss of self-control.
   2. Positive feedback from parents and teachers is crucial to development.
   3. Formal and informal peer group membership is the key in forming self-esteem.
   4. A full range of defense mechanisms is used, including rationalization and intellectualization.

   Answer: _____ Rationale: _____

   _____

   _____

13 Young and Middle Adults

PRELIMINARY READING

Chapter 13, pp. 159-172

COMPREHENSIVE UNDERSTANDING

Young Adults

1. Describe the period of life called *emerging adulthood*.

   _____

   _____

2. Summarize the physical changes that occur in young adults.

   _____

   _____

3. Briefly explain the cognitive development of the period in relation to educational, life, and occupational experiences.

   _____

   _____

4. Explain the psychosocial patterns of the following age groups.

   a. 23–28 years: _____

   _____

   b. 29–34 years: _____

   _____

   c. 35–43 years: _____

   _____

5. Briefly explain the psychosocial development of a young adult in relation to the following.

   a. Lifestyle: _____

   _____

   b. Career: _____

   _____

   c. Sexuality: _____

   _____

   d. Childbearing cycle: _____

   _____

6. Describe the following types of families.

   a. Singlehood: _____

   _____

   b. Parenthood: _____

   _____

   c. Alternative family structures and parenting: _____

   _____

Briefly explain the risk factors for young adults in regard to the following.

7. Family history: _____

   _____

8. Personal hygiene habits: _____

   _____

9. Violent death and injury: _____

   _____

10. Substance abuse: _____

   _____

11. Human trafficking: _____

   _____

12. Unplanned pregnancies: _____

   _____

13. Sexually transmitted infections: _____

   _____

14. Environmental and occupational risks: _____

   _____

Explain how you would assess the concerns of the young adult related to:

15. Job stress: _____

   _____

16. Family stress: _____

   _____

17. Infertility: _____

   _____

18. Obesity: _____

   _____

19. Exercise: _____

_____

Explain the physiological changes that occur to pregnant women and childbearing families.

20. Prenatal care: _____

_____

21. Physiological changes during pregnancy: _____

_____

  a. First trimester: _____

  _____

  b. Second trimester: _____

  _____

  c. Third trimester: _____

  _____

Middle Adults

22. Middle adulthood is the period from _____ to _____

23. Identify the major physiological changes that occur between 40 and 65 years of age.

_____

_____

24. Define the following.

  a. Perimenopause: _____

  _____

  b. Menopause: _____

  _____

  c. Climacteric: _____

  _____

Summarize the psychosocial development of middle adults in the following areas.

25. "Sandwich generation": _____

_____

26. Career transition: _____

_____

27. Sexuality: _____

_____

28. Singlehood: _____

_____

29. Marital changes: _____

_____

30. Family transitions: _____

_____

The following are health concerns for middle adults. Identify strategies for each one.

31. Stress: _____

_____

32. Obesity: _____

_____

33. Summarize two psychosocial concerns of middle adults.

    a. Anxiety: _____

    _____

    b. Depression: _____

    _____

REVIEW QUESTIONS

Select the appropriate answer and cite the rationale for choosing that particular answer.

34. The greatest cause of illness and death in the young adult population is.
    1. Violence
    2. Substance abuse
    3. Cardiovascular disease
    4. Sexually transmitted disease

Answer: _____ Rationale: _____

_____

_____

35. Which physiological change would be a normal assessment finding in a middle adult?
    1. Increased breast size
    2. Reduced auditory acuity
    3. Thickening of the waistline
    4. Increased anteroposterior diameter of the thorax

Answer: _____ Rationale: _____

_____

_____

36. In planning patient education for Mrs. Smith, a 45-year-old woman who had an ovarian cyst removed, which of the following facts is true about the sexuality of middle-aged adults?
    1. Menstruation ceases after menopause.
    2. Estrogen is produced after menopause.
    3. With removal of the ovarian cyst, pregnancy cannot occur.
    4. After reaching climacteric, a man is unable to father a child.

Answer: _____ Rationale: _____

_____

_____

14 Older Adults

PRELIMINARY READING

Chapter 14, pp. 173-194

COMPREHENSIVE UNDERSTANDING

Myths and Stereotypes

1. Older adults are persons age _____ and over.

2. Identify three myths or stereotypes regarding older adults.

   a. _____

   b. _____

   c. _____

3. *Ageism* is: _____

   _____

Developmental Tasks for Older Adults

4. List the seven developmental tasks of older adults.

   a. _____

   b. _____

   c. _____

   d. _____

   e. _____

   f. _____

   g. _____

Community-Based and Institutional Health Care Services

5. Identify the nine aspects of quality to consider when selecting a nursing home.

   a. _____

   b. _____

   c. _____

   d. _____

   e. _____

   f. _____

   g. _____

   h. _____

   i. _____

Assessing the Needs of Older Adults

6. Nurses need to take into account three key points to ensure an age-specific approach.

    a. _____

    b. _____

    c. _____

7. Identify the early indicators of an acute illness.

    a. _____

    b. _____

    c. _____

    d. _____

    e. _____

    f. _____

Match the following common physiological changes to the system.

8. _____ Integumentary
9. _____ Respiratory
10. _____ Cardiovascular
11. _____ Gastrointestinal
12. _____ Musculoskeletal
13. _____ Neurological
14. _____ Sensory
15. _____ Genitourinary
16. _____ Reproductive
17. _____ Endocrine

a. Decreased estrogen production, atrophy of vagina, uterus, and breasts
b. Decrease in saliva, gastric secretions, and pancreatic enzymes
c. Decreased ability to respond to stress
d. Pigmentation changes, glandular atrophy, thinning hair
e. 50% decrease in renal blood flow, decreased bladder capacity
f. Decreased cough reflex and vital capacity, increased airway resistance
g. Lower cardiac output, decreased baroreceptor sensitivity
h. Presbyopia, presbycusis, decreased proprioception
i. Decalcification of bones, degenerative changes, dehydration of intervertebral disks
j. Degeneration of nerve cells, decrease in neurotransmitters

18. Functional status in older adults refers to: _____

    _____

19. Explain the three common conditions that affect cognition.

    a. Delirium: _____

    _____

    b. Dementia: _____

    _____

    c. Depression: _____

    _____

20. Identify the psychosocial changes that occur in older adults.

    a. Retirement: _____

    _____

    b. Social isolation: _____

    _____

    c. Sexuality: _____

    _____

d. Housing and environment: _____

_____

e. Death: _____

_____

Addressing the Health Concerns of Older Adults

21. List the national initiative goals proposed for 2020.

a. _____

b. _____

c. _____

d. _____

e. _____

22. List general preventive measures to recommend to older adults.

a. _____

b. _____

c. _____

d. _____

e. _____

f. _____

g. _____

h. _____

i. _____

j. _____

k. _____

l. _____

Match the following health concerns.

23. _____ Heart disease
24. _____ Cancer
25. _____ Stroke
26. _____ Smoking
27. _____ Alcohol abuse
28. _____ Nutrition
29. _____ Dental problems
30. _____ Exercise
31. _____ Polypharmacy
32. _____ Falls
33. _____ Sensory impairments
34. _____ Pain
35. _____ Medication use

a. Concurrent use of many medications
b. Changes in vision, hearing, taste, and smell
c. Leading cause of death
d. Consequences can include depression, loss of appetite, sleep difficulties
e. Third leading cause of death
f. Risk factors: impaired vision, arthritis, incontinence, medication reactions
g. Risk factor in the four most common causes of death
h. Second most common cause of death
i. Situational factors and clinical conditions affect older adults' needs
j. Adverse effects include confusion, impaired balance, dizziness, and nausea
k. Caused by depression, loneliness, and lack of social support
l. Caries, gingivitis, and ill-fitting dentures
m. Maintains and strengthens functional ability and promotes well-being

Match the following interventions used to maintain the psychosocial health of older adults.

36. _____ Therapeutic communication
37. _____ Touch
38. _____ Reality orientation
39. _____ Validation therapy
40. _____ Reminiscence
41. _____ Body image

a. Assisting with grooming and hygiene
b. An alternative approach to communication with a confused adult
c. Nurse expresses attitudes of concern, kindness, and compassion
d. Technique to make older adults aware of time, place, and person
e. Can significantly lower agitation levels in older adults with dementia
f. Recalling the past

42. *Elder mistreatment* is defined as: _____

_____

43. Identify types of elder abuse.

_____

_____

Describe the following therapeutic communication tools.

44. Touch: _____

_____

45. Reality orientation: _____

_____

46. Validation therapy: _____

_____

47. Reminiscence: _____

_____

Older Adults and the Acute Care Setting

Explain why older adults are at risk for each of the following.

48. Delirium: _____

_____

49. Dehydration and malnutrition: _____

_____

50. Health care–associated infections: _____

_____

51. Transient urinary incontinence: _____

_____

52. Skin breakdown: _____

_____

53. Falls: _____

_____

Older Adults and Restorative Care

54. Summarize the two types of ongoing care for older adults.

   a. _____

   b. _____

REVIEW QUESTIONS

Select the appropriate answer and cite the rationale for choosing that particular answer.

55. Which statement describing delirium is correct?
   1. Symptoms of delirium are irreversible.
   2. The onset of delirium is slow and insidious.
   3. Symptoms of delirium are stable and unchanging.
   4. Causes include electrolyte imbalances and cerebral anoxia.

   Answer: _____ Rationale: _____

   _____

   _____

56. Ms. Dale states that she does not need the TV turned on because she cannot see very well. Normal visual changes in older adults include all of the following except:
   1. Double vision
   2. Sensitivity to glare
   3. Decreased visual acuity
   4. Decreased accommodation to darkness

   Answer: _____ Rationale: _____

   _____

   _____

57. Mr. DeLone states that he is worried about his parents' plans to retire. All of the following would be appropriate responses regarding retirement of older adults except:
   1. Retirement may affect an individual's physical and psychological functioning.
   2. Positive adjustment is often related to how much a person planned for the retirement.
   3. Reactions to retirement are influenced by the importance that has been attached to the work role.
   4. Retirement for most persons represents a sudden shock that is irreversibly damaging to self-image and self-esteem.

   Answer: _____ Rationale: _____

   _____

   _____

15 Critical Thinking in Nursing Practice

PRELIMINARY READING

Chapter 15, pp. 195–208

COMPREHENSIVE UNDERSTANDING

Clinical Judgment in Nursing Practice

1. Critical thinking involves: _____

_____

2. Define *evidenced-based knowledge.*

_____

_____

3. List the tips on how to use reflection.

   a. _____

   b. _____

   c. _____

   d. _____

   e. _____

   f. _____

Levels of Critical Thinking in Nursing

4. Three levels of critical thinking in nursing have been identified. Briefly describe each.

   a. Basic:_____

   _____

   b. Complex:_____

   _____

   c. Commitment: _____

   _____

Critical Thinking Competencies

Match the following cognitive processes to critical thinking competencies.

5. _____ Scientific method
6. _____ Problem solving
7. _____ Decision making
8. _____ Diagnostic reasoning
9. _____ Inference
10. _____ Clinical decision making
11. _____ Nursing process

a. Focuses on problem resolution
b. Process of drawing conclusions from related pieces of evidence
c. Systematic, ordered approach to gathering data and solving problems
d. Obtain information and then use the information plus what you already know to find a solution
e. Five-step clinical decision-making approach
f. Careful reasoning so the best options are chosen for the best outcomes
g. Determining a patient's health status after you have assigned meaning to the behaviors and symptoms presented

A Critical Thinking Model for Clinical Decision Making

12. Identify the concepts and behaviors of a critical thinker.

a. _____

b. _____

c. _____

d. _____

e. _____

f. _____

g. _____

Match the following attitudes with the appropriate application to practice.

13. _____ Confidence
14. _____ Thinking independently
15. _____ Fairness
16. _____ Responsibility
17. _____ Risk taking
18. _____ Discipline
19. _____ Perseverance
20. _____ Creativity
21. _____ Curiosity
22. _____ Integrity
23. _____ Humility

a. Refer to policy and procedure manual to review steps of a skill
b. Explore and learn more about a patient to make appropriate clinical judgments
c. Speak with conviction and always be prepared to perform care safely
d. Be cautious of an easy answer; look for a pattern and find a solution
e. Be willing to recommend alternative approaches to nursing care
f. Look for different approaches if interventions are not working
g. Read the nursing literature
h. Take time to be thorough and manage your time effectively
i. Do not compromise nursing standards or honesty in delivering nursing care
j. Listen to both sides in any discussion
k. Recognize when you need more information to make a decision

24. Explain the two terms below.

a. Diagnostic reasoning: _____

_____

b. Inference: _____

_____

25. Identify the two components of "knowing the patient."

a. _____

b. _____

26. List the tips suggested to foster knowing your patient.

a. _____

b. _____

c. _____

d. _____

e. _____

27. List the five steps of the nursing process.

a. _____

b. _____

c. _____

d. _____

e. _____

28. Discuss the standards for critical thinking.

a. Intellectual standards: _____

_____

b. Professional standards: _____

_____

Developing Critical Thinking Skills

29. Define *reflective journaling*.

_____

_____

30. Define *concept mapping*.

_____

_____

Managing Stress

31. Identify some ways the nurse may better manage stress.

a. _____

b. _____

c. _____

d. _____

e. _____

REVIEW QUESTIONS

Select the appropriate answer and cite the rationale for choosing that particular answer.

32. Clinical decision making requires the nurse to:
    1. Improve a patient's health
    2. Standardize care for the patient
    3. Follow the health care provider's orders for patient care
    4. Establish and weigh criteria in deciding the best choice of therapy for a patient

    Answer: _____   Rationale: _____

    _____

    _____

33. Which of the following is not one of the five steps of the nursing process?
    1. Planning
    2. Evaluation
    3. Assessment
    4. Hypothesis testing

    Answer: _____   Rationale: _____

    _____

    _____

34. Gathering, verifying, and communicating data about the patient to establish a database is an example of which component of the nursing process?
    1. Planning
    2. Evaluation
    3. Assessment
    4. Implementation
    5. Nursing diagnosis

    Answer: _____   Rationale: _____

    _____

    _____

16 Nursing Assessment

Chapter 16, pp. 209-224

COMPREHENSIVE UNDERSTANDING

A Critical Thinking Approach to Assessment

1. Identify the two steps of a nursing assessment.

   a. _____

   b. _____

2. Identify the variety of sources where data can be obtained.

   a. _____

   b. _____

   c. _____

   d. _____

   e. _____

3. List some types of nursing assessments.

   _____

   _____

4. Define the following terms.

   a. *Cue*: _____

   _____

   b. *Inference*: _____

   _____

5. List Gordon's 11 functional health patterns.

   a. _____

   b. _____

   c. _____

   d. _____

   e. _____

   f. _____

   g. _____

   h. _____

   i. _____

   j. _____

   k. _____

6. Discuss the two primary types of data.

   a. Subjective data: _____

     _____

   b. Objective data: _____

     _____

The Patient-Centered Interview

7. Describe motivational interviewing.

   _____

   _____

8. List the communication skills that are needed to effectively communicate.

   a. _____

   b. _____

   c. _____

   d. _____

9. List the three phases of all patient-centered interviews.

   a. _____

   b. _____

   c. _____

10. During an interview, the following are used. Briefly explain.

   a. Observation: _____

     _____

   b. Open-ended questions: _____

     _____

   c. Leading questions: _____

     _____

   d. Back channeling: _____

     _____

   e. Probing: _____

     _____

   f. Direct closed-ended questions: _____

     _____

Nursing Health History

Match the following basic components of the health history.

11. _____ Biographical information
12. _____ Reasons for seeking health care
13. _____ Patient expectations
14. _____ Present illness/health concerns
15. _____ Health history
16. _____ Family history
17. _____ Environmental history
18. _____ Psychosocial history
19. _____ Spiritual history
20. _____ Review of systems (ROS)

a. Represents the totality of one's being
b. Reveals the patient's support systems and coping mechanisms
c. To determine whether the patient is at risk for illnesses of a genetic or a familial nature
d. Systematic approach for collecting the patient's self-reported data on all body systems
e. Patient's understanding of why he or she is seeking health care
f. Factual demographic data about the patient
g. Chief concerns or problems
h. Essential and relevant data about the nature and onset of symptoms
i. Health care experiences and current health habits and lifestyle patterns
j. Patient's home and work, focusing on determining the patient's safety

21. Diagnostic and laboratory data provide: _____

_____

22. Define the term *data validation*:_____

_____

23. Identify some common practices related to documentation, the last part of a complete assessment.

_____

_____

24. A concept map is: _____

_____

REVIEW QUESTIONS

Select the appropriate answer and cite the rationale for choosing that particular answer.

25. The interview technique that is most effective in strengthening the nurse–patient relationship by demonstrating the nurse's willingness to hear the patient's thoughts is:
    1. Direct question
    2. Problem solving
    3. Problem seeking
    4. Open-ended question

    Answer:_____ Rationale: _____

    _____

    _____

26. While obtaining a health history, the nurse asks Mr. Jones if he has noted any change in his activity tolerance. This is an example of which interview technique?
    1. Direct question
    2. Problem solving
    3. Problem seeking
    4. Open-ended question

    Answer:_____ Rationale: _____

    _____

    _____

27. Mr. Davis tells the nurse that he has been experiencing more frequent episodes of indigestion. The nurse asks if the indigestion is associated with meals or a reclining position and asks what relieves the indigestion. This is an example of which interview technique?
    1. Direct question
    2. Problem solving
    3. Problem seeking
    4. Open-ended question

Answer: _____   Rationale: _____

_____

_____

28. The information obtained in a review of systems (ROS) is:
    1. Objective
    2. Subjective
    3. Based on the nurse's perspective
    4. Based on physical examination findings

Answer: _____   Rationale: _____

_____

_____

17 Nursing Diagnosis

PRELIMINARY READING

Chapter 17, pp. 225-239

COMPREHENSIVE UNDERSTANDING

Match the following terms that relate to diagnostic conclusions.

1. _____ Medical diagnosis
2. _____ Collaborative problem
3. _____ Defining characteristics
4. _____ Nursing diagnosis
5. _____ Risk nursing diagnosis
6. _____ Health promotion nursing diagnosis
7. _____ Problem-focused nursing diagnosis

a. Desire to increase well-being and actualize human health potential
b. The clinical criteria or assessment findings that support an actual nursing diagnosis
c. Describes human responses to health conditions or life processes that exist in an individual, family, or community
d. Identification of a disease condition
e. Actual or potential physiological complication that is monitored in collaboration with others
f. Human responses to health conditions that may possibly develop in a vulnerable individual, family, or community
g. Clinical judgment concerning an undesirable human response to a health condition or life processes

Critical Thinking and the Nursing Diagnostic Process

Define the following components of the diagnostic reasoning process.

8. Data cluster: _____

_____

9. Defining characteristics: _____

_____

10. Data interpretation: _____

_____

Explain the following components of a nursing diagnosis.

11. Diagnostic label: _____

_____

12. Related factor: _____

_____

13. PES format: _____

_____

14. Questions to consider using in making a culturally competent nursing diagnosis.

a. _____

b. _____

c. _____

d. _____

e. _____

Concept Mapping Nursing Diagnosis

15. Identify the purpose of concept mapping a nursing diagnosis.

_____

_____

Sources of Diagnostic Errors

Identify the sources of error in the steps of the nursing process related to:

16. Errors in interpretation and analysis of data: _____

_____

17. Errors in data clustering: _____

_____

18. Errors in the diagnostic statement: _____

_____

19. State the guidelines to use to reduce errors when formulating the diagnostic statement.

a. _____

b. _____

c. _____

d. _____

e. _____

f. _____

g. _____

h. _____

i. _____

j. _____

k. _____

l. _____

20. Explain how you would document a patient's nursing diagnoses.

_____

_____

REVIEW QUESTIONS

Select the appropriate answer and cite the rationale for choosing that particular answer.

21. A nursing diagnosis:
    1. Identifies nursing problems
    2. Is not changed during the course of a patient's hospitalization
    3. Is derived from the physician's history and physical examination
    4. Is a statement of a patient response to a health problem that requires nursing intervention

    Answer: _____ Rationale: _____
    _____
    _____

22. The first part of the nursing diagnosis statement:
    1. May be stated as a medical diagnosis
    2. Identifies the cause of the patient problem
    3. Identifies appropriate nursing interventions
    4. Identifies an actual or potential health problem

    Answer: _____ Rationale: _____
    _____
    _____

23. The second part of the nursing diagnosis statement:
    1. Is usually stated as a medical diagnosis
    2. Identifies the expected outcomes of nursing care
    3. Identifies the probable cause of the patient problem
    4. Is connected to the first part of the statement with the phrase "related to"

    Answer: _____ Rationale: _____
    _____
    _____

24. Which of the following is the correctly stated nursing diagnosis?
    1. Needs to be fed related to broken right arm
    2. Impaired skin integrity related to fecal incontinence
    3. Abnormal breath sounds caused by weak cough reflex
    4. Impaired physical mobility related to rheumatoid arthritis

    Answer: _____ Rationale: _____
    _____
    _____

18 Planning Nursing Care

Chapter 18, pp. 240-256

COMPREHENSIVE UNDERSTANDING

Establishing Priorities

1. Planning involves _____, _____, and
   _____

2. Nurses establish priorities in relation to importance and time. Briefly explain the following.

   a. High priority: _____

   b. Intermediate priority: _____

   c. Low priority: _____

3. Identify some factors within the health care environment that affect the ability to set priorities.

   a. _____

   b. _____

   c. _____

   d. _____

   e. _____

   f. _____

   g. _____

Critical Thinking in Setting Goals and Expected Outcomes

Match the following.

4. _____ Goal
5. _____ Patient-centered goal
6. _____ Short-term goal
7. _____ Long-term goal
8. _____ Expected outcome
9. _____ Nursing-sensitive patient outcome

a. An individual, family, or community state, behavior, or perception that is measurable in response to a nursing intervention
b. Specific and measurable behavior or response that reflects a patient's highest possible level of wellness
c. Objective behavior that is expected over a long period
d. A broad statement that describes a desired change in a patient's condition or behavior
e. Objective behavior that you expect the patient will achieve in a short time
f. A measurable criterion to evaluate goal achievement

10. The SMART approach for writing goals and outcome statement stands for: _____
    _____

Briefly explain the guidelines to follow when writing goals and expected outcomes.

11. Singular goal or outcome: _____
    _____

12. Measurable: _____

_____

13. Attainable: _____

_____

14. Realistic: _____

_____

15. Timed: _____

_____

Critical Thinking in Planning Nursing Care

There are three categories of interventions, and category selection is based on the patient's needs. Define each.

16. *Independent nursing interventions*: _____

_____

17. *Dependent nursing interventions*: _____

_____

18. *Collaborative interventions*: _____

_____

19. Identify the six factors the nurse uses to select nursing interventions for a specific patient.

    a. _____

    b. _____

    c. _____

    d. _____

    e. _____

    f. _____

Systems for Planning Nursing Care

20. Define the purposes of the *nursing care plan.*

_____

_____

Briefly explain the following types of care plans.

21. Student care plans: _____

_____

22. Interdisciplinary care plans: _____

_____

23. Explain the process of "nursing handoffs" as a practice of communication information at the end of the shift.

_____

_____

Consulting With Other Health Care Professionals

24. Consultation is a process in which: _____

    _____

25. List the six steps of the nurse's role when seeking consultation.

    a. _____

    b. _____

    c. _____

    d. _____

    e. _____

    f. _____

REVIEW QUESTIONS

Select the appropriate answer and cite the rationale for choosing that particular answer.

26. The following statement appears on the nursing care plan for an immunosuppressed patient: "The patient will remain free from infection throughout hospitalization." This statement is an example of a (an):
    1. Long-term goal
    2. Short-term goal
    3. Nursing diagnosis
    4. Expected outcome

    Answer:_____   Rationale:_____

    _____

    _____

27. The following statements appear on a nursing care plan for a patient after a mastectomy: "Incision site approximated; absence of drainage or prolonged erythema at incision site; and patient remains afebrile." These statements are examples of:
    1. Long-term goals
    2. Short-term goals
    3. Nursing diagnosis
    4. Expected outcomes

    Answer:_____   Rationale:_____

    _____

    _____

28. The planning step of the nursing process includes which of the following activities?
    1. Assessing and diagnosing
    2. Evaluating goal achievement
    3. Setting goals and selecting interventions
    4. Performing nursing actions and documenting them

    Answer:_____   Rationale:_____

    _____

    _____

19 Implementing Nursing Care

Chapter 19, pp. 257-269

COMPREHENSIVE UNDERSTANDING

1. Define the fourth step of the nursing process.

   _____

   _____

2. Define the following terms related to implementation.

   a. Direct care: _____

   b. Indirect care: _____

3. List the domains of nursing practice when intervening with patients.

   a. _____

   b. _____

   c. _____

   d. _____

   e. _____

   f. _____

   g. _____

Standard Nursing Interventions

Define the following terms.

4. Clinical practice guideline: _____

   _____

5. Standing order: _____

   _____

6. Nursing Interventions Classification (NIC) interventions: _____

   _____

Critical Thinking in Implementation

7. Briefly explain the activities for making decisions during implementation.

   a. _____

   b. _____

   c. _____

   d. _____

Implementation Process

Briefly explain the five preparatory activities for implementation of safe and effective nursing care.

8. Reassessing the patient: _____

_____

9. Reviewing and revising the existing nursing care plan: _____

_____

10. Prepare for implementation: _____

_____

11. Anticipate and prevent complications: _____

_____

12. Implementation skills: _____

_____

Direct Care

13. Define activities of daily living (ADLs).

_____

_____

14. Instrumental activities of daily living (IADLs) include: _____

_____

_____

15. Physical care techniques include: _____

_____

_____

16. Lifesaving measures are: _____

_____

_____

17. Counseling is: _____

_____

_____

18. The focus of teaching is: _____

_____

_____

19. An adverse reaction is: _____

_____

_____

20. Preventive nursing actions are: _____

_____

_____

Indirect Care

21. Define interdisciplinary care plan.

_____

_____

Achieving Patient Goals

22. Patient adherence is: _____

_____

REVIEW QUESTIONS

Select the appropriate answer and cite the rationale for choosing that particular answer.

23. Which of the following is not true of standing orders?
    1. Standing orders are commonly found in critical care and community health settings.
    2. Standing orders are approved and signed by the health care provider in charge of care before implementation.
    3. With standing orders, nurses have the legal protection to intervene appropriately in the patient's best interest.
    4. With standing orders, the nurse relies on the health care provider's judgment to determine if the intervention is appropriate.

    Answer:_____ Rationale:_____

    _____

    _____

24. The nursing care plan calls for the patient, a 300-lb woman, to be turned every 2 hours. The patient is unable to assist with turning. The nurse knows that she may hurt her back if she attempts to turn the patient by herself. The nurse should:
    1. Turn the patient by herself
    2. Ask another nurse to help her turn the patient
    3. Rewrite the care plan to eliminate the need for turning
    4. Ignore the intervention related to turning in the care plan

    Answer:_____ Rationale:_____

    _____

    _____

25. Mrs. Kay comes to the family clinic for birth control. The nurse obtains a health history and performs a pelvic examination and Pap smear. The nurse is functioning according to:
    1. Protocol
    2. Standing order
    3. Nursing care plan
    4. Intervention strategy

    Answer:_____ Rationale:_____

    _____

    _____

26. Mary Jones is a newly diagnosed patient with diabetes. The nurse shows Mary how to administer an injection. This intervention activity is:
    1. Teaching
    2. Managing
    3. Counseling

    Answer:_____ Rationale:_____

    _____

    _____

20 Evaluation

PRELIMINARY READING

Chapter 20, pp. 270-278

COMPREHENSIVE UNDERSTANDING

Critical Thinking in Evaluation

1. Briefly define the final step of the nursing process.

   _____

   _____

2. The purpose of conducting evaluative measures is: _____

   _____

3. The competencies for evaluation are:

   a. _____

   b. _____

   c. _____

   d. _____

4. Explain the purpose of the Nursing Outcomes Classification (NOC).

   _____

   _____

5. Expected outcome is: _____

   _____

6. List the steps to evaluate the degree of success in achieving the outcomes of care.

   a. _____

   b. _____

   c. _____

   d. _____

   e. _____

7. Reflection-in-action involves: _____

   _____

Briefly explain the following parts of the evaluative process.

8. Care plan revision: _____

   _____

   _____

9. Discontinuing a care plan: _____

_____

_____

10. Modifying a care plan: _____

_____

_____

Standards for Evaluation

11. The competencies for evaluation include: _____

_____

12. Successful collaboration involves: _____

_____

13. Identify the responsibilities of documenting and reporting.

_____

_____

REVIEW QUESTIONS

Select the appropriate answer and cite the rationale for choosing that particular answer.

14. Measuring the patient's response to nursing interventions and his or her progress toward achieving goals occurs during which phase of the nursing process?
    1. Planning
    2. Evaluation
    3. Assessment
    4. Nursing diagnosis

    Answer: _____ Rationale: _____

    _____

    _____

15. Evaluation is:
    1. Only necessary if the health care provider orders it
    2. An integrated, ongoing nursing care activity
    3. Begun immediately before the patient's discharge
    4. Performed primarily by nurses in the quality assurance department

    Answer: _____ Rationale: _____

    _____

    _____

16. The criteria used to determine the effectiveness of a nursing action are based on the:
    1. Nursing diagnosis
    2. Expected outcomes
    3. Patient's satisfaction
    4. Nursing interventions

    Answer: _____ Rationale: _____

    _____

    _____

17. When a patient-centered goal has not been met in the projected time frame, the most appropriate action by the nurse would be to:
    1. Rewrite the plan using different interventions.
    2. Continue with the same plan until the goal is met.
    3. Repeat the entire sequence of the nursing process to discover needed changes.
    4. Conclude that the goal was inappropriate or unrealistic and eliminate it from the plan.

    Answer: _____ Rationale: _____

    _____

    _____

21 Managing Patient Care

PRELIMINARY READING

Chapter 21, pp. 279-291

COMPREHENSIVE UNDERSTANDING

Building a Nursing Team

1. Identify the 12 characteristics of an effective nurse leader.

   a. _____

   b. _____

   c. _____

   d. _____

   e. _____

   f. _____

   g. _____

   h. _____

   i. _____

   j. _____

   k. _____

   l. _____

2. When a nurse manager uses transformational leadership they:

   a. _____

   b. _____

   c. _____

Match the following terms.

3. _____ Magnet recognition
4. _____ Team nursing
5. _____ Total patient care
6. _____ Case management
7. _____ Decentralized management
8. _____ Responsibility
9. _____ Autonomy
10. _____ Authority
11. _____ Accountability
12. _____ Interprofessional collaboration

a. Bringing representatives of various disciplines together to work with patients to improve quality of care
b. Original care delivery model of Florence Nightingale
c. Decision making is moved down to the level of the staff; managers and staff are more actively involved
d. The hospital has clinical promotion systems and research and evidence-based practice programs; nurses have professional autonomy over their practice
e. Interdisciplinary team approach developed in response to severe shortage of nursing after World War II
f. Duties and activities that an individual is employed to perform
g. Accepting the commitment to provide excellent care and the responsibility for the outcomes of the actions
h. Freedom of choice and responsibility for choices
i. Legitimate power to give commands and make final decisions specific to a given position
j. Approach that coordinates and links health care services to patients, streamlining costs and maintaining quality

13. List the responsibilities of nursing managers.

   a. _____

   b. _____

   c. _____

   d. _____

   e. _____

   f. _____

   g. _____

   h. _____

   i. _____

   j. _____

   k. _____

   l. _____

   m. _____

14. Identify the five approaches the nurse manager uses to support staff involvement.

   a. _____

   b. _____

   c. _____

   d. _____

   e. _____

Leadership Skills for Nursing Students

Summarize each of the following skills.

15. Clinical decisions: _____

_____

16. Priority setting: _____

_____

17. Organizational skills: _____

_____

18. Use of resources: _____

_____

19. Time management: _____

_____

20. Evaluation: _____

_____

21. Team communication: _____

_____

22. List the principles of time management.

    a. _____

    b. _____

    c. _____

    d. _____

    e. _____

23. Identify the five rights of delegation.

    a. _____

    b. _____

    c. _____

    d. _____

    e. _____

24. Summarize the requirements for appropriate delegation.

    a. _____

    b. _____

    c. _____

    d. _____

    e. _____

REVIEW QUESTIONS

Select the appropriate answer and cite the rationale for choosing that particular answer.

25. A student nurse practicing primary leadership skills would demonstrate all of the following except:
    1. Being sensitive to the group's feelings
    2. Recognizing others for their contributions
    3. Developing listening skills and being aware of personal motivation
    4. Assuming primary responsibility for planning, implementation, follow-up, and evaluation

Answer: _____ Rationale: _____

_____

_____

22 Ethics and Values

PRELIMINARY READING

Chapter 22, pp. 292-301

COMPREHENSIVE UNDERSTANDING

Basic Terms in Health Ethics

Match the following terms in health ethics.

1. _____ Autonomy
2. _____ Beneficence
3. _____ Nonmaleficence
4. _____ Justice
5. _____ Fidelity

a. The agreement to keep promises and the unwillingness to abandon patients
b. The best interests of the patient remain more important than self-interest
c. Fairness
d. Commitment to include patients in decisions about care
e. Avoidance of harm or hurt

Professional Nursing Code of Ethics

6. Identify the four basic principles of the code of ethics.

a. _____

b. _____

c. _____

d. _____

Values

Define the following terms.

7. Value: _____

_____

8. Values clarification: _____

_____

Ethics and Philosophy

Briefly explain the following philosophical constructs in relation to ethical systems.

9. Deontology: _____

_____

10. Utilitarianism: _____

_____

11. Feminist ethics: _____

_____

12. Ethic of care: _____

_____

13. Casuistry: _____

_____

Nursing Point of View

14. List the key steps in the resolution of an ethical dilemma.

    a. _____

    b. _____

    c. _____

    d. _____

    e. _____

    f. _____

15. Identify the purposes of the ethics committee.

_____

_____

Issues in Health Care Ethics

Briefly describe the following issues that are common in health care settings.

16. Quality of life: _____

_____

17. Disabilities: _____

_____

18. End of life care: _____

_____

REVIEW QUESTIONS

Select the appropriate answer and cite the rationale for choosing that particular answer.

19. A health care issue often becomes an ethical dilemma because:
    1. Decisions must be made based on value systems
    2. The choices involved do not appear to be clearly right or wrong
    3. Decisions must be made quickly, often under stressful conditions
    4. A patient's legal rights coexist with a health professional's obligations

Answer: _____   Rationale: _____

_____

_____

20. Which statement about an institutional ethics committee is correct?
    1. The ethics committee would be the first option in addressing an ethical dilemma.
    2. The ethics committee replaces decision making by the patient and health care providers.
    3. The ethics committee relieves health care professionals from dealing with ethical issues.
    4. The ethics committee provides education, policy recommendations, and case consultation.

Answer: _____   Rationale: _____

_____

_____

21. The nurse is working with the parents of a seriously ill newborn. Surgery has been proposed for the infant, but the chances of success are unclear. In helping the parents resolve this ethical conflict, the nurse knows that the first step is:
    1. Exploring reasonable courses of action
    2. Identifying people who can solve the difficulty
    3. Clarifying values related to the cause of the dilemma
    4. Collecting all available information about the situation

Answer: _____   Rationale: _____

_____

_____

23 Legal Implications in Nursing Practice

PRELIMINARY READING

Chapter 23, pp. 302-315

COMPREHENSIVE UNDERSTANDING

Legal Limits of Nursing

Match the following key terms.

1. _____ Nurse Practice Acts
2. _____ Regulatory law
3. _____ Common law
4. _____ Criminal laws
5. _____ Felony
6. _____ Misdemeanor
7. _____ Civil laws
8. _____ Standards of care

a. The legal guidelines for nursing practice that describe the minimum acceptable nursing care
b. Prevent harm to society and provide punishment for crimes
c. A crime of a serious nature that has a penalty of imprisonment for greater than 1 year or even death
d. Protect the rights of individual persons within our society and encourage fair and equitable treatment
e. Describe and define the legal boundaries of nursing practice within each state
f. Judicial decisions made in courts when individual legal cases are decided
g. Less serious crime that has a penalty of a fine or imprisonment for less than 1 year
h. Reflects decisions made by administrative bodies

Federal Statutory Issues in Nursing Practice

Briefly explain the following.

9. Patient Protection and Accountable Care Act (PPACA or ACO): _____

10. Americans With Disabilities Act: _____

11. Emergency Medical Treatment and Active Labor Act (EMTALA): _____

12. Mental Health Parity Act as enacted under PPACA: _____

13. Patient Self-Determination Act: _____

14. Living wills: _____

15. Durable Power of Attorney for Health Care (DPAHC): _____

16. Uniform Anatomical Gift Act: _____

17. Health Insurance Portability and Accountability Act of 1996 (HIPAA): _____

18. Health Information Technology Act (HITECH): _____

_____

19. The Joint Commission's specific guidelines for the use of restraints are:

a. _____

b. _____

c. _____

State Statutory Issues in Nursing Practice

Explain the following issues that affect nursing practice on a state level.

20. Licensure: _____

_____

21. Good Samaritan laws: _____

_____

22. Public health laws: _____

_____

23. Uniform Determination of Death Act: _____

_____

24. Physician-assisted suicide: _____

_____

Civil and Common Law Issues in Nursing Practice

Match the following terms.

25. _____ Torts
26. _____ Assault
27. _____ Battery
28. _____ False imprisonment
29. _____ Invasion of privacy
30. _____ Slander
31. _____ Libel
32. _____ Negligence
33. _____ Malpractice
34. _____ Informed consent

a. Person's agreement to allow something to happen based on disclosure of risks, benefits, and alternatives
b. Referred to as professional negligence; below the standard of care
c. When one person speaks falsely about another person
d. Civil wrong made against a person or property
e. Any intentional touching without consent
f. Written defamation of character
g. Any intentional threat to bring about harmful or offensive contact
h. Unjustified restraining of a person without legal warrant
i. The release of a patient's medical information to an unauthorized person
j. Conduct that falls below the standard of care

35. Identify the four criteria needed to establish nursing malpractice.

a. _____

b. _____

c. _____

d. _____

36. Prior to establishing a relationship, a nurse may refuse an assignment and is not considered abandonment when:

a. _____

b. _____

c. _____

d. _____

e. _____

f. _____

37. Identify what the nurse's responsibility is when he or she "floats" to another nursing unit.

_____

_____

38. What is the nurse's responsibility with health care provider's orders?

_____

_____

Risk Management and Quality Assurance

39. Risk management is: _____

_____

40. Identify the purpose of the occurrence (incident) report.

_____

_____

REVIEW QUESTIONS

Select the appropriate answer and cite the rationale for choosing that particular answer.

41. The scope of nursing practice is legally defined by:
    1. State Nurse Practice Acts
    2. Professional nursing organizations
    3. Hospital policy and procedure manuals
    4. Health care providers in the employing institutions

    Answer:_____ Rationale:_____

    _____

    _____

42. A student nurse who is employed as a nursing assistant may perform any functions that:
    1. Have been learned in school
    2. Are expected of a nurse at that level
    3. Are identified in the position's job description
    4. Require technical rather than professional skill

    Answer:_____ Rationale:_____

    _____

    _____

43. A confused patient who fell out of bed because side rails were not used is an example of which type of liability?
    1. Felony
    2. Battery
    3. Assault
    4. Negligence

    Answer:_____ Rationale:_____

    _____

    _____

44. The nurse puts restraints on a patient without the patient's permission and without a physician's order. The nurse may be guilty of:
    1. Battery
    2. Assault
    3. Neglect
    4. Invasion of privacy

    Answer:_____ Rationale:_____

    _____

    _____

45. In a situation in which there is insufficient staff to implement competent care, a nurse should:
    1. Organize a strike
    2. Refuse the assignment
    3. Inform the patients of the situation
    4. Accept the assignment but make a protest in writing to the administration

    Answer:_____ Rationale:_____

    _____

24 Communication

Chapter 24, pp. 316-335

COMPREHENSIVE UNDERSTANDING

Communication and Nursing Practice

1. Communication is: dynamic series of events that involve the transmission of meaning from sender to receiver

2. For the nurse to be able to relate to others, he or she must have the ability to:

   a. Interpret Messages

   b. Correct Misinformation

   c. Promote patient understanding

   d. Plan Patient - Centered care

   e. Critical think

3. Perceptual biases are: biases made based on Perception made from the 5 senses.

4. Emotional intelligence (EI) is: an assessment + Communication technique that allows nurses to better understand + perceive the emotions of themselves + others.

5. List some challenging communication situations that nurses may encounter.

   a. People who are silent

   b. People who are sad / depressed

   c. People who are angry

   d. People who need assistance with visual or speech

   e. People who are uncooperative

   f. People who are talkative

   g. Demanding

   h. frightened

   i. Confused

   j. No english

   k. Flirtatious or sexual

Match the following levels of communication.

6. ____C____ Intrapersonal   a. Interaction with an audience
7. ____D____ Interpersonal   b. The use of technology
8. ____E____ Small group   c. Develops self-awareness and a positive self-esteem
9. ____A____ Public   d. One-to-one interaction between a nurse and another person
10. ____B____ Electronic   e. Interaction that occurs with a small number of persons

Elements of the Communication Process

Match the following terms that address communication.

11. __G__ Referent
12. __C__ Sender
13. __f__ Receiver
14. __J__ Message
15. __L__ Channels
16. __M__ Feedback
17. __A__ Interpersonal variables
18. __H__ Environment
19. __B__ Verbal communication
20. __I__ Connotative meaning
21. __K__ Intonation
22. __N__ Timing
23. __E__ Pacing
24. __D__ Clarity and brevity

a. Factors within both the sender and the receiver that influence communication
b. Code that conveys specific meaning through the combination of words
c. Person who encodes and delivers the message
d. Simple, brief, and direct
e. Thinking before speaking and developing an awareness of the rhythm of your speech
f. Person who decodes the message
g. Motivates one person to communicate with another
h. Setting for the sender–receiver interaction
i. Interpretation of a word's meaning influenced by the thoughts and feelings that people have about the word
j. Content of the communication
k. Tone of voice
l. Means of conveying and receiving messages through the senses
m. Indicates whether the receiver understood the meaning of the sender's message
n. When a patient expresses an interest in communicating

25. State three aspects of nonverbal communication.
   a. _Voice tone_
   b. _eye contact_
   c. _Body position_

26. Identify the four zones of personal space.
   a. _Intimate zone (0-8 in)_
   b. _Personal zone (18 in – 4 feet)_
   c. _Socio-consultative zone (9-12 ft)_
   d. _Public zone (12 ft or more)_

Professional Nursing Relationships

27. List the four goal-directed phases that characterize the nurse–patient relationship.
   a. _Preinteraction_
   b. _Orientation_
   c. _Working_
   d. _Termination_

28. Motivational interviewing (MI) is a: _technique for encouraging patients to share their thoughts, beliefs, fears, & concerns with aim of changing their behavior._

Explain the focus of the following relationships.

29. Nurse–family: _To help the family & patient understand the health care. Very ~~close~~ close to one-on-ones_

30. Nurse–health care team: _Helps keep things easy and the patient & work environment safe._

31. Give some examples of lateral violence or workplace bullying: _Withholding Info_
    Snide remarks, Put downs, Back biting.

32. Identify some techniques the nurse can use when experiencing lateral violence.
    a. _Address the behavior in a calm manner_
    b. _Describe how it affects your functioning_
    c. _Ask to stop_
    d. _Notify the Manager_
    e. _Make a plan for future action._
    f. _Document Incidences_

Elements of Professional Communication

33. List the elements of professional communication.
    a. _Courtesy_
    b. _Use Names_
    c. _Trustworthiness_
    d. _Autonomy + Responsibility_
    e. _Assertiveness_

34. Define the following terms.
    a. Autonomy: _Being self-directed in accomplishing goals + advocating for others._
    b. Assertiveness: _Allows you to express feelings + Ideas without Judging or hurting others._

Nursing Process
Assessment

35. Explain the following factors that affect communication.
    a. Psychophysical context: _Physiological Status, Emotional Status Growth + development, Unmet needs. (Internal factors)_
    b. Relational context: _Trust, Social, helping, working, caring (Nature of the relationship Among Participants)_
    c. Situational context: _Goal achievement, Info exchange, Problem solving. (Reason for Communication._
    d. Environmental context: _Privacy, Noise, comfort, Distraction (Physical surroundings)_
    e. Cultural context: _Edu. level, language, expectations (Sociocultural Elements)_

36. Give some examples of how to communicate with the older adults who have a hearing loss.
    a. _Make sure they know you are talking._
    b. _Face the Patient, mouth is visible_

c. Speak clearly

d. Speak slow

e. Check patients hearing aids, glasses

f. Choose a quiet quiet environment

g. Allow patient to Respond

h. Allow patient to ask questions

i. Short t to the point.

37. Identify the implications for patient-centered care when communicating with non-English-speaking patients.

a. Understand your own cultural values & biases

b. Asses Primary language

c. Provide Professional Interpreter

d. Speak directly to patient

e. Nodding t "OK" doesn't mean they understand

f. Provide written info in English t Primary language

g. Learn about cultures

h. Put patient communication needs in care plan.

38. Gender influences communication. Explain how communication differs in regard to gender.

a. Male: Use less verbal, address Issues directly

b. Female: Disclose more personal Info, active listening, answers to keep the convo. going

Nursing Diagnosis

39. The primary diagnosis used to describe the patient with limited or no ability to communicate is: _____

Impaired verbal Communication

40. Identify the defining characteristics of the diagnosis above.

When a person can't recieve, process, transmit & use symbol to Communicate

41. Identify the related factors that contribute to the above diagnosis.

Anxiety, Social Isolation, Ineffective coping, powerless Impaired social interaction.

Planning

42. List the goals and outcomes for the patient with the above diagnosis.

a. Initiated convo about diagnosis

b. Attend the appropriate stimuli.

c. Convey clear t understandable messages

d. Express increased satisfaction with communication

Implementation

Match the following therapeutic communication techniques.

43. __E__ Active listening
44. __G__ Sharing observations
45. __M__ Sharing empathy
46. __O__ Sharing hope
47. __F__ Sharing humor
48. __A__ Sharing feelings
49. __P__ Using touch
50. __N__ Using silence
51. __L__ Providing information
52. __K__ Clarifying
53. __B__ Focusing
54. __J__ Paraphrasing
55. __I__ Asking relevant questions
56. __C__ Summarizing
57. __D__ Self-disclosure
58. __H__ Confrontation

a. Subjective feelings that result from one's thoughts and perceptions
b. Used to center on key elements or concepts of the message
c. Concise review of key aspects of an interaction
d. Subjectively true, personal experiences about self that are intentionally revealed to another
e. Being attentive to what the patient is saying both verbally and nonverbally
f. Coping strategy to adjust to stress
g. Helps the patient communicate without the need for extensive questioning
h. Helping the patient become aware of inconsistencies in his or her feelings, attitudes, beliefs, and behaviors
i. Seeking information needed for decision making
j. Restating another's message more briefly using one's own words
k. Restating an unclear or ambiguous message
l. Patients have the right to know about their health status and what is happening in their environment
m. Ability to understand and accept another person's reality
n. Useful when people are confronted with decisions that require much thought
o. "Sense of possibility"
p. Most potent form of communication

Match the following nontherapeutic communication techniques with the appropriate responses.

59. __G__ Asking personal questions
60. __K__ Giving personal opinions
61. __J__ Changing the subject
62. __F__ Autonomic responses
63. __H__ False reassurance
64. __C__ Sympathy
65. __E__ Asking for explanations
66. __D__ Approval or disapproval
67. __A__ Defensive responses
68. __I__ Passive responses
69. __B__ Arguing

a. "No one here would intentionally lie to you."
b. "How can you say you didn't sleep a wink? You were snoring all night long."
c. "I'm so sorry about your mastectomy; it must be terrible to lose a breast."
d. "You shouldn't even think about assisted suicide; it is not right."
e. "Why are you so anxious?"
f. "Older adults are always confused."
g. "Why don't you and John get married?"
h. "Don't worry; everything will be all right."
i. "Things are bad, and there's nothing I can do about it."
j. "Let's not talk about your problems with the insurance company. It's time for your walk."
k. "If I were you, I'd put your mother in a nursing home."

Briefly identify the communication techniques to use with these patients with special needs.

70. Cannot speak clearly: __Listen attentively, ask yes or no questions, visual cues__

71. Cognitively impaired: __ask one question at a time, Attentive listener, use pictures.__

72. Hearing impaired: __Check hearing Aid, Mouth visible, face patient__

73. Visually impaired: __Check glasses, speak normal, Identify self. 14 point font__

74. Unresponsive: __Call by Name, use touch, Explain Everything, Provide place & Time.__

75. Does not speak English: __Normal tone, Professional Interpreter Communication boards, Have dictionary,__

Evaluation

76. Identify what the process recording analysis reveals.

a. Whether you encouraged openness

b. Identify any missed verbal or nonverbal cues

c. Whether nursing response facilitated or blocked patient comm.

d. Whether nursing response was positive or negative.

e. Type + number of questions

f. Type + number of therapeutic communication

g. Any missed opportunities to use humor.

REVIEW QUESTIONS

Select the appropriate answer and cite the rationale for choosing that particular answer.

77. In demonstrating the method for deep breathing exercises, the nurse places his or her hands on the patient's abdomen to explain diaphragmatic movement. This technique involves the use of which communication element?
    1. Referent
    2. Message
    3. Feedback
    4. Tactile channel

    Answer: 4   Rationale: _____

78. Which statement about nonverbal communication is correct?
    1. The nurse's verbal messages should be reinforced by nonverbal cues.
    2. It is easy for a nurse to judge the meaning of a patient's facial expression.
    3. The physical appearance of the nurse rarely influences nurse–patient interaction.
    4. Words convey meanings that are usually more significant than nonverbal communication.

    Answer: 1   Rationale: _____

79. The term referring to the sender's attitude toward the self, the message, and the listener is:
    1. Denotative meaning
    2. Metacommunication
    3. Connotative meaning
    4. Nonverbal communication

    Answer: 2   Rationale: _____

80. The referent in the communication process is:
    1. Information shared by the sender
    2. The means of conveying messages
    3. That which motivates the communication
    4. The person who initiates the communication

    Answer: 3   Rationale: _____

81. A nurse is conducting an admission interview with a patient. To maintain the patient's territoriality and maximize communication, the nurse should sit:
    1. 4 to 12 feet from the patient
    2. 0 to 18 inches from the patient
    3. 12 feet or more from the patient
    4. 18 inches to 4 feet from the patient

    Answer: 4   Rationale: _____

25 Patient Education

PRELIMINARY READING

Chapter 25, pp. 336-355

COMPREHENSIVE UNDERSTANDING

Purposes of Patient Education

Briefly explain patient education in each phase of health care.

1. Maintenance and promotion of health and illness prevention: _____

_____

2. Restoration of health: _____

_____

3. Coping with impaired functions: _____

_____

Teaching and Learning

Match the following terms.

4. _____ Teaching
5. _____ Learning
6. _____ Learning objective
7. _____ Cognitive learning
8. _____ Affective learning
9. _____ Psychomotor learning
10. _____ Attentional set
11. _____ Motivation
12. _____ Self-efficacy

a. The mental state that allows the learner to focus on and comprehend a learning activity
b. A person's perceived ability to successfully complete a task
c. Interactive process that promotes learning
d. Force that acts on or within a person, causing the person to behave in a particular way
e. Integration of mental and muscular activity, ranging from perception to origination
f. Describes what the learner will be able to do after successful instruction
g. Receiving, responding, valuing, organizing, and characterizing
h. Acquisition of new knowledge, behaviors, and skills
i. Knowledge, comprehension, application analysis, synthesis, and evaluation

Summarize how each of the following influences the ability to learn.

13. Developmental capability: _____

_____

14. Learning in children: _____

_____

15. Adult learning: _____

_____

16. Physical capability: _____

_____

Nursing Process

17. Explain how the nursing process and the teaching process differ.

    a. The nursing process requires: _____

    _____

    b. The teaching process focuses on: _____

    _____

Assessment

Success in teaching the patient requires the nurse to assess the following factors. List the elements of each factor.

18. Learning needs.

    a. _____

    b. _____

    c. _____

19. Motivation to learn.

    a. _____

    b. _____

    c. _____

    d. _____

    e. _____

    f. _____

    g. _____

20. Ability to learn.

    a. _____

    b. _____

    c. _____

    d. _____

    e. _____

    f. _____

21. Teaching environment.

    a. _____

    b. _____

    c. _____

22. Resources for learning.

    a. _____

    b. _____

    c. _____

    d. _____

    e. _____

23. Define *functional illiteracy*.

_____

_____

Nursing Diagnosis

24. Describe how the nurse would define the problem.

_____

_____

Planning

The principles of teaching are techniques that incorporate the principles of learning. Explain the following principles.

25. Goals and outcomes: _____

_____

26. Setting priorities: _____

_____

27. Timing: _____

_____

28. Organizing teaching material: _____

_____

Implementation

Match the following teaching approaches.

29. _____ Telling
30. _____ Participating
31. _____ Entrusting
32. _____ Reinforcement
33. _____ One-on-one instruction
34. _____ Group instruction
35. _____ Return demonstration
36. _____ Analogies
37. _____ Role play
38. _____ Simulation

a. Economical way to teach a number of patients at one time
b. The nurse poses a pertinent problem or situation for patients to solve, which provides an opportunity to identify mistakes
c. The nurse outlines the task the patient will perform and gives explicit instructions
d. Supplement verbal instruction with familiar images
e. The nurse and patient set objectives and become involved in the learning process together
f. People play themselves or someone else
g. The chance to practice the skill
h. Most common method of instruction
i. Provides the patient with the opportunity to manage self-care
j. Using a stimulus that increases the probability for a response

Evaluation

39. Identify the nurse's responsibility in evaluating the outcomes of the teaching learning process.

_____

_____

REVIEW QUESTIONS

Select the appropriate answer and cite the rationale for choosing that particular answer.

40. An internal impulse that causes a person to take action is:
    1. Anxiety
    2. Motivation
    3. Adaptation
    4. Compliance

    Answer: _____ Rationale: _____

    _____

    _____

41. Demonstration of the principles of body mechanics used when transferring patients from bed to chair would be classified under which domain of learning?
    1. Social
    2. Affective
    3. Cognitive
    4. Psychomotor

    Answer: _____ Rationale: _____

    _____

    _____

42. Which of the following patients is most ready to begin a patient-teaching session?
    1. Ms. Hernandez, who is unwilling to accept that her back injury may result in permanent paralysis
    2. Mr. Frank, who is newly diagnosed with diabetes, who is complaining that he was awake all night because of his noisy roommate
    3. Mrs. Brown, a patient with irritable bowel syndrome, who has just returned from a morning of testing in the gastrointestinal laboratory

4. Mr. Jones, a patient who had a heart attack 4 days ago and now seems somewhat anxious about how this will affect his future

    Answer: _____ Rationale: _____

    _____

    _____

43. The nurse works with pediatric patients who have diabetes. Which is the youngest age group to which the nurse can effectively teach psychomotor skills such as insulin administration?
    1. Toddler
    2. Preschool
    3. School age
    4. Adolescent

    Answer: _____ Rationale: _____

    _____

    _____

44. Which of the following is an appropriately stated learning objective for Mr. Ryan, who is newly diagnosed with diabetes?
    1. Mr. Ryan will understand diabetes.
    2. Mr. Ryan will be taught self-administration of insulin by 5/2.
    3. Mr. Ryan will know the signs and symptoms of low blood sugar by 5/5
    4. Mr. Ryan will perform blood glucose monitoring with the EZ-Check Monitor by the time of discharge.

    Answer: _____ Rationale: _____

    _____

    _____

26 Documentation and Informatics

PRELIMINARY READING

Chapter 26, pp. 356-372

COMPREHENSIVE UNDERSTANDING

Define the following term.

1. Documentation: _____

_____

Purposes of the Medical Record

Match the following purposes of a record.

2. _____ Communication
3. _____ Legal documentation
4. _____ Diagnostic-related groups (DRGs)
5. _____ Education
6. _____ Research
7. _____ Auditing

a. Objective, ongoing reviews to determine the degree to which quality improvement standards are met
b. Learning the nature of an illness and the individual patient's responses
c. Means by which patient needs and progress, individual therapies, patient education, and discharge planning are conveyed to others in the health care team
d. Gathering of statistical data of clinical disorders, complications, therapies, recovery, and deaths
e. Describes exactly what happens to the patient and must follow agency standards
f. Classification system based on patients' medical diagnoses that supports reimbursement

8. The purpose of the electronic health record is:

   a. _____

   b. _____

Confidentiality

9. According to HIPAA (Health Insurance Portability and Accountability Act), to eliminate barriers that could delay care, providers are:

   a. _____

   b. _____

Standards

10. The standards of documentation by the Joint Commission require: _____

_____

Guidelines for Quality Documentation

Five important guidelines must be followed to ensure quality documentation and reporting. Explain each one.

11. Factual:_____

_____

12. Accurate: _____

_____

13. Complete:_____

_____

14. Current:_____

_____

15. Organized: _____

_____

Methods of Documentation

Match the following documentation systems used for recording patient data.

16. _____ Narrative
17. _____ Problem-oriented medical record (POMR)
18. _____ SOAP
19. _____ SOAPIE
20. _____ PIE
21. _____ Focus charting
22. _____ Progress notes
23. _____ Charting by exception
24. _____ Case management
25. _____ Critical pathways

a. Incorporates a multidisciplinary approach to documenting patient care
b. Focuses on deviations from the established norm or abnormal findings; highlights trends and changes
c. Database, problem list, care plan, and progress notes
d. Multidisciplinary care plans that include patient problems, key interventions, and expected outcomes
e. One of several formats or structured notes within a POMR
f. SOAP with intervention and evaluation added
g. Use of DAR (data, action, and response)
h. Problem, intervention, and evaluation with a nursing origin
i. Subjective, objective, assessment, and plan
j. Story-like format that has the tendency to have repetitious information and be time consuming

Common Record-Keeping Forms

Match the following formats used for record keeping.

26. _____ Admission nursing history forms
27. _____ Flow sheets
28. _____ Patient care summary
29. _____ Acuity records
30. _____ Standardized care plans
31. _____ Discharge summary forms

a. Includes medications, diet, community resources, and follow-up care
b. Level is based on the type and number of nursing interventions required over a 24-hour period
c. Provides current information that is accessible to all members of the health care team
d. Provides baseline data to compare with changes in the patient's condition
e. Provides the most current information that has been entered into the EHR
f. Preprinted, established guidelines used to care for the patient

Documenting Communication with Providers and Unique Events

32. List the information that needs to be documented with telephone reports.

_____

_____

33. List the guidelines the nurse should follow when receiving telephone orders from health care providers.

a. _____

b. _____

c. _____

d. _____

e. _____

34. An incident or occurrence is _____. Give some examples of incidents.

_____

_____

Informatics and Information Management in Health Care

35. Define health informatics.

_____

_____

36. Nursing informatics integrates: _____

_____

37. Identify the two nursing clinical information systems that are available.

   a. _____

   b. _____

38. Identify the advantages of a nursing clinical information system.

   a. _____

   b. _____

   c. _____

   d. _____

   e. _____

   f. _____

   g. _____

   h. _____

REVIEW QUESTIONS

Select the appropriate answer and cite the rationale for choosing that particular answer.

39. The primary purpose of a patient's medical record is to:
    1. Provide validation for hospital charges
    2. Satisfy requirements of accreditation agencies
    3. Provide the nurse with a defense against malpractice
    4. Communicate accurate, timely information about the patient

Answer: _____ Rationale: _____

_____

_____

40. Which of the following is correctly charted according to the six guidelines for quality recording?
    1. Was depressed today.
    2. Respirations rapid; lung sounds clear.
    3. Had a good day. Up and about in room.
    4. Crying. States she doesn't want visitors to see her like this.

Answer: _____ Rationale: _____

_____

_____

41. During a change-of-shift report:
    1. Two or more nurses always visit all patients to review their plan of care.
    2. The nurse should identify nursing diagnoses and clarify patient priorities.
    3. Nurses should exchange judgments they have made about patient attitudes.
    4. Patient information is communicated from a nurse on a sending unit to a nurse on a receiving unit.

    Answer: _____   Rationale: _____

    _____

    _____

42. An incident report is:
    1. A legal claim against a nurse for negligent nursing care
    2. A summary report of all falls occurring on a nursing unit
    3. A report of an event inconsistent with the routine care of a patient
    4. A report of a nurse's behavior submitted to the hospital administration

    Answer: _____   Rationale: _____

    _____

    _____

43. If an error is made while recording, the nurse should:
    1. Erase it or scratch it out
    2. Leave a blank space in the note
    3. Draw a single line through the error and initial it
    4. Obtain a new nurse's note and rewrite the entries

    Answer: _____   Rationale: _____

    _____

    _____

27 Patient Safety and Quality

PRELIMINARY READING

Chapter 27, pp. 373-406

COMPREHENSIVE UNDERSTANDING

1. Identify the Joint Commission 2015 National Patient Safety Goals for Critical Access Hospitals.

    a. Identify Patients correctly

    b. Improve staff communication

    c. use medicines safely

    d. use alarms safely

    e. prevent Infection

    f. prevent mistakes in surgery

Scientific Knowledge Base

2. Identify Maslow's hierarchy of basic needs that influence a person's safety.

    a. Oxygen

    b. Nutrition

    c. Temperature

3. List the physical hazards in the environment that threaten a person's safety.

    a. Physical Hazards

    b. Motor vehicle Accidents

    c. Poison

    d. Falls

    e. Disasters

Define the following terms.

4. Pathogen: Any microorganism capable of producing Illness

5. Immunization: reduces, prevents the transmission of disease

6. Pollutant: A harmful chemical or waste discharged into water, soil or air.

Nursing Knowledge Base

7. In addition to being knowledgeable about the environment, nurses must be familiar with:

    a. Patients developmental level

    b. Mobility, sensory, & cognitive status

c. _lifestyle choices_

d. _common safety precautions_

8. Identify the individual risk factors that can pose a threat to safety.

a. _life style_

b. _Impaired mobility_

c. _Sensory or communication Impairment_

d. _Lack of safety Awareness_

9. List the four major risks to patient safety in the health care environment.

a. _Falls_

b. _Patient - Inherent Accidents_

c. _Procedure- Related Accidents_

d. _Equipment - Related Accidents_

Nursing Process
Assessment

10. Identify the specific patient assessments to perform when considering possible threats to the patient's safety.

a. _Activity & Exercise_

b. _Medication History_

c. _History of falls_

d. _Home Maintenance & Safety_

Nursing Diagnosis

11. Identify actual or potential nursing diagnoses that apply to patients whose safety is threatened.

a. _Risk of Injury_

b. _Impaired Home Maintance_

c. _Deficient knowledge_

d. _Risk of poisoning_

e. _Risk of suffocation_

f. _Risk of trauma_

Implementation

12. Identify the strategies needed to provide safe nursing care.

a. _Effective use of technology & standardized Practice_

b. _effective use of strategies to reduce harm_

c. _use Appropriate strategies to reduce reliance on memory_

Give an example(s) of an intervention for the following developmental stages.

13. Infant and toddler: _Should be Immunized, sleep on their back_

14. Preschooler: _____

15. School-age child: _____

16. Adolescent: _____

17. Adult: _____

18. Older adult: _____

19. Nursing interventions directed at eliminating environmental threats include:

    a. _____

    b. _____

20. The Joint Commission recommends that hospitals have formal fall-reduction programs, which include a fall risk assessment of every patient conducted:

    a. _____

    b. _____

21. A physical restraint is: _____

22. A chemical restraint is: _____

23. Use of restraints must meet one of the following objectives.

    a. _____

    b. _____

    c. _____

    d. _____

24. Explain the mnemonic RACE to set priorities in case of fire.

    a. R: _____

    b. A: _____

    c. C: _____

    d. E: _____

25. Explain seizure precautions.

    _____

    _____

26. Identify the measures with which the nurse must be familiar to reduce exposure to radiation.

    _____

    _____

27. The Joint Commission (2015) requires that hospitals have an emergency management plan that addresses:

    a. _____

    b. _____

    c. _____

REVIEW QUESTIONS

Select the appropriate answer and cite the rationale for choosing that particular answer.

28. Which of the following would most immediately threaten an individual's safety?
    1. 70% humidity
    2. A sprained ankle
    3. Lack of water
    4. Unrefrigerated fresh vegetables

Answer: _____ Rationale: _____

_____

_____

29. The developmental stage that carries the highest risk of an injury from a fall is:
    1. Preschool
    2. Adulthood
    3. School age
    4. Older adulthood

Answer: _____ Rationale: _____

_____

_____

30. Mrs. Field falls asleep while smoking in bed and drops the burning cigarette on her blanket. When she awakens, her bed is on fire, and she quickly calls the nurse. On observing the fire, the nurse should immediately:
    1. Report the fire
    2. Attempt to extinguish the fire
    3. Assist Mrs. Field to a safe place
    4. Close all windows and doors to contain the fire

Answer: _____ Rationale: _____

_____

_____

CRITICAL THINKING MODEL FOR NURSING CARE PLAN FOR RISK FOR FALLS

31. Imagine that you are Mr. Key, the nurse in the care plan on p. 383 of your text. Complete the *Assessment phase* of the critical thinking model by writing your answers in the appropriate boxes of the model shown. Think about the following.
    a. As you review your assessment, what key areas did you cover?
    b. In developing Ms. Cohen's plan of care, what knowledge did Mr. Key apply?
    c. In what way might Mr. Key's previous experience assist in this case?
    d. What intellectual or professional standards were applied to Ms. Cohen?
    e. What critical thinking attitudes might have been applied in this case?

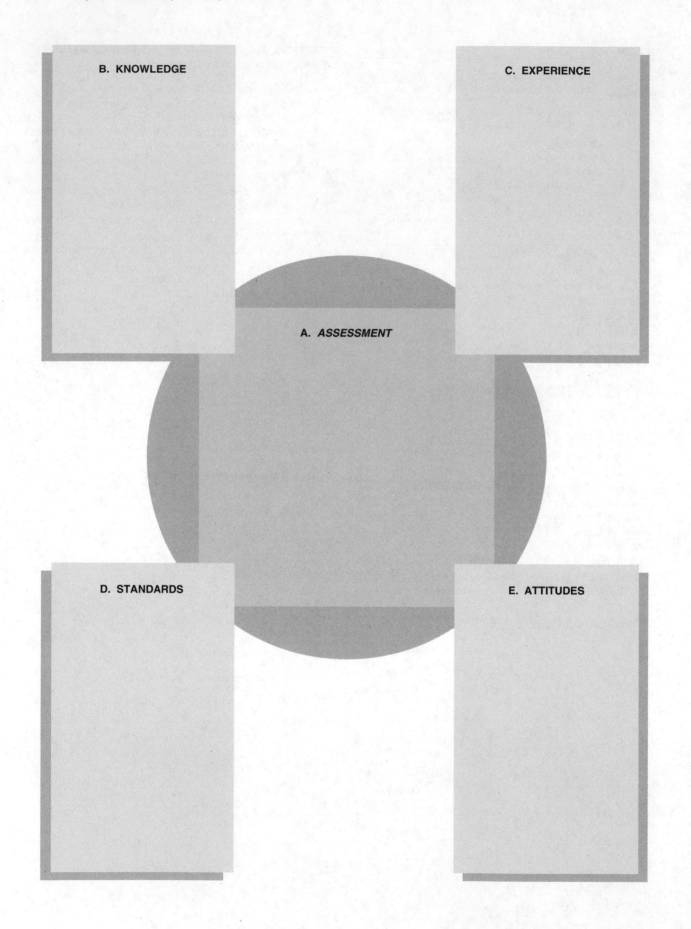

B. KNOWLEDGE

C. EXPERIENCE

A. *ASSESSMENT*

D. STANDARDS

E. ATTITUDES

28 Immobility

PRELIMINARY READING

Chapter 28, pp. 407-441

COMPREHENSIVE UNDERSTANDING

Scientific Knowledge Base

Match the following terms related to the nature of movement.

1. _____ Body mechanics
2. _____ Body alignment
3. _____ Friction
4. _____ Shear

   a. Force that occurs in a direction to oppose movement
   b. Force exerted against the skin while the skin remains stationary and the bony structures move
   c. The individual's center of gravity is stable
   d. Describes the coordinated efforts of the musculoskeletal and nervous system

Describe how the following are related to movement.

5. Joints: _____

6. Ligaments: _____

7. Tendons: _____

8. Cartilages: _____

9. Skeletal muscles: _____

10. Nervous system: _____

11. Describe how the following pathological abnormalities affect mobility.

   a. Postural: _____

   b. Muscle: _____

   c. Damage to the nervous system: _____

Nursing Knowledge Base

Define the following terms.

12. Mobility: _____

13. Immobility: _____

14. Disuse atrophy: _____

_____

15. Identify the complications of immobility in relation to the metabolic functioning of the body.

_____

_____

16. Explain the following respiratory changes that occur with immobility.

   a. Atelectasis: _____

   b. Hydrostatic pneumonia: _____

17. Explain the following cardiovascular changes that occur with immobility.

   a. Orthostatic hypotension: _____

   b. Thrombus: _____

18. Identify the complications of immobility in relation to the musculoskeletal system.

   a. _____

   b. _____

   c. _____

   d. _____

   e. _____

   f. _____

19. Identify the complications of immobility in relation to the urinary system.

   a. _____

   b. _____

20. Identify the complication of immobility in relation to the integumentary system.

_____

_____

21. Identify the psychosocial effects that occur with immobilization.

   a. _____

   b. _____

   c. _____

Briefly explain the negative outcomes of immobility to the following groups.

22. Infants, toddlers, and preschoolers: _____

_____

23. Adolescents: _____

_____

24. Adults: _____

_____

25. Older adults: _____

_____

Nursing Process
Assessment

26. Briefly describe the four major areas for assessment of patient mobility.

    a. Range of motion: _____

    b. Gait: _____

    c. Exercise and activity tolerance: _____

    d. Body alignment: _____

Describe the technique to use to assess the physiological hazards of immobility and cite an abnormal finding of each technique.

27. Metabolic: _____

_____

28. Respiratory: _____

_____

29. Cardiovascular: _____

_____

30. Musculoskeletal: _____

_____

31. Skin: _____

_____

32. Elimination: _____

_____

Nursing Diagnosis

33. List the actual or potential nursing diagnoses related to an immobilized or partially immobilized patient.

    a. _____

    b. _____

    c. _____

    d. _____

    e. _____

    f. _____

    g. _____

Planning

34. List the expected outcomes for the goal "patient skin remains intact."

    a. _____

    b. _____

Implementation

35. Identify some examples of health promotion activities that address mobility and immobility.

    a. _____

    b. _____

    c. _____

    d. _____

Identify the nursing interventions that will reduce the impact of immobility on the following body systems.

36. Metabolic system.

    a. _____

    b. _____

37. Respiratory system.

    a. _____

    b. _____

    c. _____

38. Cardiovascular system.

    a. _____

    b. _____

    c. _____

39. Musculoskeletal system.

    a. _____

    b. _____

40. Integumentary system.

    a. _____

    b. _____

41. Elimination system.

    a. _____

    b. _____

42. Psychosocial system.

    a. _____

    b. _____

43. Explain the use for the following.

    a. Trochanter roll: _____

    b. Hand rolls: _____

    c. Trapeze bar: _____

44. Give a description of the following positions.

    a. Fowler: _____

    b. Supine: _____

    c. Prone: _____

    d. Side-lying: _____

    e. Sims: _____

45. Instrumental activities of daily living (IADL) are: _____
_____

46. Describe how you would assist patients with hemiplegia or hemiparesis.

_____

_____

REVIEW QUESTIONS

Select the appropriate answer and cite the rationale for choosing that particular answer.

47. Which of the following is a potential hazard that you should assess when the patient is in the prone position?
    1. Plantar flexion
    2. Increased cervical flexion
    3. Internal rotation of the shoulder
    4. Unprotected pressure points at the sacrum and heels

    Answer: _____ Rationale: _____

    _____

    _____

48. Which of the following is a physiological effect of prolonged bed rest?
    1. An increase in cardiac output
    2. A decrease in lean body mass
    3. A decrease in lung expansion
    4. A decrease in urinary excretion of nitrogen

    Answer: _____ Rationale: _____

    _____

    _____

49. All of the following measures are used to assess for deep vein thrombosis except:
    1. Checking for a positive Homan's sign
    2. Asking the patient about the presence of calf pain
    3. Observing the dorsal aspect of lower extremities for redness, warmth, and tenderness
    4. Measuring the circumference of each leg daily, placing the tape measure at the midpoint of the knee

    Answer: _____ Rationale: _____

    _____

    _____

50. Which of the following is an appropriate intervention to maintain the respiratory system of the immobilized patient?
    1. Turn the patient every 4 hours.
    2. Maintain a maximum fluid intake of 1500 mL/day.
    3. Apply an abdominal binder continuously while the patient is in bed.
    4. Encourage the patient to deep breathe and cough every 1 to 2 hours.

    Answer: _____ Rationale: _____

    _____

    _____

29 Infection Prevention and Control

PRELIMINARY READING

Chapter 29, pp. 442-485

COMPREHENSIVE UNDERSTANDING

Scientific Knowledge Base

Match the following terms that are related to the infectious process.

1. _____ Pathogen
2. _____ Colonization
3. _____ Infectious disease
4. _____ Communicable disease
5. _____ pH
6. _____ Portal of exit
7. _____ Major route of transmission
8. _____ Virulence
9. _____ Susceptibility
10. _____ Immunocompromised
11. _____ Reservoir
12. _____ Carriers
13. _____ Aerobic bacteria
14. _____ Anaerobic bacteria
15. _____ Bacteriostasis
16. _____ Bactericidal

a. Individual's degree of resistance to pathogens
b. Persons who show no symptoms of illness but who have the pathogens that are transferred to others
c. Prevention of the growth and reproduction of bacteria by cold temperatures
d. Infectious agent
e. Bacteria that require oxygen for survival
f. Having an impaired immune system
g. Acidity of the environment
h. Bacteria that thrive with little or no free oxygen
i. A temperature or chemical that destroys bacteria
j. A place where a pathogen survives
k. Unwashed hands of a health care worker
l. An infectious disease that is transmitted directly from one person to another
m. Organism that multiplies within a host but does not cause an infection
n. Sites such as blood, mucus membranes, respiratory tract, genitourinary tract, and gastrointestinal tract
o. Illnesses such as viral meningitis or pneumonia
p. Ability to survive in the host or outside the body

17. Development of an infection occurs in a cycle that depends on the following elements.

a. _____

b. _____

c. _____

d. _____

e. _____

f. _____

18. Explain the most common modes of transmission.

a. Direct: _____

b. Indirect: _____

c. Droplet: _____

d. Airborne: _____

e. Vehicles: _____

f. Vector: _____

The Infectious Process

19. Infections follow a progressive course by four stages. List and explain each stage.

    a. _____

    b. _____

    c. _____

    d. _____

20. Describe the two types of infections.

    a. Localized: _____

    _____

    b. Systemic: _____

    _____

21. Explain the normal body defenses against infection.

    a. Normal flora: _____

    _____

    b. Body system defenses: _____

    _____

    c. Inflammation: _____

    _____

22. Acute inflammation is an immediate response to cellular injury. Explain each briefly.

    a. Vascular and cellular responses: _____

    _____

    b. Inflammatory exudate: _____

    _____

    c. Tissue repair: _____

23. Define the following types of health care–associated infections (nosocomial).

    a. Exogenous: _____

    _____

    b. Endogenous: _____

    _____

24. Identify the sites of health care–associated infections.

    a. _____

    b. _____

    c. _____

    d. _____

Nursing Knowledge Base

25. The following factors influence a patient's susceptibility to infection. Briefly explain them, giving an example of each.

a. Age: _____

_____

b. Nutritional status: _____

_____

c. Stress: _____

_____

d. Disease process: _____

_____

Nursing Process

26. Identify a cause for the following risk for infections:

a. Chronic disease: _____

b. Lifestyle behaviors: _____

c. Occupation: _____

d. Diagnostic procedures: _____

e. Heredity: _____

f. Travel history: _____

g. Trauma: _____

h. Nutrition: _____

27. Fill in the following table.

Laboratory Value	Normal (Adult) Values	Indication of Infection
WBC count		
Erythrocyte sedimentation rate		
Iron level		
Cultures of urine and blood		
Cultures and Gram stain of wound, sputum, and throat		

Laboratory Value	Normal (Adult) Values	Indication of Infection
Neutrophils		
Lymphocytes		
Monocytes		
Eosinophils		
Basophils		

Nursing Diagnosis

28. Identify some common nursing diagnoses that apply to patients at risk or who have an actual infection.

a. _____

b. _____

c. _____

d. _____

e. _____

f. _____

Planning

29. List four common goals for a patient with an actual or potential risk for infection.

a. _____

b. _____

c. _____

d. _____

Implementation

30. List the ways a nurse can teach patients and their families to prevent an infection from developing or spreading (community and health care settings).

Community settings.

a. _____

b. _____

c. _____

d. _____

Health care settings.

    e. _____

    f. _____

    g. _____

31. The nurse follows certain principles and procedures to prevent infection and to control its spread. Briefly explain each one.

    a. Concept of asepsis: _____

    b. Medical asepsis: _____

32. Explain the following methods of controlling or eliminating infectious agents.

    a. Hand hygiene: _____

    b. Alcohol-based hand antiseptics: _____

    c. Disinfection: _____

    d. Sterilization: _____

33. Effective prevention and control of infection requires the nurse to be aware of the following modes of transmission.

    a. Bathing: _____

    b. Dressing changes: _____

    c. Contaminated articles: _____

    d. Contaminated sharps: _____

    e. Bedside unit: _____

    f. Bottled solutions: _____

    g. Surgical wounds: _____

    h. Drainage bottles and bags: _____

34. The elements of respiratory hygiene or cough etiquette are:

    a. _____

    b. _____

    c. _____

    d. _____

    e. _____

    f. _____

The isolation guidelines of the Centers for Disease Control and Prevention contain a two-tiered approach. Explain each one.

35. Standard precautions (tier 1): _____

_____

36. Isolation precautions (tier 2): _____

_____

Identify the rationale for the following personal protective equipment.

37. Gowns: _____

_____

38. Respiratory protection: _____

_____

39. Protective eyewear: _____

_____

40. Gloves: _____

_____

41. Identify some common waste materials that are considered infectious.

   a. _____

   b. _____

   c. _____

   d. _____

42. List the nine responsibilities of infection control professionals.

   a. _____

   b. _____

   c. _____

   d. _____

   e. _____

   f. _____

   g. _____

   h. _____

   i. _____

43. Identify clinical situations in which a nurse would use surgical asepsis.

   a. _____

   b. _____

   c. _____

44. List the seven principles of surgical asepsis.

   a. _____

   b. _____

   c. _____

   d. _____

   e. _____

   f. _____

   g. _____

45. List in order the steps for performing a sterile procedure.

   a. _____

   b. _____

c. _____

d. _____

e. _____

f. _____

g. _____

h. _____

i. _____

j. _____

Evaluation

46. The expected outcome is the absence of signs and symptoms of infection. List some ways the nurse can monitor the patient.

a. _____

b. _____

c. _____

d. _____

REVIEW QUESTIONS

Select the appropriate answer and cite the rationale for choosing that particular answer.

47. Which of the following is not an element in the development or chain of infection?
    1. Means of transmission
    2. Infectious agent or pathogen
    3. Formation of immunoglobulin
    4. Reservoir for pathogen growth

Answer: _____ Rationale: _____

_____

_____

48. The severity of a patient's illness depends on all of the following except:
    1. Incubation period
    2. Extent of infection
    3. Susceptibility of the host
    4. Pathogenicity of the microorganism

Answer: _____ Rationale: _____

_____

_____

49. Which of the following best describes an iatrogenic infection?
    1. It results from a diagnostic or therapeutic procedure.
    2. It results from an extended infection of the urinary tract.
    3. It involves an incubation period of 3 to 4 weeks before it can be detected.
    4. It occurs when patients are infected with their own organisms as a result of immunodeficiency.

Answer: _____ Rationale: _____

_____

_____

50. The nurse sets up a nonbarrier sterile field on the patient's overbed table. In which of the following instances is the field contaminated?
    1. Sterile saline solution is spilled on the field.
    2. The nurse, who has a cold, wears a double mask.
    3. Sterile objects are kept within a 1-inch border of the field.
    4. The nurse keeps the top of the table above his or her waist.

    Answer: _____ Rationale: _____

    _____

    _____

51. When a patient on respiratory isolation must be transported to another part of the hospital, the nurse:
    1. Places a mask on the patient before leaving the room
    2. Obtains a health care provider's order to prohibit the patient from being transported
    3. Instructs the patient to cover his or her mouth and nose with a tissue when coughing or sneezing
    4. Advises other health team members to wear masks and gowns when coming in contact with the patient

    Answer: _____ Rationale: _____

    _____

    _____

30 Vital Signs

PRELIMINARY READING

Chapter 30, pp. 486-532

COMPREHENSIVE UNDERSTANDING

Guidelines for Measuring Vital Signs

1. Identify the guidelines that assist the nurse with incorporating vital sign measurements into practice.

   a. _____

   b. _____

   c. _____

   d. _____

   e. _____

   f. _____

   g. _____

   h. _____

   i. _____

   j. _____

   k. _____

   l. _____

Body Temperature

Match the following terms that address the physiology of body temperature.

2. _____ Core temperature

3. _____ Thermoregulation

4. _____ Hypothalamus

5. _____ Basal metabolic rate

6. _____ Shivering

7. _____ Nonshivering thermogenesis

8. _____ Radiation

9. _____ Conduction

10. _____ Convection

11. _____ Evaporation

a. Involuntary body response to temperature differences in the body

b. Transfer of heat from the surface of one object to the surface of another without direct contact

c. Transfer of heat away by air movement

d. Transfer of heat energy when a liquid is changed to a gas

e. The heat produced by the body at absolute rest

f. Controls body temperature

g. Vascular brown tissue is metabolized for heat production in the neonate

h. Temperature of the deep tissues

i. Transfer of heat from one object to another with direct contact

j. Mechanisms that regulate the balance between heat lost and heat produced

12. Diaphoresis is: _____

_____

13. The skin regulates temperature through:

    a. _____

    b. _____

    c. _____

14. The ability of a person to control body temperature depends on:

    a. _____

    b. _____

    c. _____

    d. _____

15. Identify the factors that affect body temperature.

    a. _____

    b. _____

    c. _____

    d. _____

    e. _____

    f. _____

    g. _____

Match the following terms that address temperature alterations.

16. _____ Pyrexia
17. _____ Pyrogens
18. _____ Hyperthermia
19. _____ Malignant hyperthermia
20. _____ Heatstroke
21. _____ Heat exhaustion
22. _____ Hypothermia
23. _____ Frostbite

a. Occurs when the body is exposed to subnormal temperatures
b. The body's inability to promote heat loss or reduce heat production
c. A dangerous heat emergency
d. Cold that overwhelms the body's ability to produce heat
e. Fever
f. Hereditary condition of uncontrolled heat production
g. Profuse diaphoresis with excess water and electrolyte loss
h. Bacteria and viruses that elevate body temperature

Nursing Process

Assessment

24. List at least one advantage and one disadvantage of each of the following temperature sites.

    a. Oral: _____

    b. Tympanic: _____

    c. Rectal: _____

    d. Axilla: _____

    e. Skin: _____

    f. Temporal artery: _____

25. State the formulas for the following conversions.

    a. Fahrenheit to Celsius: _____

    b. Celsius to Fahrenheit: _____

Nursing Diagnosis

26. Identify four nursing diagnoses related to thermoregulation.

    a. _____

    b. _____

    c. _____

    d. _____

Planning

27. Provide examples of goals for temperature alterations related to the environment.

    a. Short term: _____

    b. Long term: _____

Implementation

Health Promotion

28. Identify the patients who are at risk for hypothermia.

    _____

    _____

Acute Care

29. Explain the differences related to febrile states in each of the following.

    a. Children: _____

    b. Hypersensitive response to drugs: _____

30. Give an example of each type of fever therapy.

    a. Pharmacologic: _____

    b. Nonpharmacologic: _____

31. First aid treatment for heatstroke is: _____

    _____

32. Summarize the treatment for hypothermia.

    _____

    _____

Evaluation

33. Identify evaluative measures for temperature alterations.

    _____

    _____

Pulse

34. Identify the two common sites to assess the pulse rate.

    a. _____

    b. _____

35. Identify the measurement criteria for the following pulse sites.

    a. Temporal: _____

    b. Carotid: _____

    c. Apical: _____

    d. Brachial: _____

    e. Radial: _____

    f. Ulnar: _____

    g. Femoral: _____

    h. Popliteal: _____

    i. Posterior tibial: _____

    j. Dorsalis pedis: _____

36. List the characteristics to identify when assessing the following.

    a. Radial pulse: _____

    b. Apical pulse: _____

37. List the acceptable pulse ranges for the following.

    a. Infants: _____

    b. Toddlers: _____

    c. Preschoolers: _____

    d. School-age children: _____

    e. Adolescents: _____

    f. Adults: _____

38. Identify seven factors that may increase or decrease the pulse rate.

    a. _____

    b. _____

    c. _____

    d. _____

    e. _____

    f. _____

    g. _____

Define the following terms.

39. Tachycardia: _____

_____

40. Bradycardia: _____

_____

41. Pulse deficit: _____

_____

42. Dysrhythmia: _____

_____

Respiration

Define the following terms related to respirations.

43. Ventilation: _____

_____

44. Diffusion: _____

_____

45. Perfusion: _____

_____

46. Hypoxemia: _____

_____

47. Identify which phase of respirations is active and which is passive.

a. Inspiration: _____

b. Expiration: _____

48. Identify factors that influence the character of respirations and the mechanism of each factor.

a. _____

b. _____

c. _____

d. _____

e. _____

f. _____

g. _____

h. _____

49. Identify the acceptable range for respiratory rates for the following age groups.

a. Newborns: _____

b. Infants: _____

c. Toddlers: _____

d. Children: _____

e. Adolescents: _____

f. Adults: _____

Briefly explain the following alterations in breathing patterns.

50. Bradypnea: _____

_____

51. Tachypnea: _____

_____

52. Hyperpnea: _____

_____

53. Apnea: _____

_____

54. Hyperventilation: _____

_____

55. Hypoventilation: _____

_____

56. Cheyne–Stokes: _____

_____

57. Kussmaul: _____

_____

58. Biot: _____

_____

59. SaO_2: _____

_____

Blood Pressure

Define the following terms.

60. Blood pressure: _____

_____

61. Systolic pressure: _____

_____

62. Diastolic pressure: _____

_____

63. Pulse pressure: _____

_____

Blood pressure is reflected by the following. Briefly explain each.

64. Cardiac output: _____

_____

65. Peripheral resistance: _____

_____

66. Blood volume: _____

_____

67. Viscosity: _____

_____

68. Elasticity: _____

_____

69. List eight factors that influence blood pressure.

a. _____

b. _____

c. _____

d. _____

e. _____

f. _____

g. _____

h. _____

70. Identify the optimal blood pressure for the following ages.

a. Newborn: _____

b. 1 month: _____

c. 1 year: _____

d. 6 years: _____

e. 10 to 13 years: _____

f. 14 to 17 years: _____

g. Older than 18 years: _____

71. List some of the risk factors that are linked to hypertension.

_____

_____

72. Identify some of the risk factors for orthostatic hypotension.

_____

_____

73. Identify the following Korotkoff sounds.

First: _____

Second: _____

Third: _____

Fourth: _____

Fifth: _____

Health Promotion and Vital Signs

74. Identify at least two variations in each vital sign that are unique to older adults.

a. Temperature: _____

b. Pulse: _____

c. Blood pressure: _____

d. Respirations: _____

REVIEW QUESTIONS

Select the appropriate answer and cite the rationale for choosing that particular answer.

75. The skin plays a role in temperature regulation by:
    1. Insulating the body
    2. Constricting blood vessels
    3. Sensing external temperature variations
    4. All of the above

Answer: _____ Rationale: _____

_____

_____

76. The nurse bathes the patient who has a fever with cool water. The nurse does this to increase heat loss by means of:
    1. Radiation
    2. Convection
    3. Conduction
    4. Condensation

Answer: _____ Rationale: _____

_____

_____

77. The nurse is assessing a patient who she suspects has the nursing diagnosis hyperthermia related to vigorous exercise in hot weather. In reviewing the data, the nurse knows that the most important sign of heatstroke is:
    1. Confusion
    2. Excess thirst
    3. Hot, dry skin
    4. Muscle cramps

Answer: _____ Rationale: _____

_____

_____

78. The nurse is auscultating Mrs. McKinnon's blood pressure. The nurse inflates the cuff to 180 mm Hg. At 156 mm Hg, the nurse hears the onset of a tapping sound. At 130 mm Hg, the sound changes to a murmur or swishing. At 100 mm Hg, the sound momentarily becomes sharper, and at 92 mm Hg, it becomes muffled. At 88 mm Hg, the sound disappears. Mrs. McKinnon's blood pressure is:
    1. 130/88 mm Hg
    2. 156/88 mm Hg
    3. 180/92 mm Hg
    4. 180/130 mm Hg

Answer: _____ Rationale: _____

_____

_____

31 Health Assessment and Physical Examination

Chapter 31, pp. 533-608

COMPREHENSIVE UNDERSTANDING

Purposes of the Physical Examination

1. List the five nursing purposes for performing a physical assessment.

   a. _____

   b. _____

   c. _____

   d. _____

   e. _____

Preparation for Examination

2. List the principles related to the nurse performing daily physical examinations.

   a. _____

   b. _____

   c. _____

   d. _____

3. Proper preparation for examination should include:

   a. _____

   b. _____

   c. _____

   d. _____

   e. _____

4. List the tips to follow that will help in data collection when examining children.

   a. _____

   b. _____

   c. _____

   d. _____

   e. _____

5. List seven variations in the nurse's individual style that are appropriate when examining older adults.

   a. _____

   b. _____

   c. _____

   d. _____

e. _____

f. _____

g. _____

Organization of the Examination

6. Identify the principles to follow to keep an examination well organized.

a. _____

b. _____

c. _____

d. _____

e. _____

f. _____

g. _____

Techniques of Physical Assessment

7. Define *inspection*.

_____

_____

8. Identify the guidelines to achieve the best results during inspection.

a. _____

b. _____

c. _____

d. _____

e. _____

f. _____

9. Define *palpation*.

_____

_____

10. Explain the difference between:

a. Light palpation: _____

b. Deep palpation: _____

11. Define *percussion*.

_____

_____

12. Define *auscultation*.

_____

_____

13. The following are sounds that are described when auscultating. Please explain each one.

a. Frequency: _____

b. Amplitude: _____

c. Quality: _____

d. Duration: _____

General Survey

14. List at least 14 specific observations of the patient's general appearance and behavior that should be reviewed.

a. _____

b. _____

c. _____

d. _____

e. _____

f. _____

g. _____

h. _____

i. _____

j. _____

k. _____

l. _____

m. _____

n. _____

15. Identify some signs of patient abuse.

_____

_____

16. Identify the questions related to the following acronym.

C _____

A _____

G _____

E _____

17. List three actions that should be taken to ensure accurate weight measurement of a hospitalized patient.

a. _____

b. _____

c. _____

Skin, Hair, and Nails

18. Assessment of the skin reveals the patient's health status related to:

a. _____

b. _____

c. _____

d. _____

e. _____

19. Define *pigmentation*.

_____

_____

20. For each skin color variation, identify the mechanism that produces color change, common causes of the variation, and the optimal sites for assessment.

Color	Condition	Causes	Assessment Locations
Cyanosis			
Pallor			
Loss of pigmentation			
Jaundice			
Erythema			
Tan-brown			

21. Identify the physical findings of the skin that are indicative of substance abuse.

a. _____

b. _____

c. _____

d. _____

e. _____

f. _____

g. _____

h. _____

Define the following terms.

22. Indurated: _____

_____

23. Turgor: _____

_____

24. Vascularity: _____

_____

25. Edema: _____

_____

26. Lesions: _____

Briefly describe the following primary skin lesions and give an example of each.

27. Macule: _____

_____

28. Papule: _____

_____

29. Nodule: _____

_____

30. Tumor: _____

_____

31. Wheal: _____

32. Vesicle: _____

_____

33. Pustule: _____

_____

34. Ulcer: _____

_____

35. Atrophy: _____

_____

Explain the following skin malignancies.

36. Basal cell carcinoma: _____

_____

37. Squamous cell carcinoma: _____

_____

38. Melanoma: _____

_____

39. Define the following mnemonic to assess the skin for any type of carcinoma.

A _____

B _____

C _____

D _____

40. Name the three types of lice.

    a. _____

    b. _____

    c. _____

Briefly describe the following abnormalities of the nail bed.

41. Clubbing: _____

_____

42. Beaulines: _____

_____

43. Koilonychia: _____

_____

44. Splinter hemorrhages: _____

_____

45. Paronychia: _____

_____

Head and Neck

46. Define *hydrocephalus*.

_____

_____

Define the following common eye and visual abnormalities.

47. Hyperopia: _____

_____

48. Myopia: _____

_____

49. Presbyopia: _____

_____

50. Retinopathy: _____

_____

51. Strabismus: _____

_____

52. Cataract: _____

_____

53. Glaucoma: _____

_____

54. Macular degeneration: _____

_____

55. Examination of the eye includes assessment of five areas. Name them.

    a. _____

    b. _____

    c. _____

    d. _____

    e. _____

56. Identify the structures of the external eye that you would inspect.

    a. _____

    b. _____

    c. _____

    d. _____

    e. _____

    f. _____

    g. _____

Define the following terms related to the external eye.

57. Exophthalmos: _____

_____

58. Ectropion: _____

_____

59. Entropion: _____

_____

60. Conjunctivitis: _____

_____

61. Ptosis: _____

_____

62. PERRLA: _____

_____

63. Identify the internal eye structures that you would examine with an ophthalmoscope.

    a. _____

    b. _____

    c. _____

    d. _____

    e. _____

    f. _____

64. Identify the three parts of the ear canal and list the structures contained within each.

    a. _____

    b. _____

    c. _____

65. The normal tympanic membrane appears: _____
_____

66. Identify the three types of hearing loss.

   a. _____

   b. _____

   c. _____

67. Ototoxicity is caused by: _____
_____

Define the following terms that relate to the nose.

68. Excoriation: _____
_____

69. Polyps: _____
_____

Define the following terms that relate to the oral cavity.

70. Leukoplakia: _____
_____

71. Varicosities: _____
_____

72. Exostosis: _____
_____

73. Structures examined during assessment of the neck include:

   a. _____

   b. _____

   c. _____

   d. _____

   e. _____

   f. _____

74. List the sequence for assessing the nodes of the neck.

   1. _____

   2. _____

   3. _____

   4. _____

   5. _____

   6. _____

75. An abnormality of superficial lymph nodes may reveal the presence of infection or _____.

Thorax and Lungs

76. Identify the key landmarks of the chest.

    a. _____

    b. _____

    c. _____

    d. _____

    e. _____

    f. _____

77. Chest excursion is normally _____.

    Reduced chest excursion may be caused by _____.

78. Define *vocal* or *tactile fremitus*.

    _____

    _____

Define the following normal breath sounds heard over the posterior thorax.

79. Vesicular: _____

    _____

80. Bronchovesicular: _____

    _____

81. Bronchial: _____

    _____

82. Complete the following table of adventitious breath sounds.

Sound	Site Auscultated	Cause	Character
Crackles			
Rhonchi (sonorous wheeze)			
Wheezes (sibilant wheeze)			
Pleural friction rub			

Heart

Explain the following terms related to assessment of the heart.

83. Point of maximal impulse: _____

    _____

84. S$_1$: _____

_____

85. S$_2$: _____

_____

86. S$_3$: _____

_____

87. S$_4$: _____

_____

Identify the appropriate sites for inspection and palpation of the following.

88. Angle of Louis: _____

_____

89. Aortic area: _____

_____

90. Pulmonic area: _____

_____

91. Second pulmonic area: _____

_____

92. Tricuspid area: _____

_____

93. Mitral area: _____

_____

94. Epigastric area: _____

_____

95. Define *murmur*.

_____

_____

96. List the six factors to consider when auscultating a murmur.

    a. _____

    b. _____

    c. _____

    d. _____

    e. _____

    f. _____

97. Describe the sounds auscultated by the following murmurs.

    Grade 1 = _____

    Grade 2 = _____

    Grade 3 = _____

    Grade 4 = _____

Grade 5 = _____

Grade 6 = _____

Vascular System

98. Syncope is caused by _____ .

99. Arterial occlusion is _____ .

100. Stenosis is _____ .

101. A(n) _____ is the blowing sound caused by turbulence in a narrowed section of a blood vessel.

102. Explain the steps the nurse would use to assess venous pressure.

1. _____

2. _____

3. _____

4. _____

5. _____

103. Complete the following table by listing the signs of venous and arterial insufficiency.

Assessment Criterion	Venous	Arterial
Color		
Temperature		
Pulse		
Edema		
Skin changes		

104. Describe how you would assess for phlebitis.

_____

_____

Breasts

105. The American Cancer Society (2014) recommends the following guidelines for early detection of breast cancer.

a. _____

b. _____

c. _____

d. _____

e. _____

f. _____

106. Identify the three systematic approaches to palpation of the breast.

a. _____

b. _____

c. _____

107. When palpating abnormal masses in the breast, you should note:

a. _____

b. _____

c. _____

d. _____

e. _____

f. _____

g. _____

108. Benign (fibrocystic) breast disease is characterized by: _____
_____

Abdomen

Define the following terms related to the abdomen.

109. Striae: _____
_____

110. Hernias: _____
_____

111. Distention: _____
_____

112. Peristalsis: _____
_____

113. Borborygmi: _____
_____

114. Rebound tenderness: _____
_____

115. Aneurysm: _____
_____

Female Genitalia and Reproductive Tract

116. Chancres are: _____
_____

117. A Papanicolaou specimen is used to: _____
_____

Male Genitalia

118. Identify the common symptoms of testicular cancer.

_____

_____

Rectum and Anus

119. The purpose of digital examination is: _____

_____

Musculoskeletal System

Define the following terms.

120. Kyphosis: _____

_____

121. Lordosis: _____

_____

122. Scoliosis: _____

_____

123. Osteoporosis: _____

_____

124. Goniometer: _____

_____

Identify the correct range of motion for the following terms.

125. Flexion: _____

_____

126. Extension: _____

_____

127. Hyperextension: _____

_____

128. Pronation: _____

_____

129. Supination: _____

_____

130. Abduction: _____

_____

131. Adduction: _____

_____

132. Internal rotation: _____

_____

133. External rotation: _____

_____

134. Eversion: _____

_____

135. Inversion: _____

_____

136. Dorsiflexion: _____

_____

137. Plantar flexion: _____

_____

Define the following terms related to muscle tone and strength.

138. Hypertonicity: _____

_____

139. Hypotonicity: _____

_____

140. Atrophied: _____

_____

Neurologic System

141. The purpose of the Mini-Mental State Examination is to measure: _____

_____

142. Delirium is characterized by: _____

_____

143. The purpose of the Glasgow Coma Scale is to: _____

_____

144. Briefly explain the two types of aphasia.

a. Receptive: _____

b. Expressive: _____

145. Identify the 12 cranial nerves.

a. _____

b. _____

c. _____

d. _____

e. _____

f. _____

g. _____

h. _____

i. _____

j. _____

k. _____

l. _____

146. The sensory pathways of the central nervous system conduct what type of sensations?

a. _____

b. _____

c. _____

d. _____

e. _____

147. Identify the functions of the cerebellum.

_____

_____

_____

148. Identify the two types of normal reflexes and provide an example of each.

a. _____

b. _____

REVIEW QUESTIONS

Select the appropriate answer and cite the rationale for choosing that particular answer.

149. The component that should receive the highest priority before a physical examination is:
    1. Preparation of the equipment
    2. Preparation of the environment
    3. Physical preparation of the patient
    4. Psychological preparation of the patient

Answer: _____ Rationale: _____

_____

_____

150. The nurse assesses the skin turgor of the patient by:
    1. Inspecting the buccal mucosa with a penlight
    2. Palpating the skin with the dorsum of the hand
    3. Grasping a fold of skin on the back of the forearm and releasing
    4. Pressing the skin for 5 seconds, releasing, and noting each centimeter of depth

Answer: _____ Rationale: _____

_____

_____

151. While examining Mr. Parker, the nurse notes a circumscribed elevation of skin filled with serous fluid on his upper lip. The lesion is 0.4 cm in diameter. This type of lesion is called a:
    1. Macule
    2. Nodule
    3. Vesicle
    4. Pustule

Answer: _____ Rationale: _____

_____

_____

152. When assessing the patient's thorax, the nurse should:
    1. Complete the left side and then the right side
    2. Compare symmetrical areas from side to side
    3. Begin with the posterior lobes on the right side
    4. Change the position of the stethoscope between inspiration and expiration

Answer: _____ Rationale: _____

_____

_____

153. In a patient with pneumonia, the nurse hears high-pitched, continuous musical sounds over the bronchi on expiration. These sounds are called:
    1. Rhonchi
    2. Crackles
    3. Wheezes
    4. Friction rubs

    Answer: _____ Rationale: _____

    _____

    _____

154. The second heart sound (S_2) occurs when:
    1. Systole begins
    2. There is rapid ventricular filling
    3. The mitral and tricuspid valves close
    4. The aortic and pulmonic valves close

    Answer: _____ Rationale: _____

    _____

    _____

32 Medication Administration

Chapter 32, pp. 609-687

PRELIMINARY READING

Chapter 32, pp. 609-687

COMPREHENSIVE UNDERSTANDING

Scientific Knowledge Base

1. Briefly summarize the roles of the following in relation to the regulation of medications.

   a. Federal government: _____

   b. State government: _____

   c. Health care institutions: _____

   d. Nurse Practice Act: _____

A single medication may have three different names. Define each one.

2. Chemical name: _____
   _____

3. Generic name: _____
   _____

4. Trade name: _____
   _____

5. A medication classification indicates: _____
   _____

6. The form of the medication determines its: _____
   _____

7. Pharmacokinetics is: _____
   _____

8. Absorption is: _____
   _____

9. Identify the factors that influence drug absorption.
   a. _____
   b. _____
   c. _____
   d. _____
   e. _____

10. Identify the factors that affect the rate and extent of medication distribution.
    a. _____
    b. _____

    c. _____

    d. _____

    e. _____

11. Explain the role of metabolism.

_____

_____

12. Identify the primary organ for drug excretion, and explain what happens if this organ's function declines.

_____

_____

Define the following predicted or unintended effects of drugs.

13. Therapeutic effects: _____

_____

14. Side effects: _____

_____

15. Adverse effects: _____

_____

16. Toxic effects: _____

_____

17. Idiosyncratic reactions: _____

_____

18. Allergic reactions: _____

_____

19. Anaphylactic reactions: _____

_____

20. Medication interaction: _____

_____

21. Synergistic effect: _____

_____

Define the following terms related to medication dose responses.

22. Minimum effective concentration (MEC): _____

_____

23. Peak concentration: _____

_____

24. Trough concentration: _____

_____

25. Biological half-life: _____

_____

26. Identify the three types of oral routes.

    a. _____

    b. _____

    c. _____

27. List the four major sites for parenteral injections.

    a. _____

    b. _____

    c. _____

    d. _____

Define the following advanced techniques of medication administration.

28. Epidural: _____

    _____

29. Intrathecal: _____

    _____

30. Intraosseous: _____

    _____

31. Intraperitoneal: _____

    _____

32. Intrapleural: _____

    _____

33. Intraarterial: _____

    _____

34. Intracardiac: _____

    _____

35. Intraarticular: _____

    _____

36. Identify five methods for applying medications to mucous membranes.

    a. _____

    b. _____

    c. _____

    d. _____

    e. _____

37. Identify the benefit of the inhalation route.

    _____

    _____

38. Identify the two types of measurements used in medication therapy.

    a. _____

    b. _____

39. A solution is: _____

_____

Nursing Knowledge Base

40. Write out the formula used to determine the correct dose when preparing solid or liquid forms of medications.

_____

_____

Briefly explain the common types of medication orders.

41. Verbal: _____

_____

42. Standing or routine: _____

_____

43. prn: _____

_____

44. Single (one-time): _____

_____

45. STAT: _____

_____

46. Now: _____

_____

47. List the medication distribution systems.

a. _____

b. _____

48. Identify the common medication errors that can cause patient harm.

a. _____

b. _____

c. _____

d. _____

e. _____

49. Identify the process for medication reconciliation.

a. _____

b. _____

c. _____

d. _____

Critical Thinking

50. List the six rights of medication administration.

a. _____

b. _____

c. _____

d. _____

e. _____

f. _____

51. Briefly summarize *The Patient Care Partnership* related to medication administration.

a. _____

b. _____

c. _____

d. _____

e. _____

f. _____

g. _____

h. _____

Nursing Process
Assessment

52. Identify the areas the nurse needs to assess to determine the need for and potential response to medication therapy.

a. _____

b. _____

c. _____

d. _____

e. _____

f. _____

g. _____

h. _____

i. _____

Nursing Diagnosis

53. Identify seven of the potential nursing diagnoses used during the administration of medications.

a. _____

b. _____

c. _____

d. _____

e. _____

f. _____

g. _____

Planning

54. Identify the outcomes for a patient with newly diagnosed type 2 diabetes.

a. _____

b. _____

c. _____

d. _____

e. _____

Implementation

55. Identify factors that can influence the patient's compliance with the medication regimen.

a. _____

b. _____

c. _____

d. _____

56. Identify the components of medication orders.

a. _____

b. _____

c. _____

d. _____

e. _____

f. _____

g. _____

57. The recording of medication includes:

a. _____

b. _____

c. _____

d. _____

e. _____

58. Explain the reasons why polypharmacy happens to a patient.

_____

_____

Evaluation

59. Identify two goals for safe and effective medication administration.

a. _____

b. _____

Medication Administration

60. Identify the precautions to take when administering any oral preparation to prevent aspiration.

a. _____

b. _____

c. _____

d. _____

e. _____

f. _____

g. _____

h. _____

i. _____

j. _____

61. Identify the guidelines to ensure safe administration of transdermal or topical medications.

    a. _____

    b. _____

    c. _____

    d. _____

    e. _____

    f. _____

62. The most common form of nasal instillation is: _____

    _____

63. List four principles for administering eye instillations.

    a. _____

    b. _____

    c. _____

    d. _____

64. Failure to instill ear drops at room temperature causes:

    a. _____

    b. _____

    c. _____

65. Vaginal medications are available as:

    a. _____

    b. _____

    c. _____

    d. _____

66. Rectal suppositories are used for: _____

67. Explain the following types of inhalation inhalers:

    a. Pressurized metered-dose inhalers (pMDIs): _____

    b. Breath-actuated metered-dose inhalers (BAIs): _____

    c. Dry powder inhalers (DPIs): _____

68. Identify the aseptic techniques to use to prevent an infection during an injection.

    a. _____

    b. _____

    c. _____

    d. _____

69. Identify the factors that must be considered when selecting a needle for an injection.

   a. _____

   b. _____

70. Describe each of the following.

   a. Ampule: _____

   b. Vial: _____

71. List the three principles to follow when mixing medications from two vials.

   a. _____

   b. _____

   c. _____

72. Insulin is classified by: _____

   _____

73. Identify the principles to follow when mixing two types of insulin in the same syringe.

   a. _____

   b. _____

   c. _____

   d. _____

   e. _____

74. List the techniques used to minimize patient discomfort that is associated with injections.

   a. _____

   b. _____

   c. _____

   d. _____

   e. _____

   f. _____

   g. _____

   h. _____

75. Identify the best sites for subcutaneous injections.

   a. _____

   b. _____

   c. _____

76. What is the maximum amount of water-soluble medication given by the subcutaneous route?

   _____

   _____

77. What angles should be used when administering a subcutaneous injection, and with which needle should they be used?

   a. _____

   b. _____

78. What is the angle of insertion for an intramuscular (IM) injection?

_____

_____

79. Indicate the maximum volume of medication for an IM injection in each of the following groups.

    a. Well-developed adults: _____

    b. Older children, older adults, and thin adults: _____

    c. Older infants and small children: _____

Describe the characteristics of the following intramuscular injection sites.

80. Ventrogluteal: _____

_____

81. Vastus lateralis: _____

_____

82. Deltoid: _____

_____

83. Explain the rationale for the Z-track method in IM injections.

_____

_____

84. Explain the rationale for intradermal injections.

_____

_____

85. List the methods a nurse can use to administer medications intravenously.

    a. _____

    b. _____

    c. _____

86. Identify the advantages of the intravenous (IV) route of administration.

    a. _____

    b. _____

    c. _____

87. The disadvantages of IV bolus medications are:

    a. _____

    b. _____

88. List the advantages of using volume-controlled infusions.

    a. _____

    b. _____

    c. _____

89. What is a piggyback set?

_____

_____

90. What is a volume-control administration set?

_____

_____

91. What is a syringe pump?

_____

_____

92. List the five advantages of using intermittent venous access devices.

a. _____

b. _____

c. _____

d. _____

e. _____

REVIEW QUESTIONS

Select the appropriate answer and cite the rationale for choosing that particular answer.

93. The study of how drugs enter the body, reach their sites of action, are metabolized, and exit from the body is called:
    1. Pharmacology
    2. Pharmacopoeia
    3. Pharmacokinetics
    4. Biopharmaceutical

Answer: _____ Rationale: _____

_____

_____

94. Which statement correctly characterizes drug absorption?
    1. Most drugs must enter the systemic circulation to have a therapeutic effect.
    2. Oral medications are absorbed more quickly when administered with meals.
    3. Mucous membranes are relatively impermeable to chemicals, making absorption slow.
    4. Drugs administered subcutaneously are absorbed more quickly than those injected intramuscularly.

Answer: _____ Rationale: _____

_____

_____

95. The onset of drug action is the time it takes for a drug to:
    1. Produce a response
    2. Accelerate the cellular process
    3. Reach its highest effective concentration
    4. Produce blood serum concentration and maintenance

Answer: _____ Rationale: _____

_____

_____

96. Which of the following is not a parenteral route of administration?
    1. Buccal
    2. Intradermal
    3. Intramuscular
    4. Subcutaneous

Answer: _____ Rationale: _____

_____

_____

97. The nurse is preparing an insulin injection in which both regular and NPH will be mixed. Into which vial should the nurse inject air first?
    1. The vial of regular insulin
    2. The vial of NPH
    3. Either vial, as long as modified insulin is drawn up first
    4. Neither vial; it is not necessary to put air into vials before withdrawing medication

Answer: _____ Rationale: _____

_____

_____

33 Complementary and Alternative Therapies

Chapter 33, pp. 688-700

COMPREHENSIVE UNDERSTANDING

Complementary, Alternative, and Integrative Approaches to Health

Describe the difference between the following terms.

1. Complementary therapies: _____

   _____

2. Alternative therapies: _____

   _____

3. Explain the following biologically based therapies.

   a. Dietary supplements: _____

   b. Herbal medicines: _____

   c. Mycotherapies: _____

   d. Probiotics: _____

4. Explain the following energy therapies.

   a. Healing touch: _____

   b. Reiki therapy: _____

   c. Therapeutic touch: _____

5. Explain the following manipulative and body-based methods.

   a. Acupressure: _____

   b. Chiropractic medicine: _____

   c. Craniosacral therapy: _____

   d. Massage therapy: _____

6. Explain the following mind–body interventions.

   a. Biofeedback: _____

   b. Breathwork: _____

   c. Guided imagery: _____

   d. Meditation: _____

   e. Music therapy: _____

   f. Yoga: _____

   g. Tai chi: _____

7. Explain the following movement therapies:

   a. Dance therapy: _____

   b. Pilates: _____

8. Integrative health care emphasizes the:

   a. _____

   b. _____

   c. _____

   d. _____

Nursing-Accessible Therapies

9. Explain the cascade of changes that are associated with the stress response.

_____

_____

10. The relaxation response is: _____

_____

11. Progressive relaxation training helps to: _____

_____

12. The goal of passive relaxation is: _____

_____

13. The outcome of relaxation therapy is: _____

_____

14. Identify the limitations of relaxation therapy.

_____

_____

15. Meditation is: _____

_____

16. Identify the indications for the use of meditation.

_____

_____

17. Identify the limitations of meditation.

_____

_____

18. Imagery is: _____

_____

19. Creative visualization is: _____

_____

20. Identify the clinical applications of imagery.

_____

_____

Training-Specific Therapies

21. Biofeedback is: _____

_____

22. Identify some clinical applications for the use of biofeedback.

_____

_____

23. Identify the limitations of biofeedback.

_____

_____

24. Describe the clinical applications of acupuncture.

_____

_____

25. Identify the contraindications to acupuncture.

_____

_____

26. Explain the following terms related to acupuncture.

    a. _Qi_: _____

    b. Meridians: _____

    c. Acupoints: _____

27. Identify the five phases of therapeutic touch (TT).

    a. _____

    b. _____

    c. _____

    d. _____

    e. _____

28. Identify the clinical applications of therapeutic touch.

_____

_____

29. Identify the limitations of therapeutic touch.

_____

_____

30. What is the most important concept of traditional Chinese medicine (TCM)?

_____

_____

31. Briefly explain the following TCM therapeutic modalities.

a. Moxibustion: _____

b. Cupping: _____

c. Tai chi: _____

d. Qi gong: _____

32. Identify the clinical applications of herbal therapy.

_____

_____

33. Identify the limitations of herbal therapy.

_____

_____

The Integrative Nursing Role

34. Explain what the integrative medicine approach is.

_____

_____

REVIEW QUESTIONS

Select the appropriate answer and cite the rationale for choosing that particular answer.

35. Patients choose to use unconventional therapy because:
    1. They are willing to pay more to feel better.
    2. They are dissatisfied with conventional medicine.
    3. They want religious approval for the remedies they use.
    4. It is now widely accepted by the Food and Drug Administration.

Answer: _____ Rationale: _____

_____

_____

36. The Dietary Supplement and Health Education Act states that:
    1. The Food and Drug Administration must evaluate all herbal therapies.
    2. Herbs, vitamins, and minerals may be sold with their therapeutic advantages listed on the label.
    3. Herbs, vitamins, and minerals may be sold as long as no therapeutic claims are made on the label.
    4. In conjunction with the Food and Drug Administration, all supplements are considered safe for use.

Answer: _____ Rationale: _____

_____

_____

37. Which of the following steps should nurses take to be better informed about alternative therapies?
    1. Review herb manufacturers' literature on specific herbs.
    2. Read current books and magazines on alternative therapies.
    3. Familiarize themselves with general principles of phytotherapy.
    4. Familiarize themselves with recent case studies on alternative therapies.

Answer: _____ Rationale: _____

_____

_____

34 Self-Concept

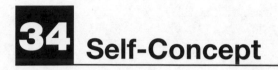

PRELIMINARY READING

Chapter 34, pp. 701-715

COMPREHENSIVE UNDERSTANDING

Scientific Knowledge Base

1. Define self-concept.

   _____

   _____

Nursing Knowledge Base

2. Self-concept is a dynamic perception that is based on the following.

   a. _____

   b. _____

   c. _____

   d. _____

   e. _____

   f. _____

   g. _____

   h. _____

   i. _____

Match the following terms.

3. _____ Identity
4. _____ Body image
5. _____ Role performance
6. _____ Self-esteem

a. Includes physical appearance, structure, and function of the body
b. The way in which individuals perceive their ability to carry out significant roles
c. Individual's overall feeling of self-worth
d. Internal sense of individuality, wholeness, and consistency of a person over time and in different situations

7. A self-concept stressor is any: _____

   _____

Match the following stressors that affect self-concept.

8. _____ Identity	a. Example: perceived inability to meet parental expectations, harsh criticism, and inconsistent discipline
9. _____ Body image	
10. _____ Role performance	b. Example: providing care to a family member with Alzheimer disease
11. _____ Role conflict	c. Example: a middle-aged woman with teenage children assuming responsibility for the care of her older parents
12. _____ Role ambiguity	
13. _____ Role strain	d. Amputation, facial disfigurement, or scars from burns
14. _____ Role overload	e. Unsuccessfully attempting to meet the demands of work and family while carving out some personal time
15. _____ Self-esteem stressors	
	f. Situational transitions
	g. An adolescent attempting to adjust to the physical, emotional, and mental changes of increasing maturity
	h. Common in adolescents and employment situations

16. List five areas the nurse must clarify and assess about him- or herself to promote a positive self-concept in patients.

a. _____

b. _____

c. _____

d. _____

e. _____

Nursing Process
Assessment

17. Identify the focus of assessing each component of self-concept.

_____

_____

18. Give some examples of behaviors suggestive of altered self-concept.

_____

_____

Nursing Diagnosis

19. Identify examples of self-concept nursing diagnoses.

a. _____

b. _____

c. _____

d. _____

e. _____

f. _____

g. _____

h. _____

Planning

20. State the expected outcomes for the nursing diagnosis Situational Low Self-Esteem related to a recent job layoff.

_____

_____

Implementation

21. List some healthy lifestyle measures that support adaptation to stress.

_____

_____

Evaluation

22. Identify the expected outcomes for a self-concept disturbance.

_____

_____

REVIEW QUESTIONS

Select the appropriate answer, and cite the rationale for choosing that particular answer.

23. Which developmental stage is particularly crucial for identity development?
    1. Infancy
    2. Young adult
    3. Adolescence
    4. Preschool age

    Answer:_____ Rationale:_____

    _____

    _____

24. Which of the following statements about body image is correct?
    1. Body image refers only to the external appearance of a person's body.
    2. Physical changes are quickly incorporated into a person's body image.
    3. Perceptions by other persons have no influence on a person's body image.
    4. Body image is a combination of a person's actual and perceived (ideal) body.

    Answer:_____ Rationale:_____

    _____

    _____

25. Robert, who is 2 years old, is praised for using his potty instead of wetting his pants. This is an example of learning a behavior by:
    1. Imitation
    2. Substitution
    3. Identification
    4. Reinforcement–extinction

    Answer:_____ Rationale:_____

    _____

    _____

26. Mrs. Watson has just undergone a radical mastectomy. The nurse is aware that Mrs. Watson will probably have considerable anxiety over:
    1. Self-esteem
    2. Body image
    3. Self-identity
    4. Role performance

    Answer:_____ Rationale:_____

    _____

    _____

CRITICAL THINKING MODEL FOR NURSING CARE PLAN FOR DISTURBED BODY IMAGE RELATED TO NEGATIVE VIEW OF SELF AFTER MASTECTOMY

27. Imagine that you are the student nurse, Susan, in the care plan on page 710-711 of your text. Complete the *Assessment phase* of the critical thinking model by writing your answers in the appropriate boxes of the model shown. Think about the following.
    - In developing Mrs. Johnson's plan of care, what knowledge did Susan apply?
    - In what way might Susan's previous experience apply in this case?
    - What intellectual or professional standards were applied to Mrs. Johnson?
    - What critical thinking attitudes did you use in assessing Mrs. Johnson?
    - As you review your assessment, what key areas did you cover?

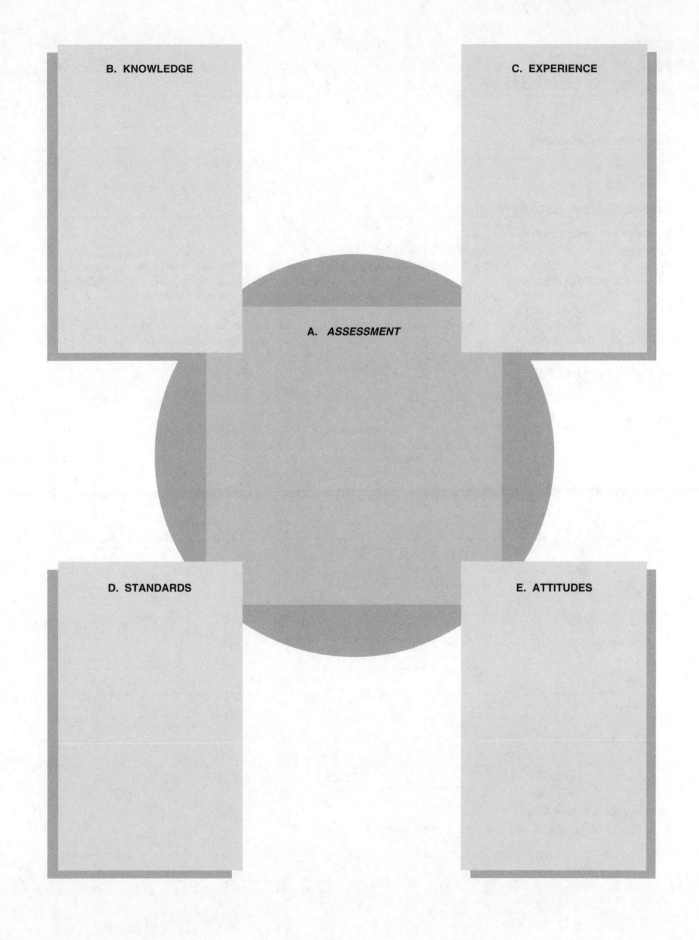

B. KNOWLEDGE

C. EXPERIENCE

A. *ASSESSMENT*

D. STANDARDS

E. ATTITUDES

35 Sexuality

Chapter 35, pp. 716-732

COMPREHENSIVE UNDERSTANDING

Scientific Knowledge Base

Match the following terms to the appropriate responses.

1. _____ Sexuality	a. Pill, intrauterine device, condoms, diaphragm, tubal ligation, vasectomy
2. _____ Sexual health	b. Changes in physical appearance lead to concerns about sexual attractiveness
3. _____ Gender roles	c. Factors that determine sexual activity include present health status, past
4. _____ Gender identity	and present life satisfaction, status of intimate relationships
5. _____ School-age children	d. Need accurate information on sexual activity, emotional responses with
6. _____ Adolescents	relationships, sexually transmitted infections, contraception, and pregnancy
7. _____ Sexual minority group	e. Have general questions regarding the physical and emotional aspects of sex
8. _____ Dyspareunia	f. Part of a person's personality and important for overall health
9. _____ Young adulthood	g. Influenced by culture
10. _____ Middle adulthood	h. State of physical, emotional, mental, and social well-being in relation to
11. _____ Older adulthood	sexuality
12. _____ Contraceptive options	i. The first 3 years are crucial for its development
	j. Lesbian, gay, bisexual, or transgender
	k. Painful intercourse
	l. Intimacy and sexuality are issues for this group

13. Identify the primary routes of human immunodeficiency virus (HIV) transmission.

    a. _____

    b. _____

    c. _____

    d. _____

    e. _____

14. List the commonly diagnosed sexually transmitted infections (STIs).

    a. _____

    b. _____

    c. _____

    d. _____

    e. _____

    f. _____

Nursing Knowledge Base

15. Identify two sociocultural dimensions of sexuality.

    a. _____

    b. _____

16. Identify three decisional issues regarding sexuality.

    a. _____

    b. _____

    c. _____

17. Identify four alterations in sexual health.

    a. _____

    b. _____

    c. _____

    d. _____

Nursing Process

Assessment

18. What factors that may affect sexuality would the nurse assess?

    a. _____

    b. _____

    c. _____

    d. _____

    e. _____

    f. _____

19. The PLISSIT assessment of sexuality stands for: _____

Nursing Diagnosis

20. Identify possible nursing diagnoses related to sexual functioning.

    a. _____

    b. _____

    c. _____

    d. _____

    e. _____

    f. _____

    g. _____

Planning

21. The expected outcomes for the nursing diagnosis Sexual Dysfunction Related to Decreased Sexual Drive are:

    a. _____

    b. _____

Implementation

22. List the sexual health issues that you would include when educating your patient.

    a. _____

    b. _____

    c. _____

    d. _____

    e. _____

23. Identify strategies that enhance sexual functioning.

a. _____

b. _____

c. _____

d. _____

e. _____

f. _____

g. _____

Acute Care

24. Identify the stressors that may affect a person's sexuality during illness.

_____

_____

Evaluation

25. Identify the follow-up discussions to determine whether the goals and outcomes were achieved.

a. _____

b. _____

REVIEW QUESTIONS

Select the appropriate answer and cite the rationale for choosing that particular answer.

26. At what developmental stage is it particularly important for children reared in single-parent families to be exposed to same-sex adults?
    1. Infancy
    2. School age
    3. Adolescence
    4. Toddlerhood and preschool years

Answer: _____ Rationale: _____

_____

_____

27. Which statement about sexual response in older adults is correct?
    1. The resolution phase is slower.
    2. The orgasm phase is prolonged.
    3. The refractory phase is more rapid.
    4. Both genders experience a reduced availability of sex hormones.

Answer: _____ Rationale: _____

_____

_____

28. The only 100% effective method to avoid contracting a disease through sex is:
    1. Abstinence
    2. Using condoms
    3. Avoiding sex with partners at risk
    4. Knowing the sexual partner's health history

Answer: _____ Rationale: _____

_____

_____

CRITICAL THINKING MODEL FOR NURSING CARE PLAN FOR SEXUAL DYSFUNCTION

29. Imagine that you are the nurse in the care plan on p. 726 of your text. Complete the *Assessment phase* of the critical thinking model by writing your answers in the appropriate boxes of the model shown. Think about the following.
    - In developing Mr. Clements' plan of care, what knowledge did the nurse apply?
    - In what way might the nurse's previous experience assist in this case?
    - What intellectual or professional standards were applied to Mr. Clements?
    - What critical thinking attitudes did you use in assessing Mr. Clements?
    - As you review your assessment, what key areas did you cover?

B. KNOWLEDGE

C. EXPERIENCE

A. *ASSESSMENT*
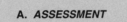

D. STANDARDS

E. ATTITUDES

36 Spiritual Health

PRELIMINARY READING

Chapter 36, pp. 733-749

COMPREHENSIVE UNDERSTANDING

Scientific Knowledge Base

1. Define *spirituality.*

_____

_____

Nursing Knowledge Base

Match the following terms.

2. _____ Transcendence   a. An energizing source that has an orientation to future goals and outcomes

3. _____ Connectedness   b. Belief that there is no known ultimate reality

4. _____ Atheist   c. Allows people to have firm beliefs despite lack of physical evidence

5. _____ Agnostic   d. Does not believe in the existence of God

6. _____ Spiritual well-being   e. Belief that there is a force outside of and greater than the person

7. _____ Faith   f. Intrapersonally, interpersonally, and transpersonally

8. _____ Religion   g. Having a vertical and horizontal dimension

9. _____ Hope   h. The system of organized beliefs and worship that a person practices

10. _____ Spiritual distress   i. Impaired ability to experience and integrate meaning and purpose in life

11. Briefly explain each of the following causes of spiritual distress.

    a. Acute illness: _____

_____

    b. Chronic illness: _____

_____

    c. Terminal illness: _____

_____

    d. Near-death experience: _____

_____

Nursing Process
Assessment

Various tools are available to assess a patient's spiritual well-being. Briefly summarize the following dimensions.

12. Faith/belief: _____

_____

13. Life/self-responsibility: _____

_____

14. Connectedness: _____

_____

15. Life satisfaction: _____

_____

16. Culture: _____

_____

17. Fellowship and community: _____

_____

18. Ritual and practice: _____

_____

19. Vocation: _____

_____

Nursing Diagnosis

20. List the nursing diagnoses that pertain to spiritual health.

    a. _____

    b. _____

    c. _____

    d. _____

    e. _____

    f. _____

    g. _____

    h. _____

    i. _____

Planning

21. Identify the three outcomes for the patient to achieve personal harmony and connections with members of his or her support system.

    a. _____

    b. _____

    c. _____

Implementation

22. Identify behaviors that establish the nurse's presence.

    _____

    _____

    _____

23. Identify the factors that are evident when a healing relationship develops between a nurse and patient.

    a. _____

    b. _____

    c. _____

Explain how the following interventions are helpful in the patient's therapeutic plan.

24. Support systems: _____

_____

_____

25. Diet therapies: _____

_____

_____

26. Supporting rituals: _____

_____

_____

27. Prayer: _____

_____

_____

28. Meditation: _____

_____

_____

29. Supporting grief work: _____

_____

_____

Evaluation

30. Identify the successful outcomes of spiritual health.

_____

_____

_____

REVIEW QUESTIONS

Select the appropriate answer and cite the rationale for choosing that particular answer.

31. When planning care to include spiritual needs for a patient of Islamic faith, the religious practices the nurse should understand include all of the following except:
    1. Strength is gained through group prayer.
    2. Family members are a source of comfort.
    3. A priest must be present to conduct rituals.
    4. Faith healing provides psychological support.

    Answer: _____   Rationale: _____

    _____

    _____

32. When consulting with the dietary department regarding meals for a patient of the Hindu religion, which of the following dietary items would not be included on the meal trays?
    1. Fruits
    2. Meats
    3. Dairy products
    4. Vegetable entrees

    Answer: _____   Rationale: _____

    _____

    _____

33. If an Islamic patient dies, the nurse should be aware of what religious practice?
    1. Last rites are mandatory.
    2. The body is always cremated.
    3. Muslims wash the body of the patient and wrap it in white cloth with the head turned to the right shoulder.
    4. Members of a ritual burial society cleanse the body.

    Answer: _____   Rationale: _____

    _____

    _____

34. If a nurse were to use a nursing diagnosis to relate concerns about spiritual health, which of the following would be used?
    1. Lack of faith
    2. Spiritual distress
    3. Inability to adjust
    4. Religious dilemma

    Answer: _____   Rationale: _____

    _____

    _____

35. Mr. Phillips was recently diagnosed with a malignant tumor. The staff had observed him crying on several occasions, and now he cries as he reads from his Bible. Interventions to help Mr. Phillips cope with his illness would include:
    1. Praying with Mr. Phillips as often as possible
    2. Asking the hospital chaplain to visit him daily
    3. Supporting his use of inner resources by providing time for meditation
    4. Engaging Mr. Phillips in diversional activities to reduce feelings of hopelessness

    Answer: _____   Rationale: _____

    _____

    _____

CRITICAL THINKING MODEL FOR NURSING CARE PLAN FOR READINESS FOR ENHANCED SPIRITUAL WELL-BEING

36. Imagine that you are the nurse in the care plan on p. 742 of your text. Complete the *Planning phase* of the critical thinking model by writing your answers in the appropriate boxes of the model shown. Think about the following.
    • In developing Lisa's plan of care, what knowledge did the nurse apply?
    • In what way might the nurse's previous experience assist in developing a plan of care for Lisa?
    • When developing a plan of care, what intellectual and professional standards were applied?
    • What critical thinking attitudes might have been applied to developing Lisa's plan?
    • How will the nurse accomplish the goals?

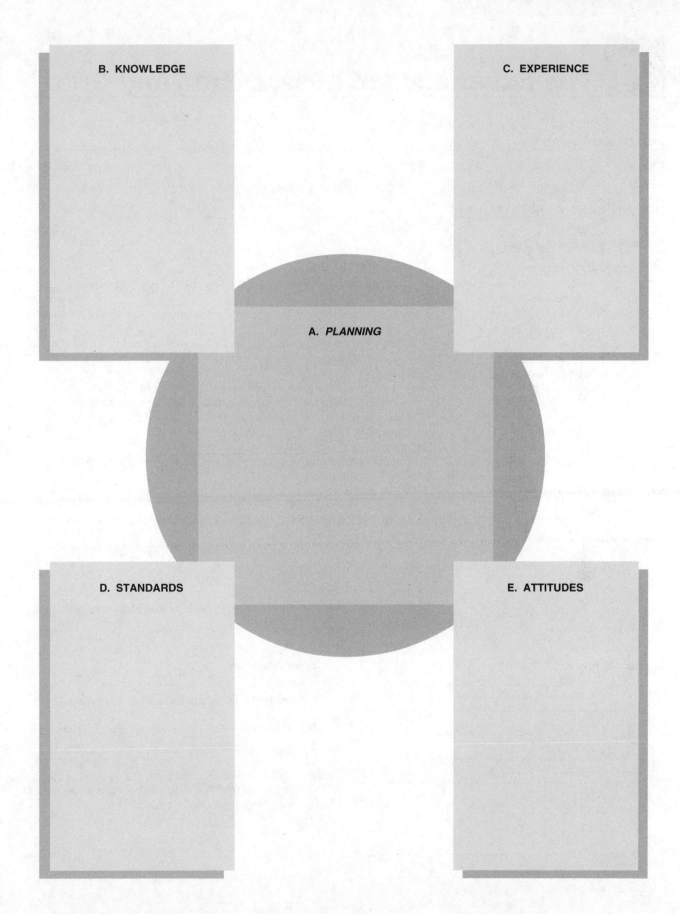

B. KNOWLEDGE

C. EXPERIENCE

A. *PLANNING*

D. STANDARDS

E. ATTITUDES

37 The Experience of Loss, Death, and Grief

PRELIMINARY READING

Chapter 37, pp. 750-770

COMPREHENSIVE UNDERSTANDING

Scientific Knowledge Base

Match the following terms.

1. _____ Maturational losses
2. _____ Situational loss
3. _____ Actual loss
4. _____ Perceived loss
5. _____ Grief
6. _____ Mourning
7. _____ Bereavement
8. _____ Normal grief
9. _____ Complicated grief
10. _____ Disenfranchised grief
11. _____ Delayed grief
12. _____ Ambiguous loss
13. _____ Exaggerated grief
14. _____ Masked grief
15. _____ Anticipatory grief

a. The unconscious process of disengaging before the actual loss or death occurs
b. Captures grief and mourning, emotional responses, and outward behaviors for a person experiencing loss
c. Difficult to process because of the lack of finality and unknown outcomes
d. Marginal or unsupported grief; the relationship may not be socially sanctioned
e. Person is unaware of disruptive behavior as a result of loss
f. Emotional response to a loss, which is unique to the individual
g. May exhibit self-destructive or maladaptive behavior, obsessions, or psychiatric disorders
h. Suppressing or postponing normal grief responses
i. Dysfunctional; the grieving person has a prolonged or significant time moving forward after a loss
j. Complex emotional, cognitive, social, physical, behavioral, and spiritual responses to loss and death
k. Outward social expression of grief and the behavior associated with loss that can be culturally influenced
l. Form of necessary loss, including all normally expected life changes across the life span
m. Can no longer feel, hear, or know a person or object
n. Sudden, unpredictable external event
o. Are uniquely defined by the person experiencing loss and are less obvious to other people

Nursing Knowledge Base

16. Identify the factors that influence loss and grief.

   a. _____

   b. _____

   c. _____

   d. _____

   e. _____

   f. _____

   g. _____

   h. _____

Nursing Process

Assessment

17. Identify the important areas of assessment.

   _____

   _____

Nursing Diagnosis

18. List the nursing diagnoses that pertain to the patient experiencing grief, loss, or death.

   a. _____

   b. _____

   c. _____

   d. _____

e. _____

f. _____

g. _____

h. _____

Planning

19. List two outcomes appropriate for a patient who has the nursing diagnosis powerlessness related to planned cancer therapy secondary to breast cancer.

a. _____

b. _____

Implementation

20. Define *palliative care.*

_____

_____

21. The World Health Organization (2015) summarizes palliative care as:

a. _____

b. _____

c. _____

d. _____

e. _____

f. _____

22. Hospice programs are built on the following core beliefs and services.

a. _____

b. _____

c. _____

d. _____

e. _____

f. _____

g. _____

h. _____

23. Identify the psychosocial care and symptom management that the nurse provides.

a. _____

b. _____

c. _____

d. _____

e. _____

f. _____

g. _____

h. _____

i. _____

24. Identify the nursing strategies for the family members to facilitate mourning.

a. _____

b. _____

c. _____

d. _____

e. _____

f. _____

g. _____

Define the following terms that relate to the care of the patient after death.

25. Organ and tissue donation: _____

_____

_____

26. Autopsy: _____

_____

_____

27. Postmortem care: _____

_____

_____

Evaluation

Identify the short- and long-term outcomes that signal a family's recovery from a loss.

28. Short term: _____

_____

_____

29. Long term: _____

_____

_____

REVIEW QUESTIONS

Select the appropriate answer and cite the rationale for choosing that particular answer.

30. Which statement about loss is accurate?
    1. Loss may be maturational, situational, or both.
    2. The degree of stress experienced is unrelated to the type of loss.
    3. Loss is only experienced when there is an actual absence of something valued.
    4. The more an individual has invested in what is lost, the less the feeling of loss.

Answer: _____ Rationale: _____

_____

_____

31. A hospice program emphasizes:
    1. Prolongation of life
    2. Hospital-based care
    3. Palliative treatment and control of symptoms
    4. Curative treatment and alleviation of symptoms

Answer: _____ Rationale: _____

_____

_____

32. Trying questionable and experimental forms of therapy is a behavior that is characteristic of which stage of dying?
    1. Anger
    2. Bargaining
    3. Depression
    4. Acceptance

Answer: _____ Rationale: _____

_____

_____

33. All of the following are crucial needs of the dying patient except:
    1. Control of pain
    2. Love and belonging
    3. Freedom from decision making
    4. Preservation of dignity and self-worth

Answer: _____ Rationale: _____

_____

_____

CRITICAL THINKING MODEL FOR NURSING CARE PLAN FOR HOPELESSNESS

34. Imagine that you are the student nurse in the care plan on page p. 758 of your text. Complete the *Evaluation phase* of the critical thinking model by writing your answers in the appropriate boxes of the model shown. Think about the following.
- In evaluating Mrs. Allison's plan of care, what did you apply?
- In what way might your previous experience influence your evaluation of Mrs. Allison's care?
- During evaluation, what intellectual and professional standards were applied to Mrs. Allison's care?
- In what way do critical thinking attitudes play a role in how you approach evaluation of Mrs. Allison's care?
- How might you adjust Mrs. Allison's care?

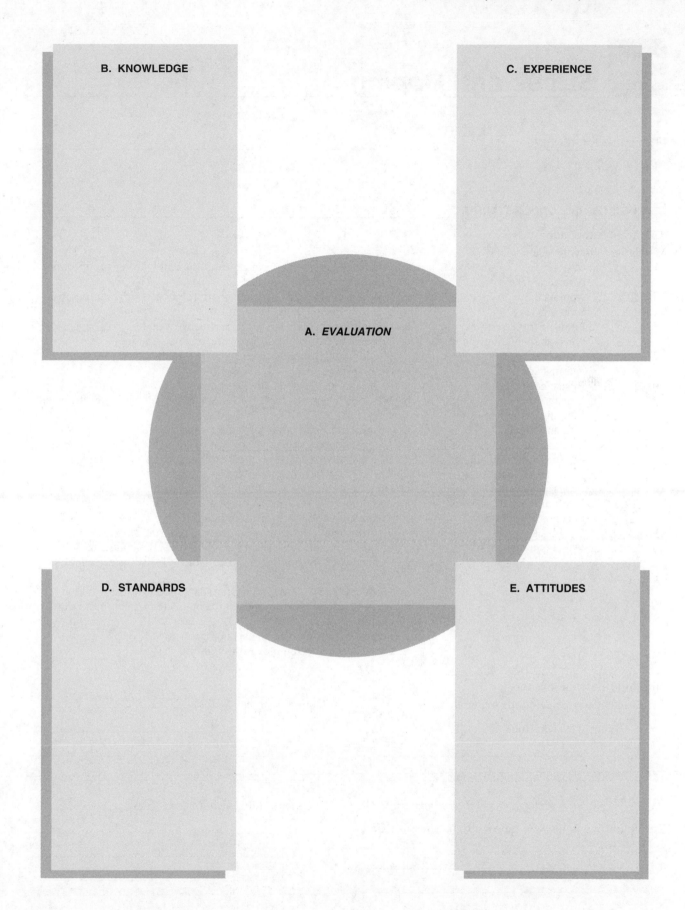

B. KNOWLEDGE

C. EXPERIENCE

A. *EVALUATION*

D. STANDARDS

E. ATTITUDES

38 Stress and Coping

PRELIMINARY READING

Chapter 38, pp. 771-786

COMPREHENSIVE UNDERSTANDING

Scientific Knowledge Base

Match the following terms.

1. _____ Stress
2. _____ Allostatic load
3. _____ Appraisal
4. _____ Stressors
5. _____ Fight-or-flight response
6. _____ General adaptation syndrome
7. _____ Crisis
8. _____ Alarm stage
9. _____ Resistance stage
10. _____ Exhaustion stage
11. _____ Medulla oblongata
12. _____ Pituitary gland
13. _____ Coping
14. _____ Ego-defense mechanisms
15. _____ Reticular formation
16. _____ Primary appraisal
17. _____ Posttraumatic stress disorder
18. _____ Secondary appraisal
19. _____ Flashbacks
20. _____ Developmental crisis

a. Monitors the physiological status of the body through connections with sensory and motor tracts
b. Person is considering possible coping strategies or resources available to help deal with the event
c. Chronic arousal that causes excessive wear and tear on the person
d. Controls heart rate, blood pressure, and respirations
e. Identifying the event or circumstance as a threat
f. A three-stage reaction to stress
g. Arousal of the sympathetic nervous system
h. A trauma occurs, and its effects sometimes last well after the event ends
i. Allow a person to cope with stress indirectly
j. An experience a person is exposed to through a stimulus or stressor
k. How people interpret the impact of the stressor on themselves
l. Recurrent or intrusive recollections of the event
m. Are tension-producing stimuli operating within or on any system
n. Symptoms of stress persist beyond the duration of a stressor
o. Rising hormone levels result in increased blood volume, blood glucose levels, epinephrine and norepinephrine amounts, heart rate, blood flow to the muscles, oxygen intake, and mental alertness
p. Occurs when the body is no longer able to resist the effects of the stressor
q. Produces hormones necessary for adaptation to stress
r. Body stabilizes and responds in the opposite manner to the alarm reaction
s. Person's effort to manage psychological stress
t. Occurs as the person moves through life's stages

Nursing Knowledge Base

21. Briefly describe the following models.

    a. Neuman systems model: _____

    _____

    b. Pender's health promotion model: _____

    _____

The following factors can potentially be stressors. Give some examples.

22. Situational factors: _____

    _____

    _____

23. Maturational factors: _____

    _____

    _____

    _____

24. Sociocultural factors: _____

    _____

    _____

    _____

Nursing Process
Assessment

25. Identify subjective areas that are used to assess a patient's level of stress.

    a. _____

    b. _____

    c. _____

    d. _____

    e. _____

26. Identify some objective findings related to stress and coping.

    a. _____

    b. _____

    c. _____

    d. _____

    e. _____

    f. _____

    g. _____

Nursing Diagnosis

27. Identify the multiple diagnoses for stress or failure of coping.

    a. _____

    b. _____

    c. _____

    d. _____

    e. _____

    f. _____

    g. _____

    h. _____

Planning

28. The nurse assesses the level and source of the existing stress and determines the appropriate points for interventions; describe each level.

    a. Primary level of prevention: _____

    _____

    b. Secondary level of prevention: _____

    _____

    c. Tertiary level of prevention: _____

    _____

Implementation

29. Identify the three primary modes of intervention to reduce stress.

    a. _____

    _____

    b. _____

    _____

    c. _____

    _____

Acute Care

30. Crisis intervention is: _____

    _____

    _____

    _____

Evaluation

31. The desired outcomes for a patient recovering from acute stress are: _____

    _____

    _____

    _____

REVIEW QUESTIONS

Select the appropriate answer and cite the rationale for choosing that particular answer.

32. Which definition does not characterize stress?
    1. Efforts to maintain relative constancy within the internal environment
    2. A condition eliciting an intellectual, behavioral, or metabolic response
    3. Any situation in which a nonspecific demand requires an individual to respond or take action
    4. A phenomenon affecting social, psychological, developmental, spiritual, and physiological dimensions

Answer: _____   Rationale: _____

_____

_____

33. Major homeostatic mechanisms are controlled by all of the following except:
    1. Thymus gland
    2. Pituitary gland
    3. Medulla oblongata
    4. Reticular formation

    Answer: _____ Rationale: _____

    _____

    _____

34. Which of the following is an example of the general adaptation syndrome?
    1. Alarm reaction
    2. Inflammatory response
    3. Fight-or-flight response
    4. Ego-defense mechanisms

    Answer: _____ Rationale: _____

    _____

    _____

35. Crisis intervention is a specific measure used for helping a patient resolve a particular, immediate stress problem. This approach is based on:
    1. An in-depth analysis of a patient's situation
    2. The ability of the nurse to solve the patient's problems
    3. Effective communication between the nurse and patient
    4. Teaching the patient how to use ego-defense mechanisms

    Answer: _____ Rationale: _____

    _____

    _____

CRITICAL THINKING MODEL FOR NURSING CARE PLAN FOR INEFFECTIVE COPING

36. Imagine that you are the nurse in the care plan on p. 779 of your text. Complete the *Evaluation phase* of the critical thinking model by writing your answers in the appropriate boxes of the model shown. Think about the following.
    - In evaluating the care of Sandra and John, what knowledge did the nurse apply?
    - In what way might the nurse's previous experience influence the evaluation of Sandra and John's care?
    - During evaluation, what intellectual and professional standards were applied to Sandra and John's care?
    - In what way do critical thinking attitudes play a role in how the nurse approaches the evaluation of Sandra and John's care?
    - How might the nurse adjust their care?

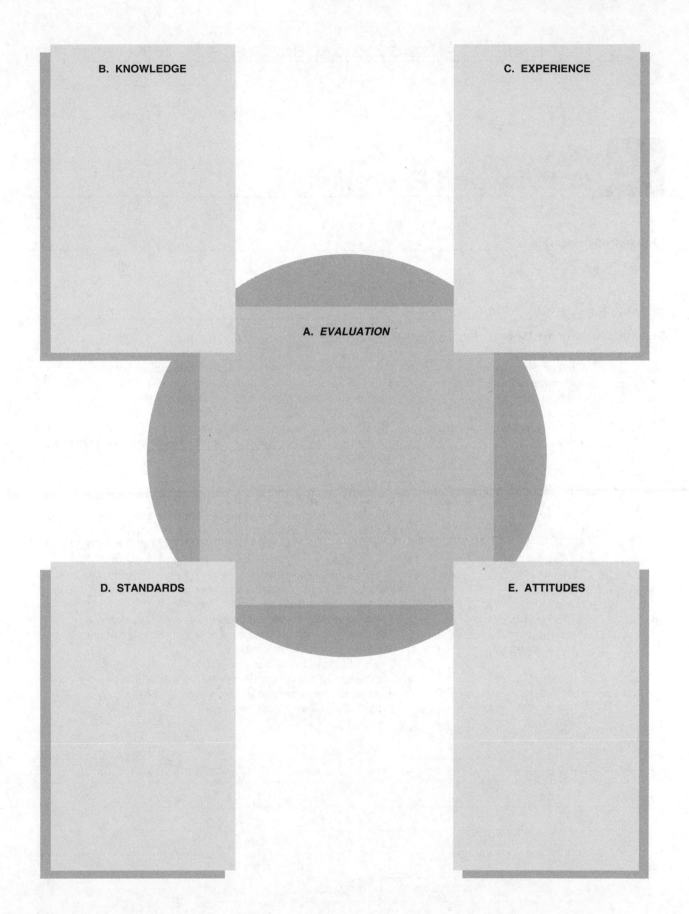

B. KNOWLEDGE

C. EXPERIENCE

A. *EVALUATION*

D. STANDARDS

E. ATTITUDES

39 Activity and Exercise

PRELIMINARY READING

Chapter 39, pp. 787-820

COMPREHENSIVE UNDERSTANDING

Scientific Knowledge Base

Match the following terms.

1. _____ Concentric tension
2. _____ Activities of daily living
3. _____ Body alignment
4. _____ Body balance
5. _____ Coordinated body movement
6. _____ Friction
7. _____ Activity tolerance
8. _____ Isotonic contractions
9. _____ Isometric contractions
10. _____ Resistive isometric exercises
11. _____ Fibrous joints
12. _____ Cartilaginous joints
13. _____ Synovial joints
14. _____ Ligaments
15. _____ Tendons
16. _____ Cartilage
17. _____ Antagonistic muscles
18. _____ Synergistic muscles
19. _____ Antigravity muscles
20. _____ Proprioception

a. The awareness of the position of the body and its parts
b. Bands of tissue that connect muscle to bone
c. Muscles that are involved with joint stabilization
d. ADLs
e. The amount of exercise or activity that the person is able to perform
f. Have little movement but are elastic and use cartilage to separate body surfaces
g. Freely movable joints
h. Nonvascular supporting tissue
i. Muscles that bring about movement of a joint
j. Muscles that contract to accomplish the same movement
k. Increased muscle contraction causes muscle shortening
l. Movement that is the result of weight, center of gravity, and balance
m. The force that occurs in a direction to oppose movement
n. Occurs with a low center of gravity and a wide, stable base of support
o. Exercises that involve tightening or tensing of muscles without moving body parts (quadriceps set exercises)
p. The relationship of one body part to another body part
q. Exercises that cause muscle contraction and change in muscle length (walking, swimming, biking)
r. Bands of fibrous tissue that bind joints and connect bones and cartilage
s. Contraction of muscles while pushing against a stationary object or resisting the movement of the object (e.g., push-ups)
t. Joints that fit closely together and are fixed

21. Identify the principles for safe patient positioning.

a. _____

b. _____

c. _____

d. _____

e. _____

f. _____

g. _____

22. Identify the pathological conditions that influence body alignment and mobility.

a. _____

b. _____

c. _____

d. _____

Nursing Knowledge Base

Identify the descriptive characteristics of body alignment and mobility related to the following developmental changes.

23. Infants: _____

_____

24. Toddlers: _____

_____

25. Adolescents: _____

_____

26. Young to middle adults: _____

_____

27. Older adults: _____

_____

Nursing Process

Assessment

Briefly explain how assessment of body alignment and posture is carried out.

28. Standing: _____

_____

29. Sitting: _____

_____

30. Recumbent: _____

_____

31. Identify the three components to assess mobility.

a. _____

b. _____

c. _____

Identify some factors that affect activity tolerance.

32. Physiological: _____

_____

33. Emotional: _____

_____

34. Developmental: _____

_____

Nursing Diagnosis

35. Identify the nursing diagnoses that are related to activity and exercise.

   a. _____

   b. _____

   c. _____

   d. _____

   e. _____

   f. _____

   g. _____

Planning

36. List three outcomes for a patient with deficits in activity and exercise.

   a. _____

   b. _____

   c. _____

Implementation

37. Explain how to calculate the patient's target heart rate (THR).

_____

_____

38. An exercise program can consist of the following. Provide examples for each one.

   a. Aerobic exercise: _____

   b. Stretching and flexibility exercises: _____

   c. Resistance training: _____

39. What is the difference between active ROM and passive ROM?

_____

_____

40. Walking helps to prevent contractures by: _____

_____

41. Identify the two types of canes that are available and their use.

   a. _____

   b. _____

42. Explain the four standard crutch gaits.

   a. Four-point gait: _____

   b. Three-point gait: _____

   c. Two-point gait: _____

   d. Swing-through gait: _____

Evaluation

43. Identify the areas to evaluate to determine the effectiveness of the nursing interventions to enhance activity and exercise.

a. _____

b. _____

c. _____

d. _____

e. _____

REVIEW QUESTIONS

Select the appropriate answer and cite the rationale for choosing that particular answer.

44. White, shiny, flexible bands of fibrous tissue binding joints together and connecting various bones and cartilage types are known as:
    1. Joints
    2. Muscles
    3. Tendons
    4. Ligaments

    Answer: _____ Rationale: _____

    _____

    _____

45. The nurse would expect all of the following physiological effects of exercise on the body systems except:
    1. Change in metabolic rate
    2. Decreased cardiac output
    3. Increased respiratory rate and depth
    4. Increased muscle tone, size, and strength

    Answer: _____ Rationale: _____

    _____

    _____

CRITICAL THINKING MODEL FOR NURSING CARE PLAN FOR ACTIVITY INTOLERANCE

46. Imagine that you are the nurse in the care plan on pp. 800-801 of your text. Complete the *Planning phase* of the critical thinking model by writing your answers in the appropriate boxes of the model shown. Think about the following.
    - In developing Mrs. Smith's plan of care, what knowledge did the nurse apply?
    - In what way might the nurse's previous experience assist in developing a plan of care for Mrs. Smith?
    - When developing a plan of care, what intellectual or professional standards were applied to Mrs. Smith?
    - What critical thinking attitudes might have been applied in developing Mrs. Smith's plan?
    - How will the nurse accomplish the goals of the plan of care?

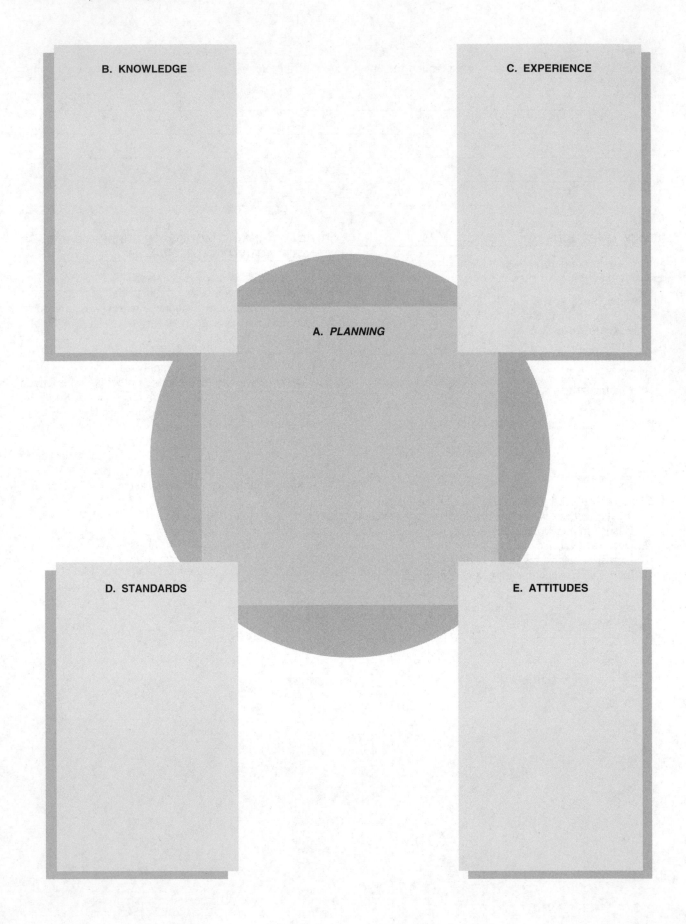

40 Hygiene

PRELIMINARY READING

Chapter 40, pp. 821-870

COMPREHENSIVE UNDERSTANDING

Scientific Knowledge Base

1. Explain the three primary layers of the skin.

   a. Epidermis: _____

   b. Dermis: _____

   c. Subcutaneous: _____

2. Identify the functions of the skin.

   a. _____

   b. _____

   c. _____

   d. _____

Nursing Knowledge Base

3. Identify the factors that influence hygiene.

   a. _____

   b. _____

   c. _____

   d. _____

   e. _____

   f. _____

   g. _____

   h. _____

Nursing Process
Assessment

4. Assessment of the skin includes: _____

   _____

5. Common skin problems can affect how hygiene is administered. Describe the hygiene provided for the following.

   a. Dry skin: _____

   _____

   b. Acne: _____

   _____

   c. Skin rashes: _____

   _____

   d. Contact dermatitis: _____

   _____

   e. Abrasion: _____

   _____

6. Identify the characteristics of the following foot and nail problems.

   a. Calluses:_____

     _____

   b. Corns: _____

     _____

   c. Plantar warts: _____

     _____

   d. Tinea pedis: _____

     _____

   e. Ingrown nails:_____

     _____

   f. Foot odors: _____

     _____

7. Halitosis is: _____

   _____

8. Identify the characteristics of the following hair and scalp conditions.

   a. Dandruff: _____

     _____

   b. Ticks: _____

     _____

   c. Pediculosis: _____

     _____

   d. Pediculosis capitis: _____

     _____

   e. Pediculosis corporis: _____

     _____

   f. Pediculosis pubis:_____

     _____

   g. Alopecia: _____

9. Give examples of patients at risk for hygiene problems.

   a. Oral problems: _____

     _____

   b. Skin problems: _____

     _____

   c. Foot problems: _____

     _____

   d. Eye care problems: _____

     _____

Nursing Diagnosis

10. List the possible nursing diagnoses that apply to patients in need of hygiene care.

   a. _____

   b. _____

   c. _____

   d. _____

   e. _____

   f. _____

   g. _____

   h. _____

Planning

11. Identify three expected outcomes for a patient who has had a cerebral vascular accident:

   a. _____

   b. _____

   c. _____

Implementation

12. List the educational tips for patients about hygiene practices.

   a. _____

   b. _____

   c. _____

   d. _____

Acute and restorative care

13. Briefly explain the following types of baths.

   a. Complete bed bath: _____

     _____

   b. Partial bed bath: _____

     _____

14. State guidelines that the nurse needs to follow regardless of the type of bath.

   a. _____

   b. _____

   c. _____

d. _____

e. _____

15. Identify the patients at risk for skin breakdown in the perineal area.

_____

_____

16. Identify the benefits of a back rub.

_____

_____

17. List the guidelines in a routine foot and nail care program.

a. _____

b. _____

c. _____

d. _____

e. _____

f. _____

g. _____

Briefly explain the benefits of the following in relation to oral hygiene.

18. Brushing: _____

19. Flossing: _____

_____

20. Denture care: _____

_____

Briefly describe the rationale for the following interventions.

21. Brushing and combing: _____

_____

22. Shampooing: _____

_____

23. Mustache and beard care: _____

_____

24. Explain how shaving should be performed and provide a rationale.

_____

_____

25. Describe basic eye care for a patient.

_____

_____

26. Describe each of the following techniques necessary in caring for an artificial eye.

a. Removal: _____

b. Cleansing: _____

c. Reinsertion: _____

d. Storage: _____

27. Describe the procedure for removal of impacted cerumen.

_____

_____

28. Describe the following types of hearing aids.

a. In-the-canal (ITC) hearing aid: _____

_____

b. In-the-ear (ITE) hearing aid: _____

_____

c. Behind-the-ear (BTE) hearing aid: _____

_____

d. Digital hearing aid: _____

_____

29. Describe the following common bed positions.

a. Fowler: _____

_____

b. Semi-Fowler: _____

_____

c. Trendelenburg: _____

_____

d. Reverse Trendelenburg: _____

_____

e. Flat: _____

_____

REVIEW QUESTIONS

Select the appropriate answer and cite the rationale for choosing that particular answer.

30. Mr. Gray is a 19-year-old patient in the rehabilitation unit. He is completely paralyzed below the neck. The most appropriate bath for Mr. Gray is a:
    1. Partial bed bath
    2. Complete bed bath
    3. Sitz bath
    4. Tepid bath

    Answer: _____   Rationale: _____

    _____

    _____

31. All of the following will help maintain skin integrity in older adults except:
    1. Environmental air that is cold and dry
    2. Use of warm water and mild cleansing agents for bathing
    3. Bathing every other day
    4. Drinking 8 to 10 glasses of water a day

    Answer: _____   Rationale: _____

    _____

    _____

32. When preparing to give complete morning care to a patient, what would the nurse do first?
    1. Gather the necessary equipment and supplies.
    2. Remove the patient's gown or pajamas while maintaining privacy.
    3. Assess the patient's preferences for bathing practices.
    4. Lower the side rails and assist the patient with assuming a comfortable position.

    Answer: _____   Rationale: _____

    _____

    _____

33. Mrs. Veech has diabetes. Which intervention should be included in her teaching plan regarding foot care?
    1. Use a pumice stone to smooth corns and calluses.
    2. File toenails straight across and square.
    3. Apply powder to dry areas along the feet and between the toes.
    4. Wear elastic stockings to improve circulation.

    Answer: _____   Rationale: _____

    _____

    _____

34. Assessment of the hair and scalp reveals that John has head lice. An appropriate intervention would be:
    1. Shave hair off the affected area.
    2. Place oil on the hair and scalp until all of the lice are dead.
    3. Shampoo with medicated shampoo and repeat 12 to 24 hours later.
    4. Shampoo with regular shampoo and dry with hair-dryer set at the hottest setting.

    Answer: _____   Rationale: _____

    _____

    _____

CRITICAL THINKING MODEL FOR NURSING CARE FOR BATHING SELF-CARE DEFICIT

35. Imagine that you are the nurse in the care plan on pp. 834-835. Complete the *Planning phase* of the critical thinking model by writing your answers in the appropriate boxes of the model shown. Think about the following.
    - In developing Mrs. White's plan of care, what knowledge did the nurse apply?
    - In what way might the nurse's previous experience apply in this case?
    - What intellectual or professional standards were applied to Mrs. White?
    - What critical thinking attitudes did you use in providing care to Mrs. White?
    - As you review your plan, what key areas did you cover?

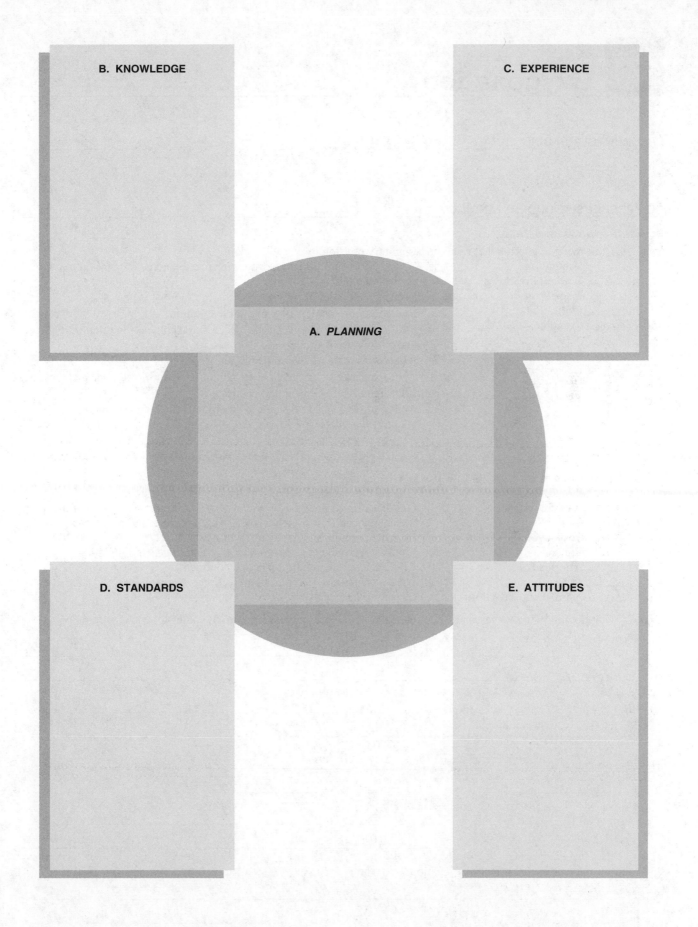

B. KNOWLEDGE

C. EXPERIENCE

A. *PLANNING*

D. STANDARDS

E. ATTITUDES

41 Oxygenation

PRELIMINARY READING

Chapter 41, pp. 871-933

COMPREHENSIVE UNDERSTANDING

Scientific Knowledge Base

Match the following key terms that relate to respiratory physiology.

1. _____ Ventilation	a.	Moves the respiratory gases from one area to another according to concentration gradients
2. _____ Work of breathing		
3. _____ Inspiration	b.	Reduced hemoglobin
4. _____ Expiration	c.	Amount of air exhaled after normal inspiration
5. _____ Compliance	d.	Pressure difference between the mouth and the alveoli in relation to the rate of flow of inspired gas
6. _____ Airway resistance		
7. _____ Respiration	e.	Process of moving gases into and out of the lungs
8. _____ Deoxyhemoglobin	f.	Is the exchange of oxygen and carbon dioxide during cellular metabolism
9. _____ Diffusion	g.	Effort required to expand and contract the lungs
10. _____ Tidal volume	h.	Ability of the lungs to distend or to expand in response to increased intraalveolar pressure
	i.	Active process stimulated by chemical receptors in the aorta
	j.	Passive process dependent on the elastic recoil properties of the lungs

Match the following cardiopulmonary physiology terms.

11. _____ Frank–Starling law	a.	Reflects the electrical activity of the conduction system
12. _____ Cardiac output	b.	End-diastolic volume
13. _____ S_1 and S_2	c.	As the myocardium stretches, the strength of the contraction increases
14. _____ Stroke volume	d.	Normal sequence on the electrocardiogram (ECG)
15. _____ Preload	e.	Amount of blood ejected from the left ventricle each minute
16. _____ Afterload	f.	Affected by preload, afterload, and contractility
17. _____ ECG	g.	The resistance to left ventricular ejection
18. _____ Normal sinus rhythm	h.	Closure of heart valves

Explain what the following waves in the conduction system represent and the normal values for each.

19. P wave: _____

_____

20. PR interval: _____

_____

21. QRS complex: _____

_____

22. QT interval: _____

_____

23. Identify the factors that affect oxygenation.

   a. _____

   b. _____

c. _____

d. _____

24. Identify conditions that affect chest wall movement and provide an example.

a. _____

b. _____

c. _____

d. _____

e. _____

f. _____

g. _____

Explain the following alterations in respiratory functioning.

25. Hyperventilation: _____

_____

26. Hypoventilation: _____

_____

27. Hypoxia: _____

_____

28. Cyanosis: _____

_____

29. Briefly describe the following dysrhythmias.

a. Tachycardia: _____

b. Bradycardia: _____

c. Atrial fibrillation: _____

30. Explain the difference between the following types of heart failure.

a. Left sided: _____

b. Right sided: _____

Describe the following disorders.

31. Myocardial ischemia: _____

_____

32. Angina pectoris: _____

_____

33. Myocardial infarction: _____

_____

Nursing Knowledge Base

Identify the cardiopulmonary risk factors for the following developmental levels.

34. Infants and toddlers:

_____

_____

35. School-age children and adolescents:

_____

_____

36. Young and middle-aged adults:

_____

_____

37. Older adults:

_____

_____

38. List the lifestyle modifications to decrease cardio-pulmonary risks.

    a. _____

    b. _____

    c. _____

    d. _____

    e. _____

39. List four occupational pollutants.

    a. _____

    b. _____

    c. _____

    d. _____

Nursing Process
Assessment

40. Explain the focus of the nursing history to meet oxygen needs for the following.

    a. Cardiac function:

    _____

    _____

    b. Respiratory function:

    _____

    _____

41. Explain the differences between the following types of chest pain.

    a. Cardiac pain:

    _____

    _____

    b. Pleuritic chest pain:

    _____

    c. Musculoskeletal pain:

    _____

Explain how the following affect oxygenation.

42. Fatigue: _____

_____

_____

43. Dyspnea: _____

_____

_____

44. Orthopnea: _____

_____

_____

45. Cough: _____

_____

_____

46. Wheezing: _____

_____

_____

Briefly explain what information is gained from the following techniques used during the physical examination to assess tissue oxygenation.

47. Inspection: _____

_____

_____

48. Palpation: _____

_____

_____

49. Percussion: _____

_____

_____

50. Auscultation: _____

_____

_____

51. Describe the following diagnostic tests used to determine the adequacy of the cardiac conduction system.

    a. Holter monitor:

    _____

    _____

    b. Exercise stress test:

    _____

    _____

    c. Thallium stress test:

    _____

    _____

    d. Electrophysiologic study (EPS):

    _____

    _____

    e. Echocardiography:

    _____

    _____

    f. Scintigraphy:

    _____

    _____

    g. Cardiac catheterization and angiography:

    _____

    _____

52. Describe the following tests used to measure the adequacy of ventilation and oxygenation.

    a. Pulmonary function tests:

    _____

    _____

    b. Peak expiratory flow rate (PEFR):

    _____

    _____

c. Bronchoscopy:

_____

_____

d. Lung scan:

_____

_____

e. Thoracentesis:

_____

_____

Nursing Diagnosis

53. List the nursing diagnoses that are appropriate for the patient with alterations in oxygenation.

    a. _____

    b. _____

    c. _____

    d. _____

    e. _____

    f. _____

    g. _____

    h. _____

Planning

54. List the specific outcomes for maintaining a patent airway.

    a. _____

    b. _____

    c. _____

    d. _____

Implementation

55. List patient and family teaching strategies to promote cardiopulmonary health.

    a. _____

    b. _____

    c. _____

    d. _____

    e. _____

    f. _____

56. List the interventions that promote mobilization of pulmonary secretions.

    a. _____

    b. _____

    c. _____

    d. _____

57. Describe the following types of cough.

    a. Cascade:

    _____

    _____

    b. Huff:

    _____

    _____

    c. Quad:

    _____

    _____

58. Postural drainage is a component of pulmonary hygiene and consists of:

    a. _____

    b. _____

59. Percussion is contraindicated in:

    a. _____

    b. _____

    c. _____

60. Suctioning techniques include:

    a. _____

    b. _____

    c. _____

61. Define the types of artificial airways.

    a. _____

    b. _____

    c. _____

    Nursing interventions that maintain or promote lung expansion include the following noninvasive techniques. Briefly explain each one.

62. Ambulation:

    _____

    _____

63. Positioning:

    _____

    _____

64. Incentive spirometry:

    _____

    _____

65. List the clinical indications for invasive mechanical ventilation.

    a. _____

    b. _____

    c. _____

    d. _____

    e. _____

    f. _____

    g. _____

66. Identify the most commonly used modes available on all ventilators.

    a. _____

    b. _____

    c. _____

67. Identify the complications of invasive mechanical ventilation.

    _____

    _____

68. Noninvasive ventilatory support can be achieved using a variety of modes. List two of them.

    a. _____

    b. _____

69. List the complications of noninvasive ventilation.

    _____

    _____

70. Identify the three reasons for inserting chest tubes.

    a. _____

    b. _____

    c. _____

71. Define the following.

    a. Hemothorax:

    _____

    _____

    b. Pneumothorax:

    _____

    _____

72. The goal of oxygen therapy is:

    _____

    _____

73. Describe the following methods of oxygen delivery.

    a. Nasal cannula: _____

    _____

    _____

    b. Face mask: _____

    _____

    _____

    c. Venturi mask: _____

    _____

    _____

74. Identify the indications for a patient to receive home oxygen therapy.

    _____

    _____

75. In cardiopulmonary resuscitation, CAB stands for:

    C: _____

    A: _____

    B: _____

76. The goal of cardiopulmonary rehabilitation for the patient to maintain an optimal level of health focuses on:

    a. _____

    b. _____

    c. _____

    d. _____

Briefly explain the following breathing techniques used to improve ventilation and oxygenation.

77. Pursed-lip breathing:

    _____

    _____

78. Diaphragmatic breathing:

    _____

    _____

REVIEW QUESTIONS

Select the appropriate answer and cite the rationale for choosing that particular answer.

79. Ventilation, perfusion, and exchange of gases are the major purposes of:
    1. Respiration
    2. Circulation
    3. Aerobic metabolism
    4. Anaerobic metabolism

Answer: _____ Rationale: _____

_____

_____

80. Afterload refers to:
    1. The resistance to left ventricular ejection
    2. The amount of blood in the left ventricle at the end of diastole
    3. The amount of blood ejected from the left ventricle each minute
    4. The amount of blood ejected from the left ventricle with each contraction

Answer: _____ Rationale: _____

_____

_____

81. The movement of gases into and out of the lungs depends on:
    1. 50% oxygen content in the atmospheric air
    2. The pressure gradient between the atmosphere and the alveoli
    3. The use of accessory muscles of respiration during expiration
    4. The amount of carbon dioxide dissolved in the fluid of the alveoli

    Answer: _____   Rationale: _____

    _____

    _____

82. Mr. Isaac comes to the emergency department complaining of difficulty breathing. An objective finding associated with his dyspnea might include:
    1. Feelings of heaviness in the chest
    2. Complaints of shortness of breath
    3. Use of accessory muscles of respiration
    4. Statements about a sense of impending doom

    Answer: _____   Rationale: _____

    _____

    _____

83. The use of chest physiotherapy to mobilize pulmonary secretions involves the use of:
    1. Hydration
    2. Percussion
    3. Nebulization
    4. Humidification

    Answer: _____   Rationale: _____

    _____

    _____

CRITICAL THINKING MODEL FOR NURSING CARE PLAN FOR INEFFECTIVE AIRWAY CLEARANCE

84. Imagine that you are the student nurse in the care plan on p. 889 of your text. Complete the *Assessment phase* of the critical thinking model by writing your answers in the appropriate boxes of the model shown. Think about the following.
    - What knowledge base was applied to Mr. Edwards?
    - In what way might your previous experience apply in this case?
    - What intellectual or professional standards were applied to Mr. Edwards?
    - What critical thinking attitudes did you use in assessing Mr. Edwards?
    - As you review your assessment, what key areas did you cover?

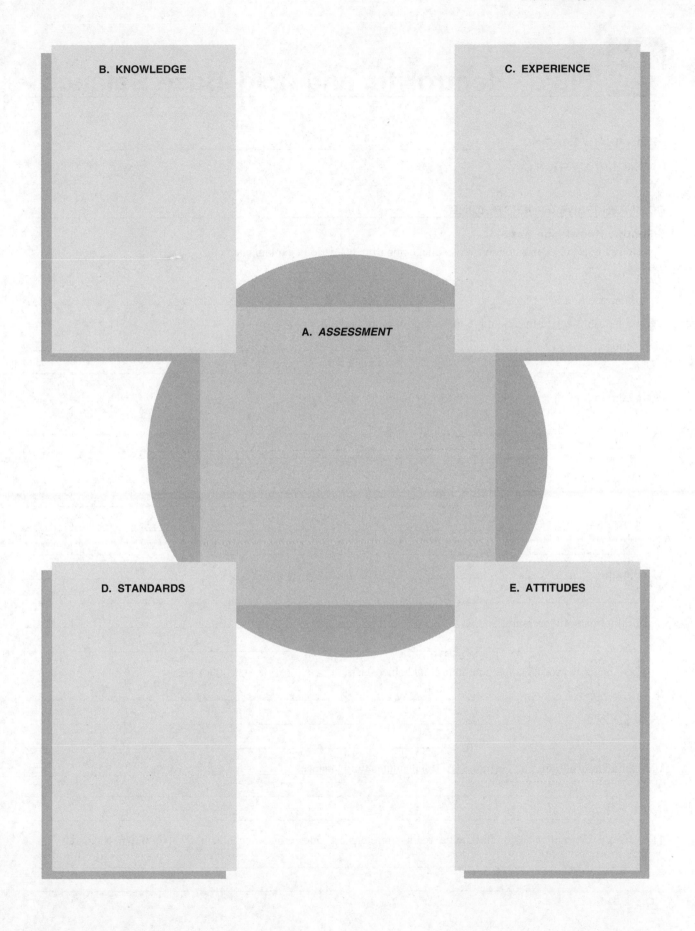

B. KNOWLEDGE

C. EXPERIENCE

A. *ASSESSMENT*

D. STANDARDS

E. ATTITUDES

42 Fluid, Electrolyte, and Acid–Base Balance

PRELIMINARY READING

Chapter 42, pp. 934-991

COMPREHENSIVE UNDERSTANDING

Scientific Knowledge Base

1. Body fluids are distributed in two distinct compartments. Briefly explain each one.

   a. Extracellular: _____

   b. Intracellular: _____

Define the following terms related to the composition of body fluids.

2. Cations: _____

3. Anions: _____

Define the following terms related to the movement of body fluids.

4. Osmosis: _____

   _____

5. Osmotic pressure: _____

   _____

6. Diffusion: _____

   _____

7. Filtration: _____

   _____

8. Colloid osmotic pressure: _____

   _____

9. List the three processes that maintain fluid homeostasis.

   a. _____

   b. _____

   c. _____

10. Define how antidiuretic hormone (ADH) regulates fluid balance.

    _____

    _____

11. Changes in renal perfusion initiate the renin–angiotension–aldosterone mechanism. Explain the mechanism.

    _____

    _____

12. What is atrial natriuretic peptide?

_____

_____

13. Explain the difference between the two types of fluid imbalances below.

    a. Extracellular fluid volume deficit: _____

    b. Extracellular fluid volume excess: _____

14. Osmolality imbalances are the following. Briefly explain.

    a. Hypernatremia: _____

    b. Hyponatremia: _____

15. Give the normal values and functions of the major body electrolytes in the following table.

Electrolyte	Values	Function
Potassium		
Ionized calcium		
Magnesium		
Phosphate		

16. For each electrolyte disturbance, identify the diagnostic laboratory finding and list at least four characteristic signs and symptoms in the following table.

Imbalance	Laboratory Finding	Signs and Symptoms
Hypokalemia		
Hyperkalemia		
Hypocalcemia		
Hypercalcemia		
Hypomagnesemia		
Hypermagnesemia		

17. Acid–base homeostasis is the dynamic interplay of three processes. Identify and explain.

    a. _____

    b. _____

    c. _____

18. The four primary types of acid–base imbalances are listed in the following table. For each acid–base imbalance, identify the diagnostic laboratory finding and list the characteristic signs and symptoms.

Acid–Base Imbalance	Laboratory Findings	Signs and Symptoms
Respiratory acidosis		
Respiratory alkalosis		
Metabolic acidosis		
Metabolic alkalosis		

Nursing Process

Assessment

Explain how the following can affect fluid, electrolyte, and acid–base balances.

19. Age: _____

    _____

20. Acute illness: _____

    _____

21. Recent surgery: _____

    _____

22. Burns: _____

    _____

23. Cancer: _____

    _____

24. Heart failure: _____

    _____

25. Gastrointestinal disturbances: _____

    _____

26. Environmental factors: _____

    _____

27. Diet: _____

_____

28. Lifestyle: _____

_____

29. Medications:

    a. Diuretics: _____

    b. Corticosteroids: _____

    c. ACE inhibitors: _____

    d. Antidepressants: _____

    e. Penicillins: _____

    f. Calcium carbonate: _____

    g. Magnesium hydroxide: _____

    h. Nonsteroidal anti-inflammatory drugs: _____

30. Indicate the possible fluid, electrolyte, or acid–base imbalances associated with each physical finding.

Assessment	Imbalances
Loss of 2.2 pounds or more in 24 hours	
Orthostatic hypotension	
Bounding pulse rate	
Full or distended neck veins	
Lung sounds: crackles or rhonchi	
Dark yellow urine	
Dependent edema in ankles	
Dry mucus membranes	
Thirst present	
Restlessness and mild confusion	
Decreased level of consciousness	
Irregular pulse and EKG changes	

Assessment	Imbalances
Increased rate and depth of respirations	
Muscle weakness	
Decreased deep tendon reflexes	
Hyperactive reflexes, muscle twitching, and cramps	
Tremors	
Abdominal distention	
Decreased bowel sounds	
Constipation	

Nursing Diagnosis

31. List potential or actual nursing diagnoses for a patient with fluid, electrolyte, or acid–base imbalances.

    a. _____

    b. _____

    c. _____

    d. _____

    e. _____

    f. _____

    g. _____

    h. _____

Planning

32. List three goals that are appropriate for a patient with deficient fluid volume.

    a. _____

    b. _____

    c. _____

Implementation

Briefly describe the rationale for the following interventions.

33. Enteral replacement of fluids: _____

34. Restriction of fluids: _____

_____

35. Parenteral replacement of fluids and electrolytes: _____
_____
_____

36. Total parenteral nutrition: _____
_____

37. Intravenous (IV) therapy: _____
_____

38. Vascular access devices: _____
_____

39. Give an example of the following types of electrolyte solutions.

    a. Isotonic: _____

    b. Hypotonic: _____

    c. Hypertonic: _____

40. A venipuncture is: _____
_____

41. Electronic infusion pumps (EIDs) are necessary for: _____
_____

42. Line maintenance involves:

    a. _____

    b. _____

    c. _____

    d. _____

43. Complete the table below describing complications of IV therapy.

Complication	Assessment Finding	Nursing Action
Infiltration		
Infection		
Phlebitis		
Circulatory overload		
Bleeding		

44. The objectives for blood transfusions are:

    a. _____

    b. _____

    c. _____

45. The ABO system includes: _____

    _____

46. The universal blood donor is: _____

    _____

47. The universal blood recipient is: _____

    _____

48. A transfusion reaction is: _____

    _____

49. Define *autotransfusion.* _____

    _____

50. Briefly describe the following acute transfusion reactions and their causes.

Reaction	Cause	Clinical Manifestations
Acute intravascular hemolytic		
Febrile, nonhemolytic		
Mild allergic		
Anaphylactic		
Circulatory overload		
Sepsis		

51. List the steps the nurse should follow if a transfusion reaction is suspected.

    a. _____

    b. _____

    c. _____

d. _____

e. _____

f. _____

g. _____

h. _____

REVIEW QUESTIONS

Select the appropriate answer and cite the rationale for choosing that particular answer.

52. The body fluids constituting the interstitial fluid and blood plasma are:
    1. Hypotonic
    2. Hypertonic
    3. Intracellular
    4. Extracellular

Answer: _____ Rationale: _____

_____

_____

53. Mrs. Green's arterial blood gas results are as follows: pH, 7.32; $PaCO_2$, 52 mm Hg; PaO_2, 78 mm Hg; HCO_3^-, 24 mEq/L. Mrs. Green has:
    1. Metabolic acidosis
    2. Metabolic alkalosis
    3. Respiratory acidosis
    4. Respiratory alkalosis

Answer: _____ Rationale: _____

_____

_____

54. Mr. Frank is an 82-year-old patient who has had a 3-day history of vomiting and diarrhea. Which symptom would you expect to find on a physical examination?
    1. Tachycardia
    2. Hypertension
    3. Neck vein distention
    4. Crackles in the lungs

Answer: _____ Rationale: _____

_____

_____

55. Which of the following is most likely to result in respiratory alkalosis?
    1. Steroid use
    2. Fad dieting
    3. Hyperventilation
    4. Chronic alcoholism

Answer: _____ Rationale: _____

_____

_____

CRITICAL THINKING MODEL FOR NURSING CARE PLAN FOR DEFICIENT FLUID VOLUME

56. Imagine that you are the nurse in the care plan on p. 953 of your text. Complete the *Evaluation phase* of the critical thinking model by writing your answers in the appropriate boxes of the model shown. Think about the following.
    - What knowledge did you apply in evaluating Mrs. Beck's care?
    - In what way might your previous experience influence your evaluation of Mrs. Beck?
    - During evaluation, what intellectual and professional standards were applied to Mrs. Beck's care?
    - In what way do critical thinking attitudes play a role in how you approach the evaluation of Mrs. Beck?
    - How might you evaluate Mrs. Beck's care?

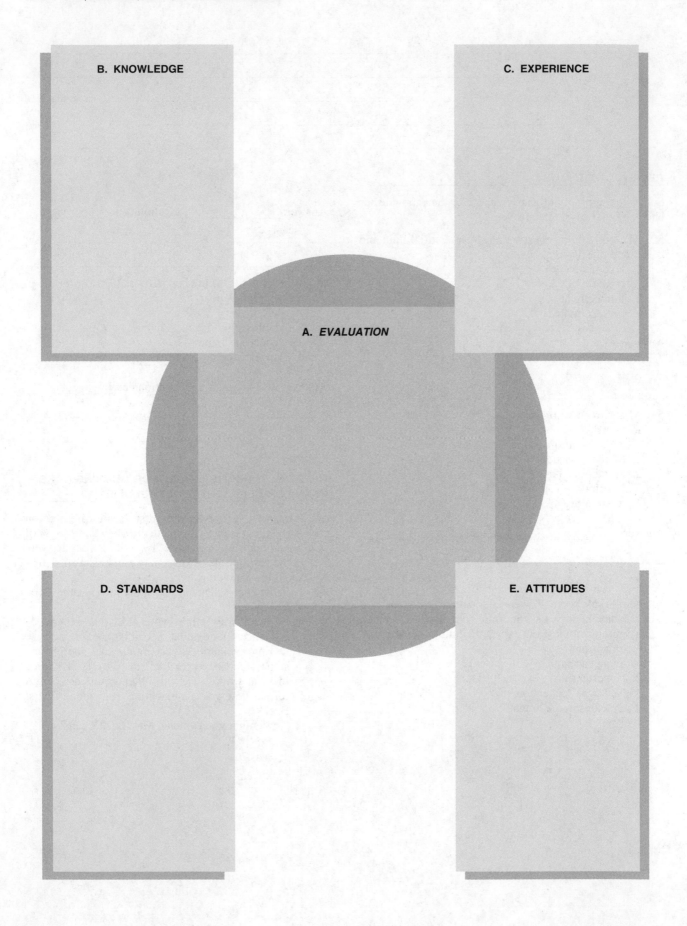

43 Sleep

PRELIMINARY READING

Chapter 43, pp. 992-1013

COMPREHENSIVE UNDERSTANDING

Scientific Knowledge Base

Match the following terms related to sleep.

1. _____Sleep
2. _____Circadian rhythm
3. _____Biological clock
4. _____NREM
5. _____REM
6. _____Dreams
7. _____Nocturia
8. _____Hypersomnolence
9. _____Polysomnogram
10. _____Insomnia
11. _____Sleep hygiene
12. _____Sleep apnea
13. _____Excessive daytime sleepiness (EDS)
14. _____Narcolepsy
15. _____Cataplexy
16. _____Sleep deprivation
17. _____Parasomnias

a. Urination during the night, which disrupts the sleep cycle
b. Involves the use of electroencephalogram (EEG), electromyogram (EMG), and electrooculogram (EOG) to monitor stages of sleep
c. Results in impaired waking function, poor work performance, accidents, and emotional problems
d. Most common sleep complaint, signaling an underlying physical or psychological disorder
e. More common in children, an example is sudden infant death syndrome (SIDS)
f. Cyclical process that alternates with longer periods of wakefulness
g. Rapid eye movement (REM) phase at the end of each sleep cycle
h. Synchronizes sleep cycles
i. Influences the pattern of major biological and behavioral functions
j. Sleep that progresses through four stages (light to deep)
k. More vivid and elaborate during REM sleep and are functionally important to learning
l. Characterized by the lack of airflow through the nose and mouth for 10 seconds or longer during sleep
m. Practices that the patient associates with sleep
n. Inadequacies in either the quantity or quality of nighttime sleep
o. Problem patients experience as a result of dyssomnia
p. Sudden muscle weakness during intense emotions at any time during the day
q. Dysfunction of mechanisms that regulate the sleep and wake states (excessive daytime sleepiness)

Nursing Knowledge Base

18. Complete the following table listing the normal sleep patterns of the following developmental stages.

Developmental Stage	Sleep Patterns
Neonates	
Infants	
Toddlers	
Preschoolers	
School-age children	
Adolescents	
Young adults	
Middle adults	
Older adults	

Describe how each of the following affects sleep and give an example of each.

19. Drugs and illicit substances: _____

_____

_____

20. Lifestyle: _____

_____

_____

21. Usual sleep patterns: _____

_____

_____

22. Emotional stress: _____

_____

_____

23. Environment: _____

_____

_____

24. Exercise and fatigue: _____

_____

_____

25. Food and caloric intake: _____

_____

_____

Nursing Process

Assessment

26. Identify sources for sleep assessment.

_____

_____

27. List the components of a sleep history.

a. _____

b. _____

c. _____

d. _____

e. _____

f. _____

g. _____

h. _____

Nursing Diagnosis

28. List the common nursing diagnoses related to sleep problems.

a. _____

b. _____

c. _____

d. _____

e. _____

f. _____

g. _____

h. _____

i. _____

Planning

29. List four goals appropriate for a patient needing rest or sleep.

a. _____

b. _____

c. _____

d. _____

Implementation

Many factors affect the ability to gain adequate rest and sleep. Briefly give examples of each of the following in relation to health promotion.

30. Environmental controls: _____

_____

_____

31. Promoting bedtime routines: _____

_____

_____

32. Promoting safety: _____

_____

_____

33. Promoting comfort: _____

_____

_____

34. Establishing periods of rest and sleep: _____

_____

_____

35. Stress reduction: _____

_____

_____

36. Bedtime snacks: _____

_____

_____

37. Pharmacologic approaches: _____

_____

_____

Acute Care

For each of the following situations, give two examples of nursing measures that will promote sleep.

38. Environmental controls:

a. _____

b. _____

39. Promoting comfort:

    a. _____

    b. _____

40. Establishing periods of rest and sleep:

    a. _____

    b. _____

41. Promoting safety:

    a. _____

    b. _____

42. Stress reduction:

    a. _____

    b. _____

Evaluation

43. With regard to sleep disturbances, the patient is the source for outcomes evaluation. List three outcomes for a patient with a sleep disturbance.

    a. _____

    b. _____

    c. _____

REVIEW QUESTIONS

Select the appropriate answer and cite the rationale for choosing that particular answer.

44. The 24-hour day–night cycle is known as:
    1. Ultradian rhythm
    2. Circadian rhythm
    3. Infradium rhythm
    4. Non-REM rhythm

    Answer: _____   Rationale: _____

    _____

    _____

45. Which of the following substances will promote normal sleep patterns?
    1. Alcohol
    2. Narcotics
    3. L-Tryptophan
    4. Beta-blockers

    Answer: _____   Rationale: _____

    _____

    _____

46. All of the following are symptoms of sleep deprivation except:
    1. Irritability
    2. Hyperactivity
    3. Decreased motivation
    4. Rise in body temperature

    Answer: _____   Rationale: _____

    _____

    _____

47. Mrs. Peterson complains of difficulty falling asleep, awakening earlier than desired, and not feeling rested. She attributes these problems to leg pain that is secondary to her arthritis. What would be the appropriate nursing diagnosis for her?
    1. Fatigue related to leg pain
    2. Insomnia related to arthritis
    3. Deficient knowledge related to sleep hygiene measures
    4. Insomnia related to chronic leg pain

    Answer: _____   Rationale: _____

    _____

    _____

48. A nursing care plan for a patient with sleep problems has been implemented. All of the following would be expected outcomes except:
    1. Patient reports satisfaction with amount of sleep.
    2. Patient falls asleep within 1 hour of going to bed.
    3. Patient reports no episodes of awakening during the night.
    4. Patient rates sleep as an 8 or above on the visual analog scale.

    Answer: _____   Rationale: _____

    _____

    _____

CRITICAL THINKING MODEL FOR NURSING CARE PLAN FOR INSOMNIA

49. Imagine that you are the nurse in the care plan on p. 1004 of your text. Complete the *Evaluation phase* of the critical thinking model by writing your answers in the appropriate boxes of the model shown. Think about the following.
    • What knowledge did you apply in evaluating Julie's care?
    • In what way might your previous experience influence your evaluation of Julie's care?
    • During evaluation, what intellectual and professional standards were applied to Julie's care?
    • In what way do critical thinking attitudes play a role in how you approach the evaluation of Julie's plan?
    • How might you evaluate Julie's plan of care?

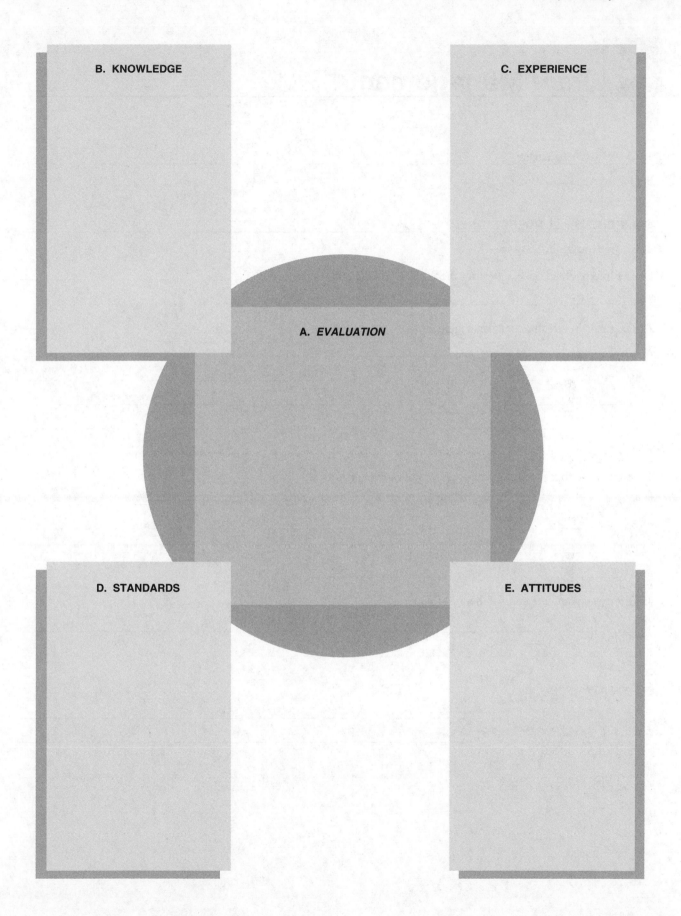

B. KNOWLEDGE

C. EXPERIENCE

A. *EVALUATION*

D. STANDARDS

E. ATTITUDES

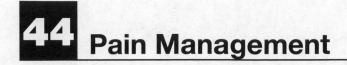# Pain Management

PRELIMINARY READING

Chapter 44, pp. 1014-1052

COMPREHENSIVE UNDERSTANDING

Scientific Knowledge Base

1. The International Association for the Study of Pain (IASP) defines pain as: _____

   _____

2. The goals of effective pain management are:

   a. _____

   b. _____

   c. _____

   d. _____

   e. _____

3. Identify the four physiological processes of normal pain. Briefly explain.

   a. _____

   b. _____

   c. _____

   d. _____

4. Briefly explain gate control theory of pain.

   _____

   _____

5. Define pain threshold.

   _____

   _____

Match the following physiological reactions to pain to the cause or effect.

Response

6. _____ Dilation of bronchial tubes and increased heart rate
7. _____ Increased heart rate
8. _____ Peripheral vasoconstriction
9. _____ Increased blood glucose level
10. _____ Increased cortisol level
11. _____ Diaphoresis
12. _____ Increased muscle tension
13. _____ Dilation of pupils
14. _____ Decreased gastrointestinal motility
15. _____ Pallor
16. _____ Nausea and vomiting
17. _____ Decreased heart rate and blood pressure
18. _____ Rapid, irregular breathing

Cause or Effect

a. Provides additional energy
b. Affords better vision
c. Heightened memory functions, a burst of increased immunity
d. Causes blood supply to shift away from periphery
e. Provides increased oxygen intake
f. Elevated blood pressure with shift of blood supply from periphery and viscera to skeletal muscles and brain
g. Vagus nerve sends impulses to chemoreceptor trigger zone in the brain
h. Results from vagal stimulation
i. Prepares muscles for action
j. Controls body temperature during stress
k. Frees energy for more immediate activity
l. Provides increased oxygen transport
m. Causes body defenses to fail under prolonged stress of pain

19. Explain the difference between the following.

    a. Acute pain: _____

    _____

    _____

    b. Chronic pain: _____

    _____

    _____

20. Define the following terms related to pain.

    a. Chronic episodic pain: _____

    _____

    _____

    b. Idiopathic pain: _____

    _____

    _____

Nursing Knowledge Base

21. List some common biases and misconceptions about pain.

    a. _____

    _____

    _____

    b. _____

    _____

    _____

c. _____

_____

_____

d. _____

_____

e. _____

_____

_____

f. _____

_____

g. _____

_____

_____

h. _____

_____

_____

i. _____

_____

_____

22. Identify the physiological factors that influence pain.

    a. _____

    b. _____

    c. _____

    d. _____

23. Identify the social factors that can influence pain.

    a. _____

    b. _____

    c. _____

    d. _____

24. Identify the psychological factors that can influence pain.

    a. _____

    _____

    _____

    b. _____

    _____

    _____

25. Explain how a person's cultural background factors affect coping with pain.

    _____

    _____

    _____

    _____

    _____

    _____

Nursing Process

Assessment

26. Identify the ABCDE clinical approach to pain assessment and management.

    a. _____

    b. _____

    c. _____

    d. _____

    e. _____

27. Identify the common characteristics of pain that the nurse would assess.

    a. _____

    b. _____

c. _____

d. _____

e. _____

f. _____

g. _____

Nursing Diagnosis

28. List potential or actual nursing diagnoses related to a patient in pain.

    a. _____

    b. _____

    c. _____

    d. _____

    e. _____

    f. _____

    g. _____

    h. _____

Planning

29. List the patient outcomes appropriate for the patient experiencing pain.

    a. _____

    b. _____

    c. _____

    d. _____

Implementation

30. Nonpharmacologic interventions include the following. Briefly explain each.

    a. Cognitive behavioral approaches: _____

    _____

    _____

    b. Physical approaches: _____

    _____

    _____

31. List the guidelines recommended for nonpharmacologic therapies in the older adult.

    a. _____

    _____

    _____

b. _____

_____

c. _____

_____

Nonpharmacologic interventions such as the following lessen pain. Briefly explain each one.

32. Relaxation: _____

_____

_____

33. Distraction: _____

_____

_____

34. Music: _____

_____

_____

35. Cutaneous stimulation: _____

_____

_____

36. Herbals: _____

_____

_____

37. Reducing pain perception and reception: _____

_____

_____

38. Identify the three types of analgesics used for pain relief.

a. _____

_____

_____

b. _____

_____

_____

c. _____

39. Define adjuvants or coanalgesics. _____

_____

_____

40. Give at least two examples of the following common opioid effects on the following systems.

a. Central nervous system: _____

_____

_____

b. Ocular: _____

_____

c. Respiratory: _____

_____

_____

d. Cardiac: _____

_____

_____

e. Gastrointestinal: _____

_____

_____

f. Genitourinary: _____

_____

_____

g. Endocrine: _____

_____

_____

h. Skin: _____

_____

_____

i. Immunological: _____

_____

_____

41. List the nursing principles for administering analgesics.

    a. _____

    _____

    _____

    b. _____

    _____

    _____

    _____

    c. _____

    _____

    d. _____

    _____

    _____

42. The main benefit of multimodal analgesia is: _____

    _____

    _____

    _____

43. What is patient-controlled analgesia (PCA)? What is the goal of PCA?

    _____

    _____

    _____

    _____

    _____

    _____

44. Explain the purpose of perineural local anesthetic infusion.

    _____

    _____

    _____

    _____

    _____

Explain the differences between the following.

45. Local anesthesia:

    _____

    _____

    _____

    _____

    _____

    _____

46. Regional anesthesia:

    _____

    _____

    _____

    _____

    _____

    _____

    _____

47. Epidural analgesia: _____

    _____

    _____

48. List the goals for the care of a patient with epidural infusions. Describe one action for each goal.

    a. _____

    _____

    _____

    b. _____

    _____

    _____

    c. _____

    _____

    _____

    d. _____

    _____

    e. _____

    _____

    _____

    f. _____

    _____

    _____

49. Identify the following types of breakthrough pain.

    a. Incident pain: _____

    _____

    _____

    b. End-of-dose failure pain: _____

    _____

    _____

    c. Spontaneous pain: _____

    _____

    _____

50. Give some examples of barriers to effective pain management.

    a. Patient: _____

    _____

    _____

    b. Health care provider: _____

    _____

    _____

    c. Health care system: _____

    _____

    _____

51. Define the following terms related to the use of opioids in pain treatment.

    a. Physical dependence: _____

    _____

    _____

    b. Drug tolerance: _____

    _____

    _____

    c. Addiction: _____

    _____

    _____

52. Define *placebo*.

    _____

    _____

    _____

    _____

    _____

Explain the purpose of the following.

53. Pain clinics: _____

    _____

    _____

    _____

    _____

54. Palliative care: _____

    _____

    _____

    _____

55. Hospice: _____

    _____

    _____

    _____

    _____

    _____

Evaluation

56. Identify some principles to evaluate related to pain management.

    _____

    _____

    _____

    _____

    _____

    _____

REVIEW QUESTIONS

Select the appropriate answer and cite the rationale for choosing that particular answer.

57. Pain is a protective mechanism warning of tissue injury and is largely a(n):
    1. Objective experience
    2. Subjective experience
    3. Acute symptom of short duration
    4. Symptom of a severe illness or disease

    Answer: _____   Rationale: _____

    _____

    _____

58. A substance that can cause analgesia when it attaches to opiate receptors in the brain is:
    1. Endorphin
    2. Bradykinin
    3. Substance P
    4. Prostaglandin

    Answer: _____   Rationale: _____

    _____

    _____

59. To adequately assess the quality of a patient's pain, which question would be appropriate?
    1. "Is it a sharp pain or a dull pain?"
    2. "Tell me what your pain feels like."
    3. "Is your pain a crushing sensation?"
    4. "How long have you had this pain?"

    Answer: _____   Rationale: _____

    _____

    _____

60. The use of patient distraction in pain control is based on the principle that:
    1. Small C fibers transmit impulses via the spinothalamic tract.
    2. The reticular formation can send inhibitory signals to gating mechanisms.
    3. Large A fibers compete with pain impulses to close gates to painful stimuli.
    4. Transmission of pain impulses from the spinal cord to the cerebral cortex can be inhibited.

    Answer: _____   Rationale: _____

    _____

    _____

CRITICAL THINKING MODEL FOR NURSING CARE PLAN FOR ACUTE PAIN

61. Imagine that you are the student nurse in the care plan on pp. 1030-1031 of your text. Complete the *Assessment phase* of the critical thinking model by writing your answers in the appropriate boxes of the model shown. Think about the following.
    - What knowledge base was applied to Mrs. Mays?
    - In what way might previous experience assist you in this case?
    - What intellectual or professional standards were applied to the care of Mrs. Mays?
    - What critical thinking attitudes did you use in assessing Mrs. Mays?
    - As you review your assessment, what key areas did you cover?

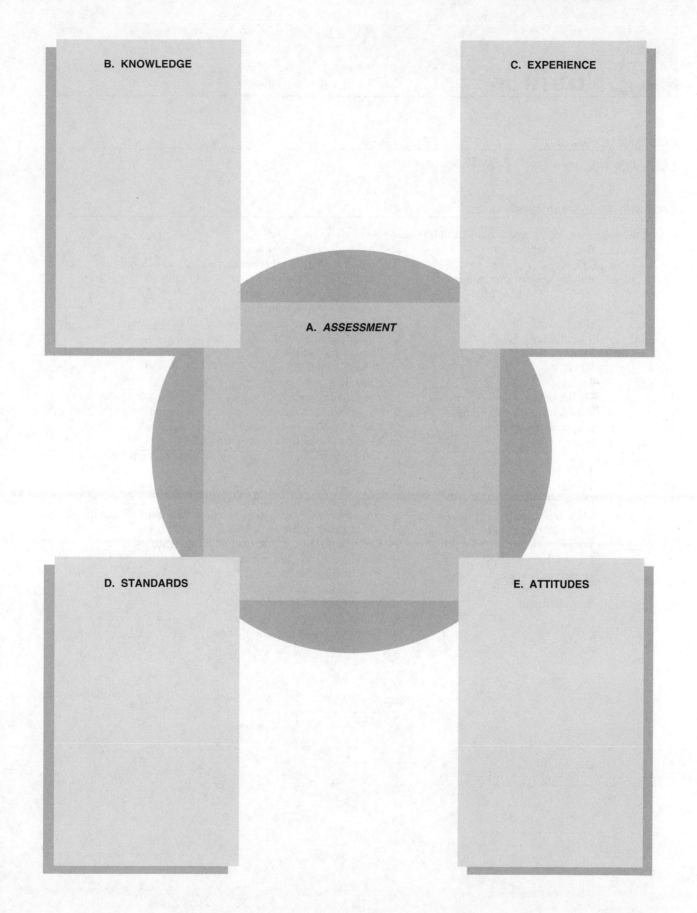

B. KNOWLEDGE

C. EXPERIENCE

A. *ASSESSMENT*

D. STANDARDS

E. ATTITUDES

45 Nutrition

PRELIMINARY READING

Chapter 45, 1053-1100

COMPREHENSIVE UNDERSTANDING

Match the following biochemical units of nutrition.

1. _____ Basal metabolic rate (BMR)
2. _____ Resting energy expenditure (REE)
3. _____ kcal
4. _____ Nutrient density
5. _____ Saccharides
6. _____ Simple carbohydrates
7. _____ Fiber
8. _____ Proteins
9. _____ Amino acid
10. _____ Indispensable amino acids
11. _____ Dispensable amino acids
12. _____ Nitrogen balance
13. _____ Lipids
14. _____ Triglycerides
15. _____ Saturated fatty acids
16. _____ Unsaturated fatty acids
17. _____ Monounsaturated fatty acids
18. _____ Polyunsaturated fatty acids
19. _____ Water
20. _____ Fat-soluble vitamins
21. _____ Hypervitaminosis
22. _____ Water-soluble vitamins
23. _____ Trace elements

a. Vitamin C and B complex
b. Inorganic elements that act as catalysts in biochemical reactions
c. Energy needed to maintain life-sustaining activities for a specific period of time at rest
d. Simplest form of a protein
e. Made up of three fatty acids attached to a glycerol
f. The intake and output of nitrogen are equal
g. Fatty acids that have two or more double carbon bonds
h. Resting metabolic rate over a 24-hour period
i. Kilocalorie
j. Are found primarily in sugars
k. Polysaccharide that does not contribute calories to the diet
l. Makes up 60% to 70% of total body weight
m. Most calorie-dense nutrient; provides 9 kcal/g
n. The proportion of essential nutrients to the number of kilocalories
o. Carbohydrate units
p. Alanine, asparagine, and glutamic acid
q. Unequal number of hydrogen atoms are attached and the carbon atoms attach to each other with a double bond
r. Each carbon has two attached hydrogen atoms
s. Histidine, lysine, and phenylalanine
t. Results from megadoses of supplemental vitamins, fortified food, and large intake of fish oils
u. Vitamins A, D, E, and K
v. A source of energy (4 kcal/g)
w. Fatty acids with one double bond

Match the following key terms related to the digestive system.

24. _____ Enzymes
25. _____ Peristalsis
26. _____ Chyme
27. _____ Active transport
28. _____ Passive diffusion
29. _____ Osmosis
30. _____ Pinocytosis
31. _____ Metabolism
32. _____ Anabolism
33. _____ Catabolism
34. _____ Glycogenolysis
35. _____ Glycogenesis
36. _____ Gluconeogenesis

a. Anabolism of glucose into glycogen for storage
b. Acidic, liquefied mass
c. Catabolism of glycogen into glucose, carbon dioxide, and water
d. Building of more complex biochemical substances by synthesis of nutrients
e. Breakdown of biochemical substances into simpler substances, occurring during a negative nitrogen balance
f. Protein-like substances that act as catalysts to speed up chemical reactions
g. Particles move from an area of greater concentration to an area of lesser concentration
h. Wave-like muscular contractions
i. Catabolism of amino acids and glycerol into glucose for energy
j. Engulfing of large molecules of nutrients by the absorbing cell
k. Movement of water through a membrane that separates solutions of different concentrations, do not need a special "carrier"
l. Force by which particles move outward from an area of greater concentration to lesser concentration
m. All biochemical reactions within the cells of the body

37. Explain the four components of the dietary reference intake (DRI).

   a. Estimated average requirement (EAR): _____

   _____

   _____

   b. Recommended dietary allowance (RDA): _____

   _____

   _____

   c. Adequate intake (AI): _____

   _____

   _____

   d. Tolerable upper intake level (UL): _____

   _____

   _____

Nursing Knowledge Base

38. List the factors to estimate a patient's nutritional requirements.

   a. _____

   b. _____

   c. _____

   d. _____

   e. _____

39. List the benefits of breastfeeding an infant.

   a. _____

   b. _____

   c. _____

   d. _____

   e. _____

   f. _____

   g. _____

Explain why the following should not be used in infant formula.

40. Cow's milk: _____

   _____

   _____

41. Honey and corn syrup: _____

   _____

42. What governs an infant's readiness to begin solid foods?

    a. _____

    b. _____

    c. _____

43. Identify the factors that contribute to childhood obesity.

    a. _____

    b. _____

    c. _____

    d. _____

    e. _____

    f. _____

44. Identify the factors that influence the adolescent's diet.

    a. _____

    b. _____

    c. _____

    d. _____

    e. _____

45. Identify the diagnostic criteria for the following eating disorders.

    a. Anorexia nervosa: _____

    _____

    b. Bulimia nervosa: _____

    _____

    _____

46. Explain the importance of folic acid intake in pregnant women.

    _____

    _____

47. List the factors that influence the nutritional status of older adults.

    a. _____

    b. _____

    c. _____

    d. _____

    e. _____

Explain the following types of vegetarian diets.

48. Ovolactovegetarian: _____

    _____

    _____

49. Lactovegetarian: _____

    _____

50. Vegan: _____

    _____

51. Fruitarian: _____

    _____

    _____

Nursing Process
Assessment

52. List the five components of a nutritional assessment and briefly explain them.

    a. _____

    b. _____

    c. _____

    d. _____

    e. _____

53. Dysphagia is: _____

    _____

    _____

54. For each assessment area, list at least two signs of poor nutrition.

    a. General appearance: _____

    _____

    b. Weight: _____

    _____

    c. Posture: _____

    _____

    d. Muscles: _____

    _____

    _____

e. Nervous system: _____

_____

_____

f. Gastrointestinal function: _____

_____

_____

g. Cardiovascular function: _____

_____

_____

h. General vitality: _____

_____

_____

i. Hair: _____

_____

_____

j. Skin: _____

_____

_____

k. Face and neck: _____

_____

_____

l. Lips: _____

_____

_____

m. Mouth, oral membranes: _____

_____

_____

n. Gums: _____

_____

_____

o. Tongue: _____

_____

_____

p. Teeth: _____

_____

_____

q. Eyes: _____

_____

_____

r. Neck: _____

_____

_____

s. Nails: _____

_____

_____

t. Legs, feet: _____

_____

_____

u. Skeleton: _____

_____

_____

Nursing Diagnosis

55. List the potential or actual nursing diagnoses for altered nutritional status.

a. _____

b. _____

c. _____

d. _____

e. _____

f. _____

g. _____

Planning

56. List the goals for a patient with nutritional problems.

a. _____

b. _____

c. _____

d. _____

e. _____

Implementation

57. Identify the food source for the following foodborne diseases.

a. Botulism: _____

_____

_____

b. *Escherichia coli*: _____

_____

_____

c. Listeriosis: _____

_____

_____

d. Perfringens enteritis: _____

_____

_____

e. Salmonellosis: _____

_____

_____

f. Shigellosis: _____

_____

_____

g. *Staphylococcus*: _____

_____

_____

58. Identify three ways to promote an appetite.

a. _____

b. _____

c. _____

59. Identify the four levels of the dysphagia diet.

a. _____

b. _____

c. _____

d. _____

60. Identify the four levels of a liquid diet.

a. _____

b. _____

c. _____

d. _____

61. Identify the following types of enteral formulas.

a. Polymeric: _____

_____

_____

b. Modular: _____

_____

_____

c. Elemental: _____

_____

_____

d. Specialty: _____

_____

_____

62. Identify the complications of enteral tube feedings and possible cause.

a. _____

b. _____

c. _____

d. _____

e. _____

f. _____

g. _____

h. _____

i. _____

j. _____

63. List the three factors on which safe administration of PN depends.

a. _____

b. _____

c. _____

64. Intravenous fat emulsions provide: _____

_____

65. Explain the goal of transition from PN to enteral nutrition (EN) or oral feeding. _____

_____

_____

66. Medical nutrition therapy is: _____

_____

_____

67. *Helicobacter pylori* is: _____

_____

Identify the nutritional interventions for the following common disease states.

68. Inflammatory bowel disease: _____

_____

_____

69. Malabsorption syndromes: _____

_____

_____

70. Diverticulitis: _____

_____

_____

71. Diabetes mellitus (DM): _____

_____

_____

72. Cardiovascular disease: _____

_____

_____

73. Cancer: _____

_____

_____

74. Human immunodeficiency virus (HIV): _____

_____

_____

Evaluation

75. Identify the ongoing evaluative measures.

_____

_____

REVIEW QUESTIONS

Select the appropriate answer and cite the rationale for choosing that particular answer.

76. Which nutrient is the body's most preferred energy source?
    1. Fat
    2. Protein
    3. Vitamin
    4. Carbohydrate

Answer: _____ Rationale: _____

_____

77. Positive nitrogen balance would occur in which condition?
    1. Infection
    2. Starvation
    3. Pregnancy
    4. Burn injury

Answer: _____ Rationale: _____

_____

_____

78. Mrs. Nelson is talking with the nurse about the dietary needs of her 23-month-old daughter, Laura. Which of the following responses by the nurse would be appropriate?
    1. "Use skim milk to cut down on the fat in Laura's diet."
    2. "Laura should be drinking at least 1 quart of milk per day."
    3. "Laura needs less protein in her diet now because she isn't growing as fast."
    4. "Laura needs fewer calories in relation to her body weight now than she did as an infant."

Answer: _____ Rationale: _____

_____

_____

79. All of the following patients are at risk for alteration in nutrition except:
    1. Patient L, whose weight is 10% above his ideal body weight
    2. Patient J, who is 86 years old, lives alone, and has poorly fitting dentures
    3. Patient M, a 17-year-old girl who weighs 90 pounds and frequently complains about her baby fat
    4. Patient K, who has been allowed nothing by mouth (NPO) for 7 days after bowel surgery and is receiving 3000 mL of 10% dextrose per day

Answer: _____ Rationale: _____

_____

_____

80. Which of the following is the most accurate method of bedside confirmation of placement of a small-bore nasogastric tube?
    1. Assess the patient's ability to speak.
    2. Test the pH of withdrawn gastric contents.
    3. Auscultate the epigastrium for gurgling or bubbling.
    4. Assess the length of the tube that is outside the patient's nose.

    Answer: _____ Rationale: _____

    _____

    _____

81. A patient who has been hospitalized after experiencing a heart attack will most likely receive a diet consisting of:
    1. Low fat, low sodium, and low carbohydrates
    2. Low fat, low sodium, and high carbohydrates
    3. Low fat, high protein, and high carbohydrates
    4. Liquids for several days, progressing to a soft and then a regular diet

    Answer: _____ Rationale: _____

    _____

    _____

CRITICAL THINKING MODEL FOR NURSING CARE PLAN FOR IMBALANCED NUTRITION: LESS THAN BODY REQUIREMENTS

82. Imagine that you are the nurse practitioner in the care plan on pp. 1071-1072 of your text. Complete the *Assessment phase* of the critical thinking model by writing your answers in the appropriate boxes of the model shown. Think about the following.
    - In developing Mrs. Cooper's plan of care, what knowledge did Maria apply?
    - In what ways might the nurse practitioner's previous experience assist in developing Mrs. Cooper's plan of care?
    - When developing a plan of care for Mrs. Cooper, what intellectual and professional standards were applied?
    - What critical thinking attitudes might have been applied in developing Mrs. Cooper's plan of care?
    - How will the nurse practitioner accomplish these goals?

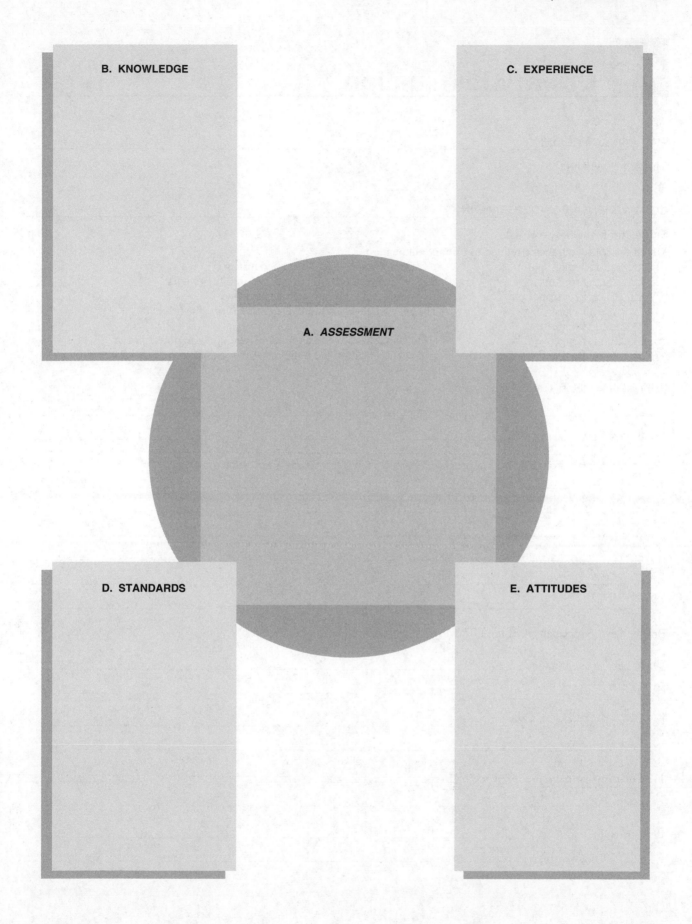

B. KNOWLEDGE

C. EXPERIENCE

A. *ASSESSMENT*

D. STANDARDS

E. ATTITUDES

46 Urinary Elimination

PRELIMINARY READING

Chapter 46, 1101-1148

COMPREHENSIVE UNDERSTANDING

Scientific Knowledge Base

Match the following terms related to urinary elimination.

1. _____ Nephron
2. _____ Proteinuria
3. _____ Erythropoietin
4. _____ Renin
5. _____ Micturition
6. _____ Urinary reflux
7. _____ Bladder

a. Two portions—trigone and a detrusor
b. Reflux of urine from the bladder into the ureters
c. Presence of large proteins in the urine
d. Functional unit of the kidneys that forms the urine
e. Back flow of urine
f. Enzyme that coverts angiotensinogen into angiotensin I
g. Functions within the bone marrow to stimulate red blood cell production

8. List nine factors that influence urination.

a. _____

b. _____

c. _____

d. _____

e. _____

f. _____

g. _____

h. _____

i. _____

Briefly describe the causes of the following types of incontinence.

9. Transient incontinence: _____

_____

10. Functional incontinence: _____

_____

11. Overflow urinary incontinence: _____

_____

12. Stress incontinence: _____

_____

13. Urgency incontinence: _____

_____

14. Reflex incontinence: _____

_____

Explain the following alterations in urinary elimination.

15. Urinary retention: _____

_____

16. Urinary tract infection (UTI): _____

_____

17. Symptoms of a lower urinary tract infection can include:
   a. _____
   b. _____
   c. _____
   d. _____
   e. _____
   f. _____
   g. _____

Briefly describe the following continent urinary diversions.

18. Urinary reservoir: _____

_____

19. Orthopedic neobladder: _____

_____

20. Ureterostomy: _____

_____

21. Nephrostomy: _____

_____

Nursing Process
Assessment
22. List the major factors to be explored during a nursing history in regard to urinary elimination.
   a. _____
   b. _____
   c. _____

Match the following common types of urinary alterations.

23. _____ Urgency
24. _____ Dysuria
25. _____ Frequency
26. _____ Hesitancy
27. _____ Polyuria
28. _____ Oliguria
29. _____ Nocturia
30. _____ Dribbling
31. _____ Incontinence
32. _____ Hematuria
33. _____ Retention
34. _____ Residual urine

a. Accumulation of urine in the bladder with the inability to empty fully
b. May be caused by stress incontinence
c. Greater than 100 mL of urine remaining after voiding
d. Caused by loss of pelvic muscle tone, fecal impaction, overactive bladder
e. Painful or difficult urination
f. Blood in the urine
g. Due to increased fluid intake, pregnancy, and diuretics
h. Large amounts of urine voided
i. Caused by prostate enlargement, anxiety, or urethral edema
j. Feeling of the need to void immediately
k. Diminished urinary output relative to intake
l. Nighttime voiding often caused by coffee or alcohol

Describe the following characteristics of normal urine.

35. Color: _____
_____

36. Clarity: _____
_____

37. Odor: _____
_____

38. Describe the following types of urine specimens collected for testing.

a. Random: _____
_____

b. Clean-voided or midstream: _____
_____

c. Sterile: _____
_____

d. Timed urine: _____
_____

Common urine tests include the following. Briefly explain each.

39. Urinalysis: _____
_____

40. Specific gravity: _____
_____

41. Urine culture: _____
_____

42. Briefly explain the purpose of each of the following noninvasive/invasive diagnostic examinations.

    a. Abdominal roentgenogram: _____

    b. Intravenous pyelogram (IVP): _____

    c. Cystoscopy: _____

    d. Computerized axial tomography (CT): _____

    e. Ultrasonography: _____

Nursing Diagnosis

43. List the potential or actual nursing diagnoses related to urinary elimination.

    a. _____

    b. _____

    c. _____

    d. _____

    e. _____

    f. _____

    g. _____

Planning

44. List the goals appropriate for a patient with a urinary elimination problem.

    a. _____

    b. _____

    c. _____

Implementation

45. List measures that promote normal micturition:

    a. _____

    b. _____

    c. _____

    d. _____

46. State the indications for the following types of catheterizations.

    a. Intermittent: _____

    b. Short- or long-term indwelling: _____

Explain the following nursing measures taken to prevent infection and maintain an unobstructed flow of urine in catheterized patients.

47. Perineal hygiene: _____

_____

48. Catheter care: _____

_____

49. Fluid intake: _____

_____

50. Irrigations and installations: _____

_____

Briefly explain the two alternatives to urinary catheterization.

51. Suprapubic catheter: _____

_____

52. External catheter: _____

_____

Explain the purpose of the following.

53. Pelvic floor muscle training (PFMT): _____

_____

_____

54. Bladder retraining: _____

_____

55. Scheduled toileting: _____

_____

Evaluation

56. Identify how the nurse would evaluate the effectiveness of the interventions used.

_____

_____

_____

REVIEW QUESTIONS

Select the appropriate answer and cite the rationale for choosing that particular answer.

57. Mrs. Rantz complains of leaking urine when she coughs and laughs. This is known as:
    1. Urge incontinence
    2. Stress incontinence
    3. Reflex incontinence
    4. Functional incontinence

Answer: _____ Rationale: _____

_____

_____

58. Ms. Hathaway has a UTI. Which of the following symptoms would you expect her to exhibit?
    1. Dysuria
    2. Oliguria
    3. Polyuria
    4. Proteinuria

Answer: _____ Rationale: _____

_____

_____

59. The nurse is working in the radiology department with a patient who is having an intravenous pyelogram. Which of the following complaints by the patient is an abnormal response?
    1. Frequent, loose stools
    2. Thirst and feeling "worn out"
    3. Shortness of breath and audible wheezing
    4. Feeling dizzy and warm with obvious facial flushing

    Answer: _____ Rationale: _____

    _____

    _____

60. The urinalysis of Ms. Hathaway reveals a high bacteria count. Ampicillin is prescribed for her UTI. The teaching plan for the prevention of a UTI should include all of the following except:
    1. Drink at least 2000 mL of fluid daily.
    2. Always wipe the perineum from front to back.
    3. Drink plenty of orange and grapefruit juices.
    4. Explain the possible side effects of medication.

    Answer: _____ Rationale: _____

    _____

    _____

CRITICAL THINKING MODEL FOR NURSING CARE PLAN FOR STRESS URINARY INCONTINENCE

61. Imagine that you are Mrs. Kay, the nurse in the care plan on pp. 1116-1117 of your text. Complete the *Assessment phase* of the critical thinking model by writing your answers in the appropriate boxes of the model shown. Think about the following.
    - What knowledge base was applied to the care of Mrs. Grayson?
    - In what way might Mrs. Kay's previous experience assist in this case?
    - What intellectual or professional standards were applied to the care of Mrs. Grayson?
    - What critical thinking attitudes did you use in assessing Mrs. Grayson?
    - As you review the assessment, what key areas did Mrs. Kay cover?

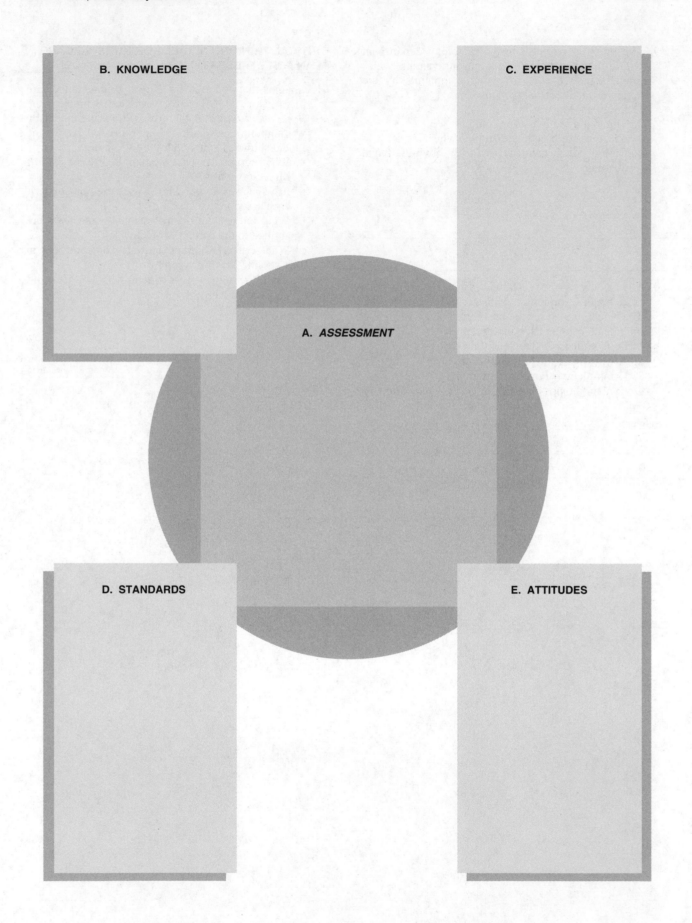

A. *ASSESSMENT*

B. KNOWLEDGE

C. EXPERIENCE

D. STANDARDS

E. ATTITUDES

47 Bowel Elimination

PRELIMINARY READING

Chapter 47, pp. 1149-1183

COMPREHENSIVE UNDERSTANDING

Scientific Knowledge Base

Summarize the functions of the following.

1. Mouth: _____

_____

2. Esophagus: _____

_____

3. Stomach: _____

_____

4. Small intestine: _____

_____

5. Large intestine: _____

_____

6. Anus: _____

_____

7. List the physiological factors essential to bowel function and defecation.

a. _____

b. _____

c. _____

d. _____

Nursing Knowledge Base

8. Identify twelve factors that can influence bowel elimination.

a. _____

b. _____

c. _____

d. _____

e. _____

f. _____

g. _____

h. _____

i. _____

j. _____

k. _____

l. _____

9. Explain how fiber affects the diet, and give some examples of good fiber sources.

_____

_____

10. Summarize how fluids can affect the character of feces.

_____

_____

11. Summarize the benefits of physical activity.

_____

_____

12. List the diseases of the gastrointestinal (GI) tract that may be associated with stress.

_____

_____

13. _____ is the normal position during defecation.

14. List conditions that may result in painful defecation.

a. _____

b. _____

c. _____

d. _____

15. Summarize the effects of anesthetic agents and peristalsis on defecation.

_____

_____

16. List four factors that place a patient at risk for constipation.

a. _____

b. _____

c. _____

d. _____

17. List the signs of constipation.

a. _____

b. _____

18. Define *fecal impaction*.

_____

_____

19. List signs and symptoms of fecal impaction.

    a. _____

    b. _____

    c. _____

    d. _____

    e. _____

20. Define *diarrhea*.

    _____

    _____

21. Name the two complications associated with diarrhea.

    a. _____

    b. _____

22. Explain *Clostridium difficile* infection: _____

    _____

23. Explain the following.

    a. Fecal incontinence: _____

    _____

    b. Flatulence: _____

    _____

24. Hemorrhoids are: _____

    _____

Define the following bowel diversions.

25. Stoma: _____

    _____

26. Ileostomy: _____

    _____

27. Colostomy: _____

    _____

Nursing Process

Assessment

28. List 14 factors that affect elimination that need to be included in a nursing history for patients with altered elimination status.

    a. _____

    b. _____

    c. _____

d. _____

e. _____

f. _____

g. _____

h. _____

i. _____

j. _____

k. _____

l. _____

m. _____

n. _____

Summarize the following steps for assessing the abdomen.

29. Inspection: _____

_____

30. Auscultation: _____

_____

31. Palpation: _____

_____

32. Percussion: _____

_____

33. Define *fecal occult blood testing (FOBT)*.

_____

_____

34. Describe the normal fecal characteristics.

a. Color: _____

b. Odor: _____

c. Consistency: _____

d. Frequency: _____

e. Amount: _____

f. Shape: _____

g. Constituents: _____

35. List the common radiologic and diagnostic tests used with a patient with altered bowel elimination.

    a. _____

    b. _____

    c. _____

    d. _____

    e. _____

    f. _____

    g. _____

    h. _____

Nursing Diagnosis

36. List the potential or actual nursing diagnoses for a patient with alteration in bowel elimination.

    a. _____

    b. _____

    c. _____

d. _____

e. _____

f. _____

g. _____

h. _____

i. _____

j. _____

Planning

37. List the overall outcomes that are appropriate for patients with elimination problems.

    a. _____

    b. _____

    c. _____

    d. _____

    e. _____

Implementation

38. List the factors to consider to promote normal defecation.

    a. _____

    b. _____

Identify the primary action of the following.

39. Cathartics and laxatives: _____

_____

40. Antidiarrheals: _____

_____

41. Enemas: _____

_____

Briefly describe the following types of enemas.

42. Cleansing enema: _____

_____

43. Tap water enema: _____

_____

44. Normal saline: _____

_____

45. Hypertonic solution: _____

_____

46. Soapsuds: _____

_____

47. Oil retention: _____

_____

48. Explain the purpose of a carminative enema.

_____

_____

_____

49. List the complications of excessive rectal manipulation.

a. _____

b. _____

c. _____

50. List the purposes of nasogastric (NG) intubation.

a. _____

b. _____

c. _____

d. _____

51. Explain how the nurse would provide comfort to a patient with an NG tube.

_____

_____

_____

52. List the measures included for a successful bowel training program.

a. _____

b. _____

c. _____

d. _____

e. _____

f. _____

g. _____

h. _____

i. _____

Evaluation

53. Identify some positive outcomes for a patient with alterations in bowel elimination.

_____

_____

REVIEW QUESTIONS

Select the appropriate answer and cite the rationale for choosing that particular answer.

54. Most nutrients and electrolytes are absorbed in the:
    1. Colon
    2. Stomach
    3. Esophagus
    4. Small intestine

    Answer: _____ Rationale: _____

    _____

    _____

55. Which of the following should be included in the teaching plan for the patient who is scheduled for an upper GI series?
    1. The patient will be allowed nothing by mouth (NPO) after midnight.
    2. General anesthetic is usually used for the procedure.
    3. Moderate abdominal pain is common after the procedure.
    4. A cleansing enema will be given the evening before the procedure.

    Answer: _____ Rationale: _____

    _____

    _____

56. Mrs. Anthony is concerned about her breastfed infant's stool, stating that it is yellow instead of brown. The nurse explains to Mrs. Anthony that:
    1. The stool is normal for an infant.
    2. A change to formula may be necessary.
    3. It will be necessary to send a stool specimen to the laboratory.
    4. Her infant is dehydrated, and she should increase his fluid intake.

    Answer: _____ Rationale: _____

    _____

    _____

57. After positioning a patient on the bedpan, the nurse should:
    1. Leave the head of the bed flat.
    2. Raise the head of the bed 30 degrees.
    3. Raise the bed to the highest working level.
    4. Raise the head of the bed to a 90-degree angle.

    Answer: _____ Rationale: _____

    _____

    _____

58. The health care provider has ordered a cleansing enema for 7-year-old Michael. The nurse realizes the maximum volume to be given would be:
    1. 100 to 150 mL
    2. 150 to 250 mL
    3. 300 to 500 mL
    4. 600 to 700 mL

    Answer: _____ Rationale: _____

    _____

    _____

CRITICAL THINKING MODEL FOR NURSING CARE PLAN FOR CONSTIPATION

59. Imagine that you are Javier, the home care nurse in the care plan on p. 1159 of your text. Complete the *Planning phase* of the critical thinking model by writing your answers in the appropriate boxes of the model shown. Think about the following.
    • In developing Mr. Johnson's plan of care, what knowledge did Javier apply?
    • In what way might Javier's previous experience assist in developing a plan of care for Mr. Johnson?
    • When developing a plan of care, what intellectual and professional standards were applied?
    • What critical thinking attitudes might have been applied in developing a plan for Mr. Johnson?
    • How will Javier accomplish the goals?

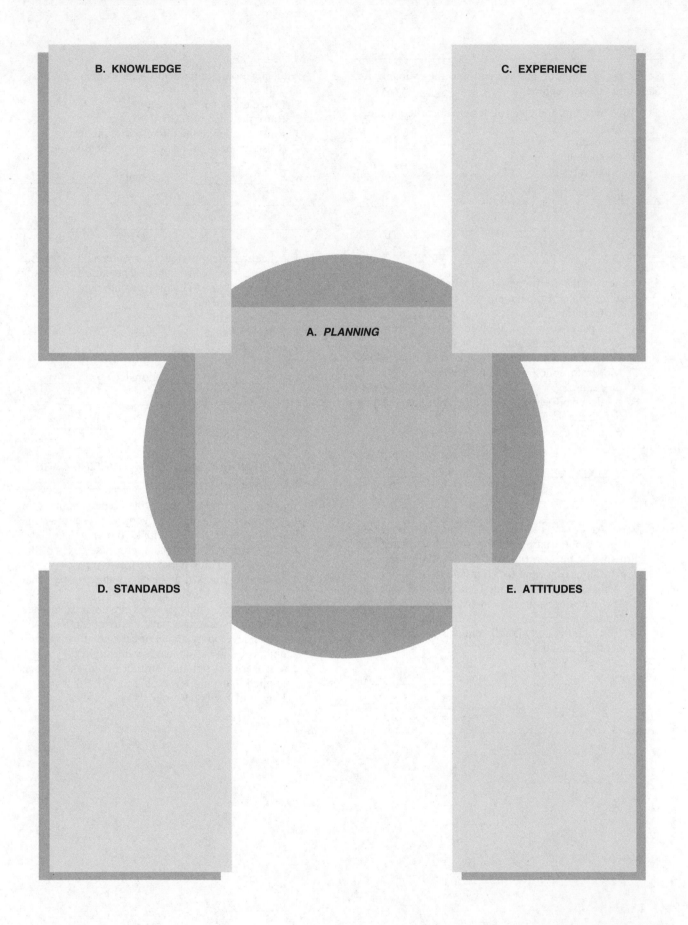

B. KNOWLEDGE

C. EXPERIENCE

A. *PLANNING*

D. STANDARDS

E. ATTITUDES

48 Skin Integrity and Wound Care

PRELIMINARY READING

Chapter 48, pp. 1184-1240

COMPREHENSIVE UNDERSTANDING

Scientific Knowledge Base

Match the following key terms related to skin integrity.

1. _____ Epidermis   a. Tough, fibrous protein
2. _____ Dermis   b. Localized injury to the skin and underlying tissue over a body prominence
3. _____ Collagen   c. Does not blanch
4. _____ Pressure ulcer   d. Normal red tones of light-skinned patients are absent
5. _____ Blanching   e. Top layer of the skin
6. _____ Darkly pigmented skin   f. Inner layer of the skin that provides tensile strength and mechanical support

7. Identify the pressure factors that contribute to pressure ulcer development.

    a. _____

    b. _____

    c. _____

    d. _____

    e. _____

    f. _____

8. Identify the risk factors that predispose a patient to pressure ulcer formation.

    a. _____

    b. _____

    c. _____

9. Staging systems for pressure ulcers are based on the depth of tissue destroyed. Briefly describe each stage.

    I. _____

    II. _____

    III. _____

    IV. _____

Define the following terms related to wound healing.

10. Granulation tissue: _____

_____

_____

11. Slough: _____

_____

_____

12. Eschar: _____

_____

_____

13. Exudate: _____

_____

_____

Describe the physiological process involved with wound healing.

14. Primary intention: _____

_____

_____

15. Secondary intention: _____

_____

_____

_____

16. Identify the three components involved in the healing process of a partial-thickness wound.

a. _____

_____

_____

b. _____

_____

_____

c. _____

_____

_____

17. Explain the four phases involved in the healing process of a full-thickness wound.

a. Hemostasis: _____

_____

_____

b. Inflammatory phase: _____

_____

c. Proliferative phase: _____

_____

d. Maturation: _____

_____

_____

18. Briefly explain the following complications of wound healing.

a. Hemorrhage: _____

_____

_____

b. Hematoma: _____

_____

_____

c. Health care–associated infection: _____

_____

_____

d. Dehiscence: _____

_____

_____

e. Evisceration: _____

_____

_____

Nursing Knowledge Base

19. The Braden Scale was developed for assessing pressure ulcer risks. Identify the subscales of this tool.

a. _____

b. _____

c. _____

d. _____

e. _____

f. _____

20. List the factors that influence pressure ulcer formation.

    a. _____

    b. _____

    c. _____

    d. _____

    e. _____

Nursing Process

Assessment

21. Explain the following factors that place a patient at risk for a pressure ulcer.

    a. Mobility: _____

    _____

    _____

    b. Nutritional status: _____

    _____

    _____

    c. Body fluids: _____

    _____

    _____

    d. Pain: _____

    _____

    _____

22. Identify the following types of emergency setting wounds.

    a. Abrasion: _____

    _____

    _____

    b. Laceration: _____

    _____

    c. Puncture: _____

    _____

    _____

Explain how the nurse assesses the following.

23. Wound appearance: _____

    _____

    _____

24. Character of wound drainage: _____

    _____

    _____

25. Complete the table below describing the types of wound drainage.

Type	Appearance
Serous	
Purulent	
Serosanguineous	
Sanguineous	

26. Drains: _____

_____

_____

27. Wound closures: _____

_____

_____

Nursing Diagnosis

28. List the potential or actual nursing diagnoses related to impaired skin integrity.

a. _____

b. _____

c. _____

d. _____

e. _____

f. _____

g. _____

h. _____

Planning

29. List possible goals to achieve wound improvement.

a. _____

b. _____

c. _____

Implementation

30. Identify the three major areas of nursing interventions for preventing pressure ulcers.

a. _____

b. _____

c. _____

Acute Care

31. List the principles to address to maintain a healthy wound environment.

a. _____

b. _____

c. _____

d. _____

e. _____

f. _____

g. _____

h. _____

32. Explain the rationale for debriding a wound.

_____

_____

_____

_____

_____

_____

33. Identify the four methods of debridement.

a. _____

_____

_____

b. _____

_____

c. _____

_____

d. _____

_____

First aid for wounds includes the following. Briefly explain each one.

34. Hemostasis: _____

_____

_____

35. Cleansing: _____

_____

_____

36. Protection: _____

_____

_____

37. List the purposes of dressings.

a. _____

b. _____

c. _____

d. _____

e. _____

f. _____

38. List the clinical guidelines to use when selecting the appropriate dressing.

    a. _____

    b. _____

    c. _____

    d. _____

    e. _____

    f. _____

39. List the advantages of a transparent film dressing.

    a. _____

    b. _____

    c. _____

    d. _____

    e. _____

    f. _____

40. List the functions of hydrocolloid dressings.

    a. _____

    b. _____

    c. _____

    d. _____

    e. _____

    f. _____

    g. _____

41. List the advantages of the hydrogel dressing.

    a. _____

    b. _____

    c. _____

    d. _____

42. List the guidelines to follow during a dressing change procedure.

    a. _____

    b. _____

    c. _____

    d. _____

43. Summarize the principles of packing a wound.

    _____

    _____

    _____

_____

_____

_____

44. Briefly describe how the wound vacuum-assisted closure (wound VAC) device works.

    _____

    _____

    _____

    _____

    _____

    _____

45. Identify three principles that are important when cleaning an incision.

    a. _____

    _____

    _____

    b. _____

    _____

    c. _____

    _____

46. Summarize the principles of wound irrigation.

    _____

    _____

    _____

    _____

    _____

    _____

47. Explain the purpose for drainage evacuation.

    _____

    _____

    _____

    _____

    _____

    _____

48. Explain the benefits of binders and bandages.

   a. _____

   _____

   _____

   b. _____

   _____

   _____

   c. _____

   _____

   _____

   d. _____

   _____

   _____

   e. _____

   _____

   _____

   f. _____

   _____

   _____

49. List the nursing responsibilities when applying a bandage or binder.

   a. _____

   _____

   _____

   b. _____

   _____

   _____

   c. _____

   _____

   _____

   d. _____

   _____

   _____

50. Describe the physiological responses to the following.

   a. Heat applications: _____

   _____

   _____

   b. Cold applications: _____

   _____

   _____

51. List the factors that influence heat and cold tolerance.

   a. _____

   _____

   _____

   b. _____

   _____

   _____

   c. _____

   _____

   _____

   d. _____

   _____

   _____

   e. _____

   _____

   _____

   f. _____

   _____

   _____

   g. _____

   _____

   _____

Explain the rationale for the following types of applications.

52. Warm, moist compresses: _____

_____

_____

53. Warm soaks: _____

_____

_____

54. Sitz baths: _____

_____

_____

55. Commercial hot packs: _____

_____

_____

56. Cold, moist, and dry compresses: _____

_____

_____

57. Cold soaks: _____

_____

_____

58. Ice bags or collars: _____

_____

_____

Evaluation

59. List the questions to ask if the identified outcomes were not met.

a. _____

_____

_____

b. _____

_____

_____

c. _____

_____

_____

REVIEW QUESTIONS

Select the appropriate answer and cite the rationale for choosing that particular answer.

60. Mr. Post is in a Fowler position to improve his oxygenation status. The nurse notes that he frequently slides down in the bed and needs to be repositioned. Mr. Post is at risk for developing a pressure ulcer on his coccyx because of:
    1. Friction
    2. Maceration
    3. Shearing force
    4. Impaired peripheral circulation

    Answer: _____ Rationale: _____

    _____

    _____

61. Which of the following is not a subscale on the Braden Scale for predicting pressure ulcer risk?
    1. Age
    2. Activity
    3. Moisture
    4. Sensory perception

    Answer: _____ Rationale: _____

    _____

    _____

62. Which of these patients has a nutritional risk for pressure ulcer development?
    1. Patient A has an albumin level of 3.5.
    2. Patient B has a hemoglobin level within normal limits.
    3. Patient C has a protein intake of 0.5 g/kg/day.
    4. Patient D has a body weight that is 5% greater than his ideal weight.

    Answer: _____ Rationale: _____

    _____

    _____

63. Mr. Perkins has a stage II ulcer of his right heel. What would be the most appropriate treatment for this ulcer?
    1. Apply a heat lamp to the area for 20 minutes twice daily.
    2. Apply a hydrocolloid dressing and change it as necessary.
    3. Apply a calcium alginate dressing and change when strikethrough is noted.
    4. Apply a thick layer of enzymatic ointment to the ulcer and the surrounding skin.

    Answer: _____ Rationale: _____

    _____

    _____

CRITICAL THINKING MODEL FOR NURSING CARE PLAN FOR IMPAIRED SKIN INTEGRITY

64. Imagine that you are the nurse in the care plan on pp. 1201-1202 of your text. Complete the *Assessment phase* of the critical thinking model by writing your answers in the appropriate boxes of the model shown. Think about the following.
    • What knowledge base was applied to Mrs. Stein?
    • In what way might your previous experience assist you in this case?
    • What intellectual or professional standards were applied to Mrs. Stein?
    • What critical thinking attitudes did you use in assessing Mrs. Stein?
    • As you review your assessment, what key areas did you cover?

B. KNOWLEDGE

C. EXPERIENCE

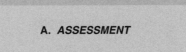

A. *ASSESSMENT*

D. STANDARDS

E. ATTITUDES

49 Sensory Alterations

PRELIMINARY READING

Chapter 49, pp. 1241-1260

COMPREHENSIVE UNDERSTANDING

Scientific Knowledge Base

Match the following key terms related to sensations.

1. _____ Auditory		a.	Enables a person to be aware of position and movement of body parts
2. _____ Tactile		b.	Taste
3. _____ Olfactory		c.	Hearing
4. _____ Gustatory		d.	Smell
5. _____ Kinesthetic		e.	Recognition of an object's size, shape, and texture
6. _____ Stereognosis		f.	Touch

Match the following terms related to the common sensory deficits.

7. _____ Presbyopia	a.	Numbness and tingling of the affected area, stumbling gait
8. _____ Cataract	b.	Results from vestibular dysfunction, vertigo
9. _____ Dry eyes	c.	Decreased accommodation of the lens to see near objects clearly
10. _____ Glaucoma	d.	Blurring of reading matter, distortion or loss of central vision and vertical lines
11. _____ Diabetic retinopathy	e.	Caused by clot, hemorrhage, or emboli to the brain
12. _____ Macular degeneration	f.	Opaque areas of the lens that cause glaring and blurred vision
13. _____ Presbycusis	g.	Decrease in salivary production, leading to thicker mucus and dry mouth
14. _____ Cerumen accumulation	h.	Decreased tear production that results in itching and burning
15. _____ Disequilibrium	i.	Progressive hearing disorder in older adults
16. _____ Xerostomia	j.	Increase in intraocular pressure resulting in peripheral visual loss, halo effect around lights
17. _____ Peripheral neuropathy	k.	Buildup of earwax, causing conduction deafness
18. _____ Stroke	l.	Blood vessel changes of the retina, decreased vision, and macular edema

19. Sensory overload causes: _____

_____

Nursing Knowledge Base

20. Identify the factors that influence the capacity to receive or perceive stimuli.

a. _____

b. _____

c. _____

d. _____

e. _____

f. _____

Nursing Process
Assessment

21. Identify the groups that are at high risk for sensory alterations.

_____

_____

22. List the two questions that a nurse could ask the family to assess any recent changes in a patient's behavior.

a. _____

b. _____

23. Complete the following table by describing at least one assessment technique for the identified sensory function and the behaviors for an adult and child that would indicate a sensory deficit.

Sense	Assessment Technique	Child Behavior	Adult Behavior
Vision			
Hearing			
Touch			
Smell			
Taste			

24. Identify some common home hazards.

a. _____

b. _____

c. _____

d. _____

e. _____

f. _____

g. _____

25. Explain the following types of aphasia.

a. Expressive: _____

b. Receptive: _____

Nursing Diagnosis

26. List the actual or potential nursing diagnoses for a patient with sensory alterations.

a. _____

b. _____

c. _____

d. _____

e. _____

f. _____

g. _____

h. _____

Planning

27. List outcomes that would be appropriate for patients with alteration in hearing acuity.

    a. _____

    b. _____

    c. _____

Implementation

28. List the three recommended screening interventions to prevent eye diseases.

    a. _____

    b. _____

    c. _____

    d. _____

29. The most common visual problem is: _____

    _____

30. Risk factors for children at risk for hearing impairment include:

    a. _____

    b. _____

    c. _____

    d. _____

    e. _____

31. Complete the following table by filling in the sensory deficits that occur, and explain how the nurse can minimize the loss.

Senses	Common Sensory Deficits	Interventions to Minimize Loss
Vision		
Hearing		
Taste and smell		
Touch		

32. Identify methods to promote communication in the following.

    a. Patients with aphasia: _____

    b. Patients with an artificial airway: _____

    c. Patients with a hearing impairment: _____

Acute Care

33. Identify the approaches to maximize sensory function and give an example of each.

a. _____

b. _____

c. _____

d. _____

34. List the principles for reducing loneliness.

a. _____

b. _____

c. _____

d. _____

e. _____

f. _____

g. _____

h. _____

Evaluation

35. Explain how the nurse would evaluate whether the measures improved the patient's ability to interact within the environment.

_____

_____

REVIEW QUESTIONS

Select the appropriate answer and cite the rationale for choosing that particular answer.

36. Mr. Green, a 62-year-old farmer, has been hospitalized for 2 weeks for thrombophlebitis. He has no visitors, and the nurse notices that he appears bored, restless, and anxious. The type of alteration occurring because of sensory deprivation is:
    1. Affective
    2. Cognitive
    3. Receptual
    4. Perceptual

Answer: _____ Rationale: _____

_____

_____

37. Which of the following would not provide meaningful stimuli for a patient?
    1. Interesting magazines and books
    2. A clock or calendar with large numbers
    3. Family pictures and personal possessions
    4. A television that is kept on all day at a low volume

Answer: _____ Rationale: _____

_____

_____

38. Patients with existing sensory loss must be protected from injury. What determines the safety precautions taken?
    1. The existing dangers in the environment
    2. The financial means to make needed safety changes
    3. The nature of the patient's actual or potential sensory loss
    4. The availability of a support system to enable the patient to exist in his or her present environment

    Answer: _____   Rationale: _____

    _____

    _____

39. A patient who is unable to name common objects or express simple ideas in words or writing has:
    1. Global aphasia
    2. Receptive aphasia
    3. Mental retardation
    4. Expressive aphasia

    Answer: _____   Rationale: _____

    _____

    _____

CRITICAL THINKING MODEL FOR NURSING CARE PLAN FOR RISK FOR INJURY

40. Imagine that you are the community health nurse in the care plan on p. 1251 of your text. Complete the *Planning phase* of the critical thinking model by writing your answers in the appropriate boxes of the model shown. Think about the following.
    • In developing Ms. Long's plan of care, what knowledge did you apply?
    • In what way might your previous experience assist in developing a plan of care for Ms. Long?
    • When developing a plan of care, what intellectual and professional standards were applied?
    • What critical thinking attitudes might have been applied in developing Ms. Long's plan?
    • How will you accomplish the goals?

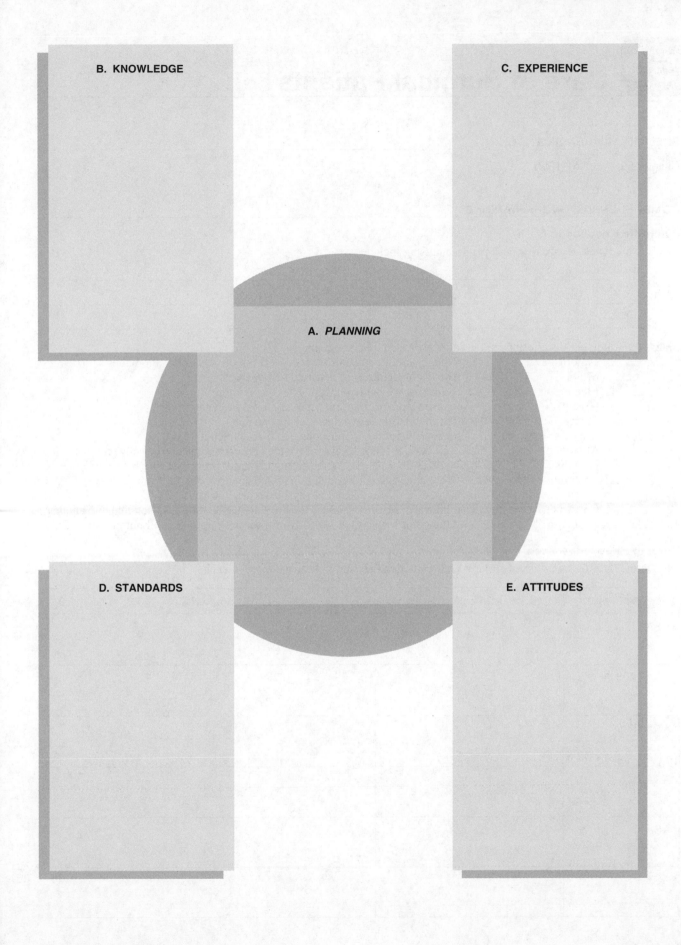

B. KNOWLEDGE

C. EXPERIENCE

A. *PLANNING*

D. STANDARDS

E. ATTITUDES

50 Care of Surgical Patients

Chapter 50, pp. 1261-1306

COMPREHENSIVE UNDERSTANDING

Scientific Knowledge Base

1. List the types of care that perioperative nursing includes.

   a. _____

   b. _____

   c. _____

Match the following descriptions to the surgical procedure classifications.

2. _____ Major
3. _____ Minor
4. _____ Elective
5. _____ Urgent
6. _____ Emergency
7. _____ Diagnostic
8. _____ Ablative
9. _____ Palliative
10. _____ Restorative
11. _____ Procurement
12. _____ Constructive
13. _____ Cosmetic

a. Restores function lost or reduced as result of congenital anomalies
b. Excision or removal of diseased body part
c. Not necessarily emergency
d. Extensive reconstruction, poses great risks to well-being
e. Performed to improve personal appearance
f. Restores function or appearance to traumatized tissues
g. Must be done immediately to save life or preserve function of body part
h. Involves minimal risks compared with major procedures
i. Exploration that allows diagnosis to be confirmed
j. Is not essential and is not always necessary for health
k. Removal of organs or tissues from a dead person for transplantation into another
l. Relieves or reduces the intensity of disease symptoms; will not produce cure

Nursing Knowledge Base

14. Define the following physical status (PS) classifications and give an example of each.

ASA Class	Definition	Characteristics
ASA I		
ASA II		
ASA III		
ASA IV		
ASA V		
ASA VI		

15. List the surgical risk factors that can affect a patient at any point in the perioperative experience.

    a. _____

    b. _____

    c. _____

    d. _____

    e. _____

    f. _____

    g. _____

    h. _____

    i. _____

16. Identify the physiological factors that place the older adult at risk during surgery and give an example of each.

    a. Cardiovascular system: _____

    b. Integumentary system: _____

    c. Pulmonary system: _____

    d. Gastrointestinal system: _____

    e. Renal system: _____

    f. Neurologic system: _____

    g. Metabolic system: _____

Preoperative Surgical Phase
Assessment

17. The goal of the preoperative assessment is to: _____

18. Give an example of how the following medical conditions increase risks of surgery.

    a. Thrombocytopenia: _____

_____

    b. Diabetes: _____

_____

_____

    c. Heart disease: _____

_____

_____

    d. Hypertension: _____

_____

_____

    e. Obstructive sleep apnea: _____

_____

_____

    f. Upper respiratory infection: _____

_____

_____

_____

    g. Liver disease: _____

_____

_____

    h. Fever: _____

_____

_____

_____

    i. Chronic respiratory disease: _____

_____

_____

j. Immunologic disorders: _____

_____

_____

_____

k. Alcohol and street drugs: _____

_____

_____

_____

l. Chronic pain: _____

_____

_____

_____

19. Explain how the following drug classes affect the patient during surgery.

a. Antibiotics: _____

_____

_____

_____

b. Antidysrhythmics: _____

_____

_____

_____

c. Anticoagulants: _____

_____

_____

_____

d. Anticonvulsants: _____

_____

_____

_____

e. Antihypertensives: _____

_____

_____

_____

f. Corticosteroids: _____

_____

_____

g. Insulin: _____

_____

_____

_____

h. Diuretics: _____

_____

_____

_____

i. Nonsteroidal antiinflammatory drugs (NSAIDs):

_____

_____

_____

j. Herbal therapies: _____

_____

_____

_____

20. Explain how the following habits affect the patient.

a. Smoking: _____

_____

_____

_____

b. Alcohol and substance use: _____

_____

_____

_____

21. A comprehensive pain assessment includes:

a. _____

b. _____

c. _____

Briefly explain each of the following factors that need to be assessed in order to understand the impact of surgery on a patient's and family's emotional health.

22. Self-concept: _____

_____

23. Body image: _____

_____

24. Coping resources: _____

_____

25. The physical examination of the patient before surgery includes:

   a. _____

   b. _____

   c. _____

   d. _____

   e. _____

   f. _____

   g. _____

26. Complete the following table of common lab tests for surgical patients.

Test	Normal Values	Low (Significance)	High (Significance)
Hgb			
Hct			
Platelet count			
WBC count			
Na			
K			
Cl			
CO_2			
BUN			
Glucose			
Creatinine			
INR			
PT			
PTT			
Activated PT			

Nursing Diagnosis

27. List the potential or actual nursing diagnoses appropriate for the preoperative patient.

a. _____

b. _____

c. _____

d. _____

e. _____

f. _____

g. _____

h. _____

i. _____

j. _____

k. _____

l. _____

m. _____

Planning

28. Identify the expected outcomes for a patient to verbalize the significance of postoperative exercises.

a. _____

b. _____

c. _____

d. _____

Implementation

29. Identify what the informed consent for surgery involves.

_____

_____

_____

_____

30. Structured teaching throughout the perioperative period influences the following. Briefly explain how.

a. Ventilatory function: _____

_____

b. Physical functional capacity: _____

_____

c. Sense of well-being: _____

_____

d. Length of hospital stay: _____

_____

e. Anxiety about pain: _____

_____

31. List the topics developed by the Association of periOperative Registered Nurses 2015 (AORN) that should be covered to ensure comprehensive preoperative instruction.

a. _____

b. _____

c. _____

d. _____

e. _____

f. _____

g. _____

h. _____

i. _____

Acute Care

32. Identify the interventions to physically prepare the patient for surgery.

a. _____

b. _____

c. _____

33. List the responsibilities of a nurse caring for a patient on the day of surgery.

a. _____

b. _____

c. _____

d. _____

e. _____

f. _____

g. _____

h. _____

i. _____

j. _____

Intraoperative Surgical Phase

34. Explain the responsibilities for the following operating room nurses.

    a. Circulating nurse: _____

    _____

    b. Scrub nurse: _____

    _____

35. Identify the nursing diagnosis for the patient during the intraoperative period.

    a. _____

    b. _____

    c. _____

    d. _____

    e. _____

    f. _____

Explain the following four types of anesthesia.

36. General: _____

    _____

    _____

37. Regional: _____

    _____

    _____

38. Local: _____

    _____

    _____

39. Conscious sedation: _____

    _____

    _____

Postoperative Surgical Phase

40. Identify the two phases of the postoperative course.

    a. _____

    b. _____

41. Identify the responsibilities of the nurse in the postanesthesia care unit (PACU).

    _____

    _____

    _____

    _____

42. Identify the outcomes for discharge from the PACU.

    _____

    _____

    _____

    _____

Postoperative Recovery and Convalescence
Assessment

43. Describe the frequency of vital sign assessment in the immediate postoperative period.

    _____

    _____

    _____

    _____

44. List the factors that contribute to airway obstruction in the postoperative patient.

    a. _____

    b. _____

    c. _____

    d. _____

45. List the areas the nurse would assess to determine a postoperative patient's circulatory status.

    _____

    _____

    _____

    _____

46. List the complications of malignant hyperthermia.

    _____

    _____

    _____

    _____

47. List the areas the nurse assesses to determine fluid and electrolyte alterations.

    a. _____

    b. _____

    c. _____

    d. _____

    e. _____

48. List the areas of assessment that help to determine a postoperative patient's neurologic status.

   a. _____

   b. _____

   c. _____

   d. _____

49. Explain the following complications related to the skin postoperatively.

   a. Rash: _____

   _____

   b. Abrasions or petechiae: _____

   _____

   c. Burns: _____

   _____

50. Explain the reasons why distention of the abdomen may occur.

   a. _____

   b. _____

Nursing Diagnosis

51. List the potential nursing diagnoses that are common in a postoperative patient.

   a. _____

   b. _____

   c. _____

   d. _____

   e. _____

   f. _____

   g. _____

   h. _____

   i. _____

   j. _____

Planning

52. List the typical postoperative orders prescribed by surgeons.

   a. _____

   b. _____

   c. _____

   d. _____

   e. _____

   f. _____

   g. _____

   h. _____

   i. _____

   j. _____

53. Identify the expected outcomes for the postoperative patient.

   a. _____

   b. _____

   c. _____

Implementation

54. List the measures that the nurse would use to promote expansion of the lungs.

   a. _____

   b. _____

   c. _____

   d. _____

   e. _____

   f. _____

   g. _____

   h. _____

   i. _____

   j. _____

55. Define the following complications and give the cause of each.

   a. Atelectasis: _____

   _____

   b. Pneumonia: _____

   _____

   c. Hypoxemia: _____

   _____

   d. Pulmonary embolism: _____

   _____

   e. Hemorrhage: _____

   f. Hypovolemic shock: _____

   _____

g. Thrombophlebitis: _____

_____

h. Thrombus: _____

_____

i. Embolus: _____

_____

j. Paralytic ileus: _____

_____

k. Abdominal distention: _____

_____

l. Nausea and vomiting: _____

_____

m. Urinary retention: _____

_____

n. Urinary tract infection: _____

_____

o. Wound infection: _____

_____

p. Wound dehiscence: _____

_____

q. Wound evisceration: _____

_____

r. Skin breakdown: _____

_____

s. Intractable pain: _____

_____

t. Malignant hyperthermia: _____

_____

56. List the measures the nurse would use to prevent circulatory complications.

a. _____

b. _____

c. _____

d. _____

e. _____

f. _____

57. Identify possible sources of a surgical patient's pain.

_____

_____

_____

_____

58. List the measures the nurse would provide to promote the return of normal elimination.

a. _____

b. _____

c. _____

d. _____

e. _____

f. _____

59. Identify the measures the nurse would provide to promote normal urinary elimination.

a. _____

b. _____

c. _____

d. _____

60. Identify the measures the nurse would use to promote the patient's self-concept.

a. _____

b. _____

c. _____

d. _____

e. _____

f. _____

REVIEW QUESTIONS

Select the appropriate answer and cite the rationale for choosing that particular answer.

61. Mrs. Young, a 45-year-old patient with diabetes, is having a hysterectomy in the morning. Because of her history, the nurse would expect:
    1. Impaired wound healing
    2. Fluid and electrolyte imbalances
    3. An increased risk of hemorrhaging
    4. Altered elimination of anesthetic agents

Answer: _____ Rationale: _____

_____

_____

62. The purposes of the nursing history for the patient who is to have surgery include all of the following except:
    1. Deciding whether surgery is indicated
    2. Identifying the patient's perception and expectations about surgery
    3. Obtaining information about the patient's past experience with surgery
    4. Understanding the impact surgery has on the patient's and family's emotional health

    Answer: _____ Rationale: _____

    _____

    _____

63. All of the following patients are at risk for developing serious fluid and electrolyte imbalances during and after surgery except:
    1. Patient F, who is 1 year old and having a cleft palate repair
    2. Patient H, who is 79 years old and has a history of congestive heart failure
    3. Patient G, who is 55 years old and has a history of chronic respiratory disease
    4. Patient E, who is 81 years old and having emergency surgery for a bowel obstruction after 4 days of vomiting and diarrhea

    Answer: _____ Rationale: _____

    _____

    _____

64. The purpose of postoperative leg exercises is to:
    1. Maintain muscle tone
    2. Promote venous return
    3. Assess range of motion
    4. Exercise fatigued muscles

    Answer: _____ Rationale: _____

    _____

    _____

65. The PACU nurse notices that the patient is shivering. This is most commonly caused by:
    1. Cold irrigations used during surgery
    2. Side effects of certain anesthetic agents
    3. Malignant hypothermia, a serious condition
    4. The use of a reflective blanket on the operating room table

    Answer: _____ Rationale: _____

    _____

    _____

CRITICAL THINKING MODEL FOR NURSING CARE PLAN FOR DEFICIENT KNOWLEDGE

66. Imagine that you are the nurse in the care plan on pp. 1276-1277 of your text. Complete the *Evaluation phase* of the critical thinking model by writing your answers in the appropriate boxes of the model shown. Think about the following.
    - What knowledge did you apply in evaluating Mrs. Campana's care?
    - In what way might your previous experience influence your evaluation of Mrs. Campana's care?
    - During evaluation, what intellectual and professional standards were applied to Mrs. Campana's care?
    - In what way do critical thinking attitudes play a role in how you approach evaluation of Mrs. Campana's care?
    - How might you adjust Mrs. Campana's care?

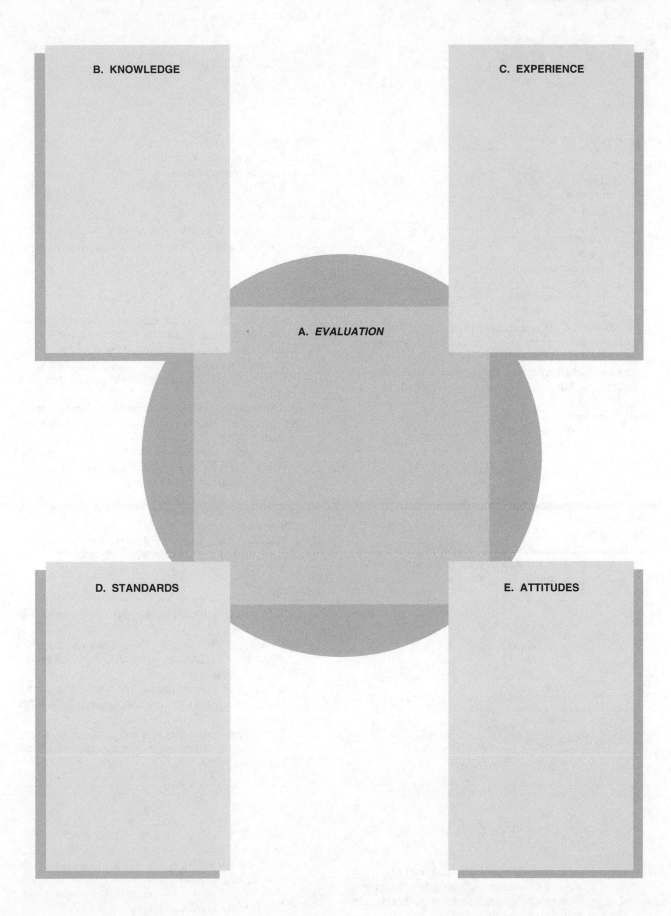

B. KNOWLEDGE

C. EXPERIENCE

A. *EVALUATION*

D. STANDARDS

E. ATTITUDES

Answer Key

CHAPTER 1

1. a. Novice
    b. Advanced beginner
    c. Competent
    d. Proficient
    e. Expert
2. a. Assessment
    b. Diagnosis
    c. Outcome identification
    d. Planning
    e. Implementation
    f. Evaluation
3. Nursing is the protection, promotion, and optimization of health and abilities; prevention of illness and injury; alleviation of suffering through the diagnosis and treatment of human response; and advocacy in the care of individuals, families, communities, and populations.
4. a. Ethics
    b. Education
    c. Evidence-based practice and research
    d. Quality of practice
    e. Communication
    f. Leadership
    g. Collaboration
    h. Professional practice evaluation
    i. Resources
    j. Environmental health
5. The nursing code of ethics is the philosophical ideals of right and wrong that define the principles you will use to provide care to your patients.
6. b
7. d
8. n
9. g
10. c
11. f
12. m
13. i
14. k
15. j
16. l
17. h
18. e
19. a
20. She saw the role of nursing as being in charge of a patient's health based on the knowledge of how to put the body in such a state as to be free of disease or to recover from disease.
21. d
22. c
23. b
24. a
25. a. Nurse's self-care
    b. Affordable Care Act and rising health care costs
    c. Demographic changes of the population
    d. Human rights
    e. Increased number of medically underserved
26. A term to describe burnout and secondary traumatic stress, which impact the health and wellness of nurses and the quality of care provided to patients

27. a. Teamwork and collaboration
    b. Evidence-based practice
    c. Quality improvement
    d. Safety
    e. Informatics
28. *Genomics* describes the study of all the genes in a person, as well as interactions of those genes with each other and with that person's environment
29. c
30. d
31. b
32. e
33. a
34. g
35. f
36. The purpose is to regulate the scope of nursing practice and protect public health, safety, and welfare.
37. A standardized minimum knowledge base for nurses
38. That the nurse may choose to be certified in a specific area of practice by meeting the practice requirements
39. To improve the standards of practice, expand nursing roles, and foster the welfare of nurses within the specialty areas
40. 3. Nursing is a combination of knowledge from the physical sciences, humanities, and social sciences along with clinical competencies.
41. 1. Candidates are eligible to take the NCLEX-RN to become registered nurses in the state in which they will practice.
42. 2. The ANA's purpose is to improve the professional development and general welfare of nurses.

CHAPTER 2

1. a. To practice to the full extent of their education and training
    b. To achieve high levels of education and training through an education system that provides seamless progression
    c. To become full partners, with physicians and health care providers in redesigning the health care system
    d. To improve data collection and information infrastructure for effective workforce planning and policy making
2. c
3. a
4. b
5. e
6. f
7. d
8. g
9. Illness; health of a community and the environment
10. IDNs include a set of providers and services organized to deliver a continuum of care to a population of patients at a capitated cost in a particular setting.
11. a. Prenatal and well-baby care, nutrition counseling, family planning, exercise classes

b. Blood pressure and cancer screening, immunizations, mental health counseling and crisis prevention, community legislation

c. Emergency care, acute medical-surgical care, radiologic procedures

d. Intensive care, subacute care

e. Cardiovascular and pulmonary rehab, sports medicine, spinal cord injury programs, home care

f. Assisted living, psychiatric, and older adult day care

12. a. Focuses on health outcomes for an entire population. Health promotion programs lower the overall costs of health care, reducing the incidence of disease, minimizing complications, and reducing the need to use more expensive health care resources.

b. Preventive care is more disease oriented and focused on reducing and controlling risk factors for disease through activities.

13. Most common and expensive service of the health care delivery system

14. a. Emergency departments
b. Urgent care centers
c. Critical care units
d. Medical–surgical units

15. Work design

16. The moment a patient is admitted to a health care facility

17. Discharge planning

18. a. Make a referral as soon as possible
b. Give the receiving provider as much information as possible about the patient
c. Involve the patient and family in the process
d. Determine what the care provider receiving the referral recommends for patient's care

19. a. Safe and effective use of medications and medical equipment
b. Instruction and counseling on food–drug interactions, nutrition, and modified diets
c. Rehabilitation techniques
d. Access to appropriate community resources
e. When and how to obtain further treatment
f. The responsibilities of the patient and the families with ongoing health care needs
g. When to notify their health care provider for changes in functioning or new symptoms

20. a. Usually nurses care for only one to two patients at a time.
b. Treatments and procedures required

21. The goal of restorative care is to help individuals regain maximal functional status and to enhance quality of life through promotion of independence and self-care.

22. a. Nursing
b. Medical and social services
c. Physical, occupational, speech, and respiratory therapy
d. Nutritional therapy

23. a. Monitoring of vital signs
b. Administration of parenteral or enteral nutrition and medications
c. IV or blood therapy

d. Wound care
e. Respiratory care

24. Rehabilitation

25. b

26. c

27. a

28. d

29. e

30. f

31. g

32. a. Developed to coordinate medical care by primary care and specialty physicians, hospitals, and other providers with the goal of coordination
b. Make care for patients more efficient, effective, continuous, comprehensive, patient-centered, and coordinated

33. Aging baby boomer generation, slow growth in nursing school enrollments, nursing faculty shortages, space limitations, clinical site availability

34. a. Recognize and respect differences in patients' values, preferences, and needs; relieve pain and suffering; coordinate continuous care; communicate with and educate patients
b. Cooperate, collaborate, and communicate; integrate care to ensure that care is continuous and reliable
c. Integrate best research with clinical practice, practice in research activities
d. Identify errors and hazards in care; practice using basic safety design principles; measure quality in relation to structure, process, and outcomes; design and test interventions to change processes
e. Information technology to communicate, manage knowledge, reduce error, and support decision making

35. a. Care is based on continuous healing relationships.
b. Individualized based on needs and values
c. Patient is the source of control, participating in shared decision making.
d. Knowledge is shared.
e. Decision making is evidence based.
f. Safety is a system property and is focused on reducing errors.
g. Transparency through sharing information
h. Needs are anticipated through planning.
i. Waste is continuously decreased.
j. Cooperation and communication among clinicians are a priority.

36. The degree to which health services for individuals and populations increase the likelihood of desired health outcomes and are consistent with current professional knowledge.

37. The goal is to reward excellence through financial incentives to motivate change to achieve measurable improvements.

38. A standardized survey developed to measure patient perceptions of their hospital experience

39. a. Respect and dignity
b. Sharing of information
c. Participation in care and care decisions
d. Collaboration

40. a. Quality patient care
b. Nursing excellence
c. Innovations in professional practice

41. a. Transformational leadership
    b. Structural empowerment
    c. Exemplary professional practice
    d. New knowledge, innovations, and improvements
    e. Empirical quality outcomes
42. Nurse-sensitive outcomes are patient outcomes and select nursing workforce characteristics that are directly related to nursing. Examples include changes in patient symptom experiences, functional status, safety, psychological distress, Registered Nurse (RN) job satisfaction, total nursing hours per patient day, and costs.
43. Nursing informatics
44. Increased connectedness of the world's economy, culture, and technology
45. a. Children
    b. Women
    c. Older adults
46. a. An approach to continuous study and improvement of the processes of providing health care services to meet the needs of patients and others to inform health care policy
    b. Organization analyzes and evaluates current performance and uses the results to develop focused improvement actions.
47. 4. Reduce the incidence of disease, minimize complications, and reduce the need to use more expensive health care resources.
48. 1. Initially focuses on the prevention of complications related to the illness or injury. After the condition stabilizes, rehabilitation helps to maximize the patient's level of independence.
49. 2. Where they receive supportive care until they are able to move back into the community
50. 1. The focus is palliative care, not curative treatment.

CHAPTER 3

1. Health promotion, disease prevention, and restorative care
2. Focuses on primary rather than institutional or acute care, and provides knowledge about health and health promotion and models of care to the community.
3. Political policy, the Affordable Care Act (ACA), social determinants of health, increases in health disparities, and economics
4. Gathering information on incident rates for identifying and reporting new infections or diseases, adolescent pregnancy rates, motor vehicle accidents (MVAs) by teenage drivers
5. Biological, socioeconomic, psychosocial, behavioral, or social in nature
6. Preventable differences in the burden of disease, injury, violence, or opportunities to achieve optimal health that are experienced by socially disadvantaged populations
7. a. Focus requires understanding the needs of a population (e.g., high-risk infants, older adults, or cultural groups).
   b. It is a nursing practice in the community, with the primary focus on the health care of individuals, families, and groups in the community.

8. In community settings such as the home or a clinic, where the focus is on the needs of the individual or family
9. a. Patients who are more likely to develop health problems as a result of excess risks
   b. Patients who have limits in access to health care services
   c. Patients who are dependent on others for care
10. Access to health care is limited because of lack of benefits, resources, language barriers, and transportation.
11. They live in hazardous environments, work at high-risk jobs, eat less nutritious foods, and have multiple stressors.
12. Mental health problems, substance abuse, socioeconomic stressors, dysfunctional relationships
13. Homeless or live in poverty and lack the ability to maintain employment or to care for themselves
14. They suffer from chronic diseases and have a greater demand for health care services.
15. Together with the family, you develop a caring partnership to recognize actual and potential health care needs and identify community resources.
16. The ability to establish an appropriate plan of care based on assessment of patients and families and to coordinate needed resources and services for the patient's well-being across a continuum of care
17. Acts to empower individuals and their families to creatively solve problems or become instrumental in creating change within a health care agency
18. Often is the one who presents the patient's point of view to obtain appropriate resources
19. Mutual trust and respect for each professional's abilities and contributions, clarifying roles, and developing a plan of care
20. Assists patients in identifying and clarifying health problems and in choosing appropriate courses of action
21. Establishes relationships with community service organizations and assesses patients' learning needs and readiness to learn within the context of the individual, the systems with which the individual interacts, and the resources available for support
22. May be involved in case finding, health teaching, and tracking incident rates
23. a. Structure (geographical boundaries, emergency services, housing, economic status)
    b. Population (age and sex distribution, growth trends, education level, ethnic and religious groups)
    c. Social (education and communication systems, government, volunteer programs, welfare system)
24. 3. They are usually jobless and do not have the advantage of shelter and cope with finding a place to sleep at night and finding food.
25. 4. The coordinating of activities of multiple providers and payers in different settings throughout a patient's continuum of care
26. 3. Observe the community's design, location of services, and locations where the residents meet

CHAPTER 4

1. e
2. f
3. a
4. d
5. h
6. i
7. j
8. c
9. g
10. b
11. c
12. d
13. e
14. g
15. f
16. a
17. b

18. A phenomenon specific to the discipline that developed the theory
19. a. Input: The data that come from a patient's assessment
    b. Output: End product of a system (whether the patient's health improves, declines, or remains stable)
    c. Feedback: The outcomes reflect the patient's responses to nursing interventions
    d. Content: Information about the nursing care for patients with specific health care problems
20. d
21. e
22. g
23. a
24. c
25. b
26. f
27. h
28. a. Uses logic to explore relationships between phenomena
    b. Determines how accurately a theory describes a nursing phenomenon
29. 1. See Table 4-3, p. 47.
30. 4. Person: The recipient of nursing care, level of health, environment; all are possible causes

CHAPTER 5

1. Evidence-based practice is a problem-solving approach to clinical practice that integrates the conscientious use of best evidence in combination with a clinician's expertise, patient preferences, and values in making decisions about patient care.
2. a. Cultivate a spirit of inquiry.
   b. Ask a clinical question in PICOT format.
   c. Search for the most relevant evidence.
   d. Clinically appraise the evidence.
   e. Integrate all the evidence with one's clinical expertise, patient preferences, and values.
   f. Evaluate the outcomes of practice decision or change.
   g. Share the outcomes of evidence-based practice (EBP) changes with others.
3. a. P = Patient or population of interest
   b. I = Intervention of interest
   c. C = Comparison of interest
   d. O = Outcome
   e. T = Time
4. a. Agency policy and procedure manuals
   b. Quality improvement data
   c. Existing clinical practice guidelines
   d. Computerized databases

5. Accuracy, validity, and rigor are approved for publication by experts before it is published.
6. Clinical guidelines are systematically developed statements about a plan of care for a specific set of clinical circumstances involving a specific patient population.
7. RCTs
8. Summarizes the purpose of the study or clinical query, the major themes or findings, and the implications for nursing practice
9. Contains information about its purpose and the importance of the topic for the reader
10. A detailed background of the level of science or clinical information that exists about the topic of the article
11. A clinical article can contain a description of the population, the health alteration, how patients are affected, or a new therapy or technology.
12. a. Purpose statement: The intent or focus of the study
    b. Methods or design: How it was organized and conducted
    c. Results or conclusions: Summary section
    d. Clinical implications
13. Nursing research is a way to identify new knowledge, improve professional education and practice, and use resources effectively.
14. Outcomes research is research designed to assess and document the effectiveness of health care services and interventions.
15. The scientific method is a systematic step-by-step process that ensures that the findings from a study are valid, reliable, and generalizable to subjects.
16. a. The problem area to be studied is identified.
    b. The steps of planning and conducting the study are systematic and orderly.
    c. External factors that may influence a relationship between the phenomena that are being studied are controlled.
    d. Empirical data are gathered.
    e. The goal is to apply the knowledge from a study to a broader group of patients.
17. The conditions are tightly controlled to eliminate bias and to ensure that findings can be generalizable to similar subjects.
18. Describe, explain, or predict; a case–control study
19. Information is obtained from populations regarding the frequency, distribution, and interrelation of variables among the subjects.
20. Evaluation involves finding out how well a program, practice, procedure, or policy is working.
21. The study of phenomena that are difficult to quantify or categorize such as patients' perceptions or quality of life
22. a. Assessment
    b. Diagnosis
    c. Planning
    d. Implementation
    e. Evaluation
23. Informed consent is when research subjects are given full and complete information about the purpose of the study, procedures, data collection, harms,

and benefits; are capable of fully understanding the research and implications of participation; and have the power of free choice to voluntarily consent or decline and understand how the researcher maintains confidentiality or anonymity.

24. 3. Together, the abstract and introduction tell you if the topic of the article is similar to your PICOT question or related closely enough to provide you with useful information.

25. 3. The summary details the results of the study and explains whether a hypothesis is supported. The results of other studies are not presented.

26. 1. Clinical guidelines are systemically developed statements about a plan of care for a specific set of clinical circumstances involving a specific patient population.

CHAPTER 6

1. a. Attain high-quality, longer lives free of preventable disease, disability, injury, and premature death
   b. Achieve health equity, eliminate disparities, and improve health of all groups
   c. Create social and physical environments
   d. Promote quality of life, healthy development, and healthy behaviors across all life stages

2. Health is a state of complete physical, mental, and social well-being.

3. a. Positive: Immunizations, proper sleep patterns, adequate exercise, stress management, and nutrition
   b. Negative: Smoking, drug or alcohol abuse, poor diet, refusal to take necessary medications

4. a. An individual's perception of susceptibility to an illness
   b. An individual's perception of the seriousness of the illness
   c. The likelihood that a person will take preventive action

5. a. The individual characteristics and experiences
   b. Behavior-specific knowledge and affect
   c. Behavioral outcomes

6. Nurses using the holistic nursing model recognize the natural healing abilities of the body and incorporate complementary and alternative interventions because they are effective, economical, noninvasive, nonpharmacological complements to traditional medical care.

7. a. Developmental stage (a person's thought and behavior patterns change throughout life; the nurse must consider the patient's level of growth and development when using his or her health beliefs and practices as a basis for planning care)
   b. Intellectual background (a person's beliefs about health are shaped in part by the person's knowledge, lack of knowledge, or incorrect information about body functions and illnesses, educational background, and past experiences)
   c. Perception of functioning (subjective data about the way the patient perceives physical functioning such as level of fatigue, shortness of breath, or pain; also obtain objective data about actual functioning, such as blood pressure, height measurements, and lung sound assessment)
   d. Emotional (the patient's degree of stress, depression, or fear can influence health beliefs and practices)
   e. Spiritual factors (how a person lives his or her life, including the values and beliefs exercised, the relationships established with family and friends, and the ability to find hope and meaning in life)

8. a. Family practice (the way in which patients' families use health care services generally affects their health practices)
   b. Psychosocial variables (the stability of the person's marital or intimate relationship, lifestyle habits, and occupational environment)
   c. Cultural background (influences beliefs, values, and customs that influence their personal health practices, their approach to the system, and the nurse–patient relationship)

9. Health promotion includes activities such as routine exercise and good nutrition that help patients maintain or enhance their present levels of health.

10. Wellness includes strategies that are designed to help persons achieve new understanding and control over their lives.

11. Illness prevention includes activities that motivate people to avoid declines in health or functional levels.

12. In passive strategies, individuals gain from the activities of others without acting themselves. In active strategies, individuals are motivated to adopt specific health programs.

13. a. Is true prevention; it precedes disease
    b. Focuses on the individuals who are experiencing health problems or illnesses and who are at risk for developing complications or worsening conditions
    c. Occurs when a defect or disability is permanent and irreversible; it involves minimizing the effects of the illness or disability

14. A risk factor is any situation, habit, social or environmental condition, physiological or psychological condition, developmental or intellectual condition, or spiritual or other variable that increases the vulnerability of an individual or group to an illness or accident.

15. a. Pregnant or overweight, diabetes mellitus, cancer, heart disease, kidney disease, or mental illness
    b. Premature infant, heart disease, and cancer with increased age
    c. Industrial workers are exposed to certain chemicals or when people live near toxic waste disposal sites
    d. Habits that have risk factors (sunbathing, overweight)

16. a. Not intending to make changes within the next 6 months
    b. Considering a change within the next 6 months
    c. Making small changes in preparation for a change in the next month
    d. Actively engaged in strategies to change behavior
    e. Sustained change over time
17. Illness is a state in which a person's physical, emotional, intellectual, social, developmental, or spiritual functioning is diminished or impaired compared with the previous experience.
18. a. Usually has a short duration and is severe; symptoms appear abruptly, are intense, and often subside after a relatively short period
    b. Usually lasts longer than 6 months; can also affect functioning in any dimension
19. How people monitor their bodies, define and interpret their symptoms, take remedial actions, and use the health care system
20. a. Their perceptions of symptoms and the nature of their illness, such as a person experiencing chest pain in the middle of the night seeking assistance
    b. The visibility of symptoms, social group, cultural background, economic variables, accessibility of the system, and social support
21. a. Depend on the nature of the illness, the patient's attitude toward it, the reaction of others to it, and the variables of the illness behavior
    b. Reaction to the changes in body image depend on the type of changes, their adaptive capacity, the rate at which changes takes place, and the support services available
    c. Depends in part on body image and roles but also includes other aspects of psychology and spirituality
    d. Role reversal can lead to stress, conflicting responsibilities for the adult or child, or direct conflict over decision making.
    e. Is the process by which the family functions, makes decisions, gives support to individual members, and copes with everyday changes and challenges
22. 4. Internal variables include all of the ones cited.
23. 1. Any situation, habit, or social or environmental condition that increases the vulnerability of the individual to an illness
24. 1. The health belief model helps nurses understand factors influencing patients' perceptions, beliefs, and behavior.

CHAPTER 7

1. Caring is a universal phenomenon influencing the ways in which people think, feel, and behave in relation to one another.
2. Leininger's concept of care defines care as the essence and central, unifying, and dominant domain that distinguishes nursing from other health disciplines. Care is the essential human need and is necessary for the health and survival of all individuals.
3. Watson's transpersonal caring looks beyond the patient's disease and its treatment by conventional means. It looks for deeper sources of inner healing to protect, enhance, and preserve a person's dignity, humanity, wholeness, and inner harmony.
4. The focus is on carative behaviors and the nurse–patient caring relationship. The relationship influences both the nurse and the patient for better or worse.
5. a. Knowing: Striving to understand an event as it has meaning in the life of the other
   b. Being with: Being emotionally present to the other
   c. Doing for the other as he or she would do for him- or herself if it were at all possible
   d. Enabling: Facilitating the other's passage through life transitions
   e. Maintaining belief: Sustaining faith in the other's capacity to get through an event or transition and face a future with meaning
6. a. Human interaction or communication
   b. Mutuality
   c. Appreciating the uniqueness of individuals
   d. Improving the welfare of patients and their families
7. The nurse is the patient's advocate, solving ethical dilemmas by attending to relationships and by giving priority to each patient's unique personhood.
8. Having presence in a person-to-person encounter conveys a closeness and a sense of caring. Presence involves both "being there" and "being with."
9. a. Alleviating suffering
   b. Decreasing a sense of isolation and vulnerability
   c. Personal growth
10. a. Task oriented: When performing a task or a procedure, the skillful and gentle performance of a nursing procedure conveys security and a sense of competence.
    b. Caring: A form of nonverbal communication, which successfully influences the patient's comfort and security, enhances self-esteem, and improves reality orientation
    c. Protective: Used to protect the nurse, patient, or both, it can be positively or negatively viewed
11. Listening involves taking in what a patient says, as well as an interpretation and understanding of what the patient is saying, and giving back that understanding to the person who is speaking.
12. a. Continuity of care
    b. Clinical expertise
13. a. Organizational structure
    b. Economic constraints
14. a. Provide honest, clear, and accurate information
    b. Listen to patient and family concerns, complaints, and fears
    c. Advocating for the patient's care preferences
    d. Asking permission before doing something to the patient
    e. Providing comfort
    f. Reading the patient passages from religious texts, favorite books, cards, or mail

g. Provide for and maintain patient privacy

h. Keep the patient informed about the types of nursing services

i. Assure the patient that nursing services will be available

j. Help patients do as much for themselves as possible

k. Teach the family how to keep the relative physically comfortable

15. Nurses are torn between the human caring model and the task-oriented biomedical model and the institutional demands that consume their practice.

16. 2. Even though human caring is a universal phenomenon, the expressions, processes, and patterns of caring vary among cultures.

17. 4. There is a mutual give and take that develops as nurse and patient begin to know and care for one another.

18. 3. Listening involves paying attention to the individual's words and the tone of his or her voice.

19. 4. It depends on the family's willingness to share information about the patient, their acceptance and understanding of therapies, whether the interventions fit the family's daily practices, and whether the family supports and delivers the therapies recommended.

CHAPTER 8

1. a. Increased risk for developing a second cancer is the result of cancer treatment, genetic or other susceptibility, or an interaction between treatment and susceptibility.

   b. Osteoporosis, congestive heart failure, diabetes, amenorrhea, sterility, impaired immune function, paresthesias, and hearing loss

   c. Treatment for the cancer or the cancer itself can cause pain and neuropathy, especially with high doses of chemotherapy.

   d. Associated sleep disturbances are the most frequent and disturbing complaints that may last months to years after treatments.

   e. In systemic cancer treatment, including chemotherapy or biotherapy, there are generalized, subtle effects ranging from small deficits in information.

2. a. Fear of cancer recurrence is common among cancer survivors. Survivors with more negative intrusive thoughts about their illness have higher levels of this fear.

   b. Cancer survivors experience symptoms of post-traumatic stress disorder (PTSD) (e.g., grief, intrusive thoughts about the disease, nightmares, relational difficulties, or fear). Being unmarried or less educated or having a lower income and less social and emotional support increases the risk for PTSD.

   c. The disabling effects of chronic cancer symptoms disrupt family and personal relationships, impair individuals' work performance, and often isolate survivors from normal social activities.

3. a. Cancer alters a young person's social skills, sexual development, body image, and the ability to think about and plan for the future.

   b. When a member of the family is diagnosed with cancer, every family member's roles, plans, and abilities change. This can mean added job responsibilities for the spouse; changes in sexuality, intimacy, and fertility; employment opportunities are affected; and economic burdens.

   c. Older adults with cancer may retire prematurely, facing a fixed income, limitations of Medicare reimbursement, retirement residences, and isolation from social supports.

4. Family members are distressed; do not know, understand, or respond supportively to other family members; try to cope with both the impact of the cancer and the tension in the family; and struggle to maintain their core functions as a long-term survivor.

5. Some examples may be: Tell me how your disease most affects you right now. What are the biggest problems that you are having from cancer? What can I do to help you at this point?

6. a. Self-caregiving: Patients are mostly independent with caregivers in a standby role.

   b. Collaborative care: Patients and caregivers share care activities and respond together to illness demands.

   c. Family caregiving: Patients are unable to perform independently and require extensive caregiver involvement.

7. Effects of cancer and cancer treatment, health care provider's explanations of the risks related to their cancer and treatment, what they need to self-monitor, what to discuss with health care providers in the future, potential for treatment effects, increased risk for developing a second cancer or chronic illness, lifestyle behaviors, and ongoing screening practices

8. a. Prevention and detection of new cancers and recurrent cancer

   b. Surveillance for cancer spread, recurrence, or second cancers

   c. Intervention for consequences of cancer and its treatments

   d. Coordination between specialists and primary care providers

9. 4. Cognitive changes can occur during all phases of the cancer experience, from small deficits in information processing to acute delirium.

10. 4. Many older adults have very limited Medicare reimbursement.

11. 2. Coordination should be between the specialists and the primary care providers for ongoing clinical care.

CHAPTER 9

1. A particular type of health difference that is closely linked with social, economic, and/or environmental disadvantage

2. The conditions in which people are born, grow, live, work, and age shaped by money, power, and resources at global, national, and local levels

3. Differences among populations in the availability, accessibility, and quality of health care services aimed at prevention, treatment, and management of diseases and their complications

4. c
5. f
6. a
7. h
8. b
9. e
10. i
11. g
12. j
13. d

14. Developmental process that evolves overtime in relation to level of awareness, knowledge, and skills
15. The ability of an organization and its staff to communicate effectively and convey information in a manner that is easily understood by diverse audiences
16. a. Open-ended
    b. Focused
    c. Contrast
    d. Ethnohistory
    e. Sexual orientation and gender identity
    f. Social organization
    g. Socioeconomic status
    h. Bicultural ecology and health risks
    i. Language and communication
    j. Caring beliefs and practices
17. a. Plan your approach
    b. Use handouts, pictures, and models
    c. Clarify
    d. Practice
18. a. Provide language services at all points of contact free of charge to all patients who speak limited English or are deaf
    b. Notify patients both verbally and in writing of their right to receive language assistance services
    c. Take steps to provide auxiliary aids and services
    d. Ensure that interpreters are competent in medical terminology and understand issues of confidentiality
19. Key quality indicators that help health care institutions improve performance, increase accountability, and reduce costs
20. a. Recognize disparities and commit to reducing them
    b. Implement a basic quality improvement structure and process
    c. Make equity an integral component of quality improvement efforts
    d. Design the intervention
    e. Implement, evaluate, and adjust the intervention
    f. Sustain the intervention
21. 2. Nurses need to determine how much an individual's life patterns are consistent with his or her heritage.
22. 2. Caused by the changing demographic profile of the United States in relation to immigration and significant culturally diverse populations
23. 1. Because different cultural groups have distinct linguistic and communication patterns

CHAPTER 10

1. a. Durability is the intrafamilial system of support and structure that extends beyond the walls of the household.
    b. Resiliency is the ability of the family to cope with expected and unexpected stressors.
    c. Diversity is the uniqueness of each family unit; each person has specific needs, strengths, and important developmental considerations.
2. A family is defined biologically, legally, or as a social network with personally constructed ties and ideologies.
3. a. A nuclear family consists of the husband and the wife (and perhaps one or more children).
    b. An extended family includes relatives in addition to the nuclear family.
    c. In a single-parent family, one parent leaves the nuclear family because of death, divorce, or desertion or a single person decides to have or adopt a child.
    d. In a blended family, parents bring unrelated children from prior or foster-parenting relationships into a new, joint living situation.
    e. Alternative families include multiadult households, skip-generation families, and communal groups with children, nonfamilies, cohabiting partners, and homosexual partners.
4. a. Families at the lower end of the income scale have been particularly affected, and single-parent families are especially vulnerable; losing a job; lack of education; lack of food or shelter.
    b. Homelessness severely affects the functioning, health, and well-being of the family and its members. Children of homeless families are often in fair or poor health and have higher rates of asthma, ear infections, stomach problems, and mental illness.
    c. Emotional, physical, and sexual abuse occurs toward spouses, children, and older adults across all social classes. Factors are complex and may include stress, poverty, social isolation, psychopathology, and learned family behavior.
    d. Hospitalization is stressful for the whole family, environments are foreign, physicians and nurses are strangers, medical language is difficult to understand or interpret, and family members become separated.
5. a. Family members need to cope with the challenges of a severe, life-threatening event that includes many stressors and may impact the family's functioning and decision making.
    b. The family's need for information, support, assurance, and presence are great. The more you know about the family, how they interact, and their strengths and their weaknesses, the better.
6. Each stage has its own challenges, needs, and resources and includes tasks that need to be completed before the family is able to successfully move on to the next stage.

7. a. A rigid structure dictates who is able to accomplish a task and may limit the number of persons outside the immediate family who assumes these tasks.
    b. An open or extremely flexible structure and consistent patterns of behavior that lead to automatic action do not exist, and enactment of roles is overly flexible.
8. Communication among family members, goal setting, conflict resolution, caregiving, nurturing, and use of internal and external resources
9. a. Interactive
    b. Developmental
    c. Coping
    d. Integrity
    e. Health
10. a. Hardiness is the internal strengths and durability of the family unit.
    b. The family's ability to return to a previous, healthy level of functioning after a disruptive or stressful event has occurred
11. The primary focus is on the health and development of an individual member existing within a specific environment.
12. Family processes and relationships are the primary focus of nursing care. There is a need to focus on family patterns versus individual characteristics.
13. Use both family as context and family as patient simultaneously
14. a. Assess all individuals within the family context
    b. Assess the family as patient
    c. Assess the family as a system
15. a. Interactive processes: Family relationships, family communication, family nurturing, intimacy expression, social support, conflict resolution, and roles
    b. Developmental processes: Current family transitions, family stage task completion, individual developmental issues and health issues
    c. Coping processes: Problem solving, use of resources, family stressors, coping strategies, past experiences with crises, and resistance resources
    d. Integrity processes: Family values and beliefs, family meaning, rituals, spirituality, culture, and practices
    e. Health processes: Health beliefs and behaviors, health patterns and management activities, caretaking responsibilities, consequences for the family, relationship with health care providers, and system access
16. a. Understand the family life
    b. Understand the current changes within it
    c. Understand the family's overall goals
    d. Understand the family's expectations
17. a. Discharge planning requires an accurate assessment of what will be needed for care at the time of discharge along with any shortcomings in the home setting.

    b. Cultural diversity requires recognizing not only the diverse ethnic, cultural, and religious backgrounds of patients but also the differences and similarities within the same family.
18. a. Family caregiving: Finding resources, providing personal care, monitoring for complications or side effects of an illness or treatments, providing instrumental activities of daily living
    b. Health promotion: Interventions to improve or maintain the physical, social, emotional, and spiritual well-being of the family unit and its members
    c. Acute care: Be aware of the implications of early discharge for patients and their families
    d. Restorative care: To maintain patients' functional abilities within the context of the family
19. 3. Ongoing membership of the family and the pattern of relationships, which are often numerous and complex
20. 4. Is critical in forming an understanding of family life, current changes in family life, overall goals and expectations, and planning family-centered care
21. 3. Very rigid structures impair functioning.

CHAPTER 11

1. Gesell's theory of development is that although each child's pattern of growth is unique, this pattern is directed by gene activity.
2. The theory explains development as primary unconscious and influenced by emotion. These unconscious conflicts influence development through universal stages experienced by all individuals.
3. a. (oral) Sucking and oral satisfaction are not only vital to life but also pleasurable.
    b. (anal) Children become increasingly aware of the pleasurable sensations of this body region with interest in the products of their effort.
    c. (phallic) The genital organs become the focus of pleasure.
    d. (latency) Sexual urges are repressed and channeled into productive activities that are socially acceptable.
    e. (genital) Earlier sexual urges reawaken and are directed to an individual outside the family circle.
4. b   8. c
5. d   9. g
6. a   10. f
7. e   11. h
12. Temperament is a behavioral style that affects the individual's emotional interactions with others.
13. a. Easy child (regular and predictable)
    b. Difficult child (highly active, irritable, and has irregular habits)
    c. Slow-to-warm-up child (reacts negatively with mild intensity to new stimuli)
14. a. Tasks that surface because of physical maturation
    b. Tasks that evolve from personal values
    c. Tasks that are a result of pressures from society

15. A contemporary life-span approach considers the individual's personal circumstances, how the person views and adjusts to changes, and the current social and historical context in which the individual is living.

16. a. Period I: Sensorimotor (birth to 2 years)
    b. Period II: Preoperational (2 to 7 years)
    c. Period III: Concrete operations (7 to 11 years)
    d. Period IV: Formal operations (11 years to adulthood)

17. Level I: The person reflects on moral reasoning based on personal gain.
    a. Stage 1: Punishment and obedience orientation (in terms of absolute obedience to authority and rules)
    b. Stage 2: Instrumental relativist orientation (more than one right view)

18. Level II: Sees moral reasoning based on his or her own personal internalization of societal and others' expectations
    a. Stage 3: Good boy–nice girl orientation (good motives, showing concern for others, and keeping mutual relationships)
    b. Stage 4: Society-maintaining orientation (expand their focus from a relationship with others to societal concerns)

19. Level III: Balance between human rights and obligations and societal rules and regulations
    a. Stage 5: Social contract orientation (follows the societal law but recognizes the possibility of changing the law to improve society)
    b. Stage 6: Universal ethical principle orientation (right by the decision of conscience in accord with self-chosen ethical principles)

20. 1. Children achieve the ability to perform mental operations.

21. 2. Puberty, marked preoccupation with appearance and body image

22. 2. The adult focuses on supporting future generations and the ability to expand one's personal and social involvement.

23. 4. Level I: Preconventional reasoning
    Stage 1: Punishment and obedience orientation

CHAPTER 12

1. a. Preembryonic stage (first 14 days)
   b. Embryonic stage (day 15 until the eighth week)
   c. Fetal stage (end of the eighth week until birth)

2. Nausea and vomiting, breast tenderness, urinary frequency, heartburn, constipation, ankle edema, and backache

3. a. Heart rate
   b. Respiratory effort
   c. Muscle tone
   d. Reflex irritability
   e. Color

4. Open airway, stabilizing and maintaining body temperature, protecting the newborn from infection

5. Close body contact, often including breastfeeding, is a satisfying way for most families to start bonding.

6. d   10. f
7. c   11. b
8. h   12. g
9. e   13. a

14. 1 month, 1 year of age

15. Size increases rapidly during the first year of life; birth weight doubles (5 months) and triples (12 months). Height increases an average of 1 inch every 6 months until 12 months.

16. The infant learns by experiencing and manipulating the environment (sensorimotor period). Developing motor skills and increasing mobility expand an infant's environment and with developing visual and auditory skills enhance cognitive development.

17. By age 1 year, infants not only recognize their own names but are also able to say three to five words and understand 100 words. The nurse can promote language development by encouraging parents to name objects on which the infant is focusing.

18. a. Infants are unaware of the boundaries of self, but they learn where the self ends and the external world begins.
    b. Much of the play is exploratory as they use their senses to observe and examine their own bodies and objects of interest in their surroundings.

19. a. Injury prevention focuses on MVA, aspiration, suffocation, falls, and poisoning.
    b. Children of any age can experience maltreatment, but the youngest are the most vulnerable. A combination of signs and symptoms or a pattern of injury should arouse suspicion.

20. a. Breastfeeding is recommended for infant nutrition because breast milk contains the essential nutrients of protein, fats, carbohydrates, and immunoglobulins that bolster the ability to resist infection. If breastfeeding is not possible or if the parent does not desire it, an acceptable alternative is iron-fortified commercially prepared formula.
    b. After 6 months, iron-fortified cereal is generally an adequate supplemental source in breastfed infants. Because iron in formula is less readily absorbed than that in breast milk, formula-fed infants need to receive iron-fortified formula throughout the first year.
    c. It is recommended that the administration of the primary series begin after birth and be completed during early childhood.
    d. Infants are nocturnal and sleep between 9 and 11 hours, averaging 15 hours a day.

21. 12 months (1 year), 36 months (3 years)

22. The rapid development of motor skills allows the child to participate in self-care activities such as feeding, dressing, and toileting.

23. Toddlers possess an increased ability to remember events and begin to put thoughts into words (2 years).

24. An 18-month-old child uses approximately 10 words. A 24-month-old child has a vocabulary of up to 300 words and is generally able to speak in two-word sentences.
25. Toddlers develop a sense of autonomy; strong wills are frequently exhibited in negative behavior.
26. Children continue to engage in solitary play during toddlerhood but also begin to participate in parallel play.
27. Newly developed locomotion abilities and insatiable curiosity increase injury risks for toddlers. Poisoning, drowning, and MVA are all risks.
28. a. Nutrition: To prevent obesity and its associated chronic illnesses, toddlers need a balanced daily intake of bread and grains, vegetables, fruit, dairy products, and proteins. Limit milk intake to two to three cups per day.
    b. Toilet training: Recognizing the urge to urinate and/or defecate is crucial in determining the child's mental readiness.
29. 3 years, 5 years
30. Children gain about 5 lb per year. Preschoolers grow 2.5 to 3 inches per year, double their birth length around 4 years, and stand an average of 43 inches tall by their fifth birthday.
31. Preschoolers demonstrate their ability to think in a more complex manner by classifying objects, increased social interaction, cause-and-effect relationships; the world remains closely linked to concrete experiences; their greatest fear is bodily harm.
32. a. Curiosity and developing initiative lead to the active exploration of the environment, development of new skills, and making of new friends.
    b. Preschoolers' vocabularies continue to increase rapidly, and by the age of 6 years, children have 8000 to 14,000 words.
33. Play shifts from parallel to associative play, and children engage in similar if not identical activity; there is no division of labor or rigid organization or rules.
34. a. The quality of food is more important than the quantity.
    b. Preschoolers average 12 hours of sleep a night. They take infrequent naps.
    c. Vision should be checked at regular intervals; early detection and treatment of strabismus is essential by age 4 years.
35. 6 years, 12 years (puberty)
36. Around the age of 12 signals the end of middle childhood.
37. Rate of growth is slow and consistent; average height is 2 inches per year; weight increase is 4 to 7 lb.
38. School-age children have the ability to think in a logical manner about the here and now and to understand the relationship between things and ideas. The thoughts of school-age children are no longer dominated by their perceptions; thus, their ability to understand the world greatly expands.
39. a. Psychosocial changes: Strive to acquire competence and skills necessary to function as adults; developing self-esteem
    b. Peers: Become more important; play involves peers and the pursuit of group goals

    c. Sexual: Great deal of curiosity, but their play is usually transitory
    d. Stress: From parental expectations, peer expectations, school environment, violence in the community
40. Accidents and injuries (MVAs and bicycle injuries), infections
41. a. Perception of wellness is based on readily observable facts such as presence or absence of illness and adequacy of eating or sleeping.
    b. Promotion of good health practices; teaching children about their bodies and the choices they make
    c. Immunizations, screenings, and dental care; parents need to be encouraged to discuss pubertal changes (10 years); routine vaccination for human papilloma virus (HPV) in girls 11 to 12 years of age.
    d. At this age, encourage children to take responsibility for their own safety.
    e. Promoting healthy lifestyle habits in selection of foods
42. 13 years, 20 years
43. a. Increased growth rate of skeleton, muscle, and viscera
    b. Sex-specific changes
    c. Alteration in distribution of muscle and fat
    d. Development of the reproductive system and secondary sex characteristics
44. Menarche is the onset of menstruation.
45. Adolescents possess the ability to determine possibilities, rank and solve problems, and make decisions through logical operations. They can think abstractly and deal effectively with hypothetical problems. They can move beyond the physical or concrete properties of a situation and use reasoning powers to understand the abstract.
46. Do not avoid discussing sensitive issues. Ask open-ended questions. Look for meaning behind the words or actions. Be alert to clues to their emotional state. Involve other individuals and resources.
47. a. Puberty enhances sexual identity; physical evidence of maturity encourages the development of masculine and feminine behaviors.
    b. Similarity in dress or speech and popularity are major concerns.
    c. Movement toward stronger peer relationships is contrasted with adolescents' movement away from their parents.
    d. They evaluate their own health according to feelings of well-being, ability to function normally, and absence of symptoms.
48. a. Accidents
    b. Homicide
    c. Suicide
49. a. Decrease in school performance
    b. Withdrawal
    c. Loss of initiative
    d. Loneliness, sadness, and crying
    e. Appetite and sleep disturbances
    f. Verbalization of suicidal thought

50. a. Anorexia nervosa is a clinical syndrome with both physical and psychosocial components that involve the pursuit of thinness through starvation.
   b. Bulimia nervosa is most identified with binge eating and behaviors to prevent weight gain (vomiting, laxatives, exercise).

51. a. Screen for use and inform of the risks for use. Those who are at higher risk are from dysfunctional families.
   b. All sexually active adolescents need to be screened for STIs even if they have no symptoms.
   c. Pregnant teens need special attention to nutrition, as well as health supervision and psychological support.

52. Minority adolescents are at greater risk for learning or emotional difficulties, death related to violence, unintentional injuries, an increased rate of adolescent pregnancy, poverty, and limited access to health care services.

53. The nurse may help the adolescent construct a safety plan before telling his or her family or friends in case the response is not supportive.

54. 4. Toddlers often develop food jags or the desire to eat one food repeatedly; continue to offer a variety of nutritious foods.

55. 1. Do not understand what is right or wrong, but they do understand positive and negative reinforcement, thus learning self-control

56. 2. The school and home influence growth and development. If they are positively recognized for success, they feel a sense of worth.

CHAPTER 13

1. Age 18 to 25
2. Young adults usually complete physical growth by age 20 years. An exception to this is pregnant or lactating women.
3. Formal and informal educational experiences, general life experiences, and occupational opportunities increase conceptual problem-solving and motor skills.
4. a. The person refines self-perception and ability for intimacy.
   b. The person directs enormous energy toward achievement and mastery of the world.
   c. This is a time of vigorous examination of life goals and relationships.
5. a. Identification of modifiable factors that increase the risk for health problems and provide education and support to reduce unhealthy lifestyle behaviors
   b. Successful employment offers both economic security as well as fulfillment; identify stressors in a two-career family—for example, transfers, increase expenditures of physical, emotional or mental energy, child care demands or household needs
   c. Young adults who have failed to achieve the developmental task of personal integration sometimes develop relationships that are superficial and stereotyped; encourage adults to explore various aspects of their sexuality and be aware that their sexual needs and concerns change.
   d. Conception, pregnancy, birth, and the puerperium are the major phases that have complex phases.
6. a. Many young adults do not marry until their late 20s or early 30s or they remain single. Parents and siblings become the nucleus of the family. Close friends and associates may be considered family.
   b. Availability of contraception, social pressures, economic considerations, general health status, and age all factor into the decision of when and if the young adult wishes to start a family.
   c. There is greater acceptance of cohabitation without marriage. About 1.5 million parents are gay or lesbian.
7. The presence of certain chronic illnesses in the family increases the patient's risk of developing a disease.
8. Poor hygiene (sharing utensils, poor dental hygiene) is a risk factor.
9. Mortality or health risks can be attributable to poverty, family breakdown, child abuse and neglect, repeated exposure to violence, and access to guns.
10. Substance abuse health risks include intoxicated MVAs, dependence on stimulant or depressive drugs, and excessive caffeine use.
11. Human trafficking, runaways, and homeless youth
12. Unplanned pregnancies are a continued source of stress that may result in adverse health outcomes for the mother, infant, and family.
13. Sexually transmitted infections can lead to major health problems, chronic disorders, infertility, or death.
14. Exposure to work-related hazards or agents, which can cause disease and cancer
15. Job assessment includes conditions and hours, duration of employment, changes in sleep or eating habits, and evidence of increased irritability or nervousness.
16. Family assessment includes a review of environmental and familial factors, including support and coping mechanisms commonly used by family members.
17. Comprehensive history of both the male and female partners to determine factors that affect fertility as well as pertinent physical findings
18. Obesity assessment involves a review of diet and physical activity and counsel about the benefits of a healthful diet and physical activity.
19. Conduct a thorough musculoskeletal assessment and exercise history to develop a realistic exercise plan.
20. Prenatal care is routine thorough physical examination of the pregnant woman.
21. a. Women commonly have morning sickness, breast enlargement and tenderness, and fatigue.
   b. Growth of the uterus and fetus results in some of the physical signs of pregnancy.
   c. Increases in Braxton Hicks contractions (irregular, short contractions), fatigue, and urinary frequency occur.
22. 35 to 64
23. The most visible changes are graying of the hair, wrinkling of the skin, thickening of the waist, and

decreases in hearing and visual acuity, which may have an impact on self-concept and body image.

24. a. Perimenopause is the period during which ovulation declines, resulting in a diminished number of ova and irregular menstrual cycles.
    b. Menopause is the disruption of this cycle, primarily because of the inability of the neurohormonal system to maintain its periodic stimulation of the endocrine system.
    c. Climacteric occurs in men in their late 40s or early 50s because of decreased levels of androgens.

25. Middle adults having the responsibility of raising their own children while caring for aging parents.

26. Changes occur by choice or as a result of changes in the workplace or society (limited upward mobility, decreasing availability of jobs, need for challenge).

27. Couples recultivate their relationships. The onset of menopause and the climacteric affect sexual health.

28. Choice and freedom; delayed marriage and delayed parenthood, adoption

29. Death of a spouse, separation, divorce, and the choice of remarrying or remaining single

30. Departure of the last child is a stressor, leading to a readjustment phase.

31. The goal of wellness guides patients to evaluate health behaviors, lifestyle, and environment by minimizing the frequency of stress-producing situations, increasing stress resistance, and avoiding physiological response to stress.

32. Continued focus on the goal of wellness assists patients in evaluating health behaviors and lifestyle that contribute to obesity during the middle adult years. Counseling related to physical activity and nutrition is an important component of the plan of care for overweight and obese patients.

33. a. Anxiety can be related to change, conflict, and perceived control of environment, which may motivate the adult to rethink his or her life goals and stimulate creativity or precipitate psychosomatic illness and preoccupation with death.
    b. Depression is a mood disorder that manifests itself in many ways. Although the most frequent age of onset is between ages 25 and 44 years, it is common among adults in the middle years and has many causes.

34. 1. Factors that predispose include poverty, family breakdown, child abuse and neglect, repeated exposure to violence, and access to guns.

35. 3. The most visible changes are the graying of hair, wrinkling of the skin, and thickening of the waist.

36. 1. Menopause is the disruption of the menstrual cycle primarily because of the inability of the neurohormonal system to maintain its periodic stimulation of the endocrine system

CHAPTER 14

1. 65

2. a. Ill, disabled, and physically unattractive
   b. Forgetful, confused, rigid, bored, and unfriendly
   c. Mistaken ideas about living arrangements and finances

3. Discrimination against people because of increasing age, which undermines self-confidence of older adults, limits their access to care, distorts caregivers' understanding of the uniqueness of each older adult

4. a. Adjusting to decreasing health and physical strength
   b. Adjusting to retirement and reduced or fixed income
   c. Adjusting to the death of a spouse
   d. Accepting oneself as an aging person
   e. Maintaining satisfactory living arrangements
   f. Redefining relationships with adult children
   g. Finding ways to maintain quality of life

5. a. It should not feel like a hospital.
   b. Is Medicare and Medicaid certified
   c. Has adequate, qualified staff members who have passed criminal background checks
   d. Provides quality care, assistance with ADLs, social and recreational activities
   e. Offers quality food and mealtimes
   f. Welcomes family when they visit the facility
   g. Is clean
   h. Active communication from staff to patient
   i. Attends quickly to resident requests

6. a. The interrelation between physical and psychosocial aspects of aging
   b. The effects of disease and disability on functional status
   c. Tailoring the assessment to an older person

7. a. Change in mental status
   b. Falls
   c. Dehydration
   d. Decrease in appetite
   e. Loss of function
   f. Dizziness and incontinence

8. d   13. j
9. f   14. h
10. g   15. e
11. b   16. a
12. i   17. c

18. Functional status refers to the capacity and safe performance of activities of daily living and is a sensitive indicator of health and illness.

19. a. Delirium is an acute confusional state that is potentially reversible and often has a physiological cause.
    b. Dementia is a generalized impairment of intellectual functioning that interferes with social and occupational functioning.
    c. Depression is not a normal part of aging. It is treatable with medication, psychotherapy, or a combination of both.

20. a. The stage of life characterized by transitions and role changes (health status, option to continue working, sufficient income)
    b. By choice (desire not to interact with others) or a response to conditions that inhibit the ability or the opportunity to interact with others
    c. Whether a person is healthy or frail, there is a need to express sexual feelings (love, warmth, sharing, and touching).

d. The ability to live independently strongly determines housing choices (social roles, family responsibilities, health status).

e. The death of a spouse affects more older women than men.

21. a. Increase the number of older adults with one or more chronic conditions who report confidence in maintaining their conditions

b. Reduce the proportion of older adults who have moderate to severe functional limitations

c. Increase the proportion of older adults with reduced physical or cognitive function who engage in physical activities

d. Increase the proportion of older adults who receive diabetes self-management benefits

e. Increase the proportion of the health care workforce with geriatric certification

22. a. Participation in screening activities

b. Regular exercise

c. Weight reduction

d. Moderate alcohol use

e. Balanced diet

f. Regular dental visits

g. Smoking cessation

h. Stress management

i. Socialization

j. Good handwashing

k. Regular checkups with health care providers

l. Immunizations

23. c	33. b
24. h	34. d
25. e	35. j
26. g	36. c
27. k	37. e
28. i	38. d
29. l	39. b
30. m	40. f
31. a	41. a
32. f	

42. Intentional actions that cause harm or create serious risk of harm (whether harm is intended) to a vulnerable elder by a caregiver or other person who is in a trusting relationship to the elder

43. Physical abuse, emotional abuse, financial exploitation, sexual abuse, neglect, and abandonment

44. Provides sensory stimulation, induces relaxation, provides physical and emotional comfort, and conveys warmth

45. Restores a sense of reality, improves the level of awareness, promotes socialization, elevates independent functioning, and minimizes physical regression

46. Accepts the description of time and place as stated by the adult; you do not challenge or argue with statements or behaviors

47. Recalling the past to bring meaning and understanding to the present and resolve current conflicts

48. The risk for delirium increases when hospitalized patients experience immobilization, sleep deprivation, infection, dehydration, pain, sensory impairment, drug interactions, anesthesia, and hypoxia.

49. The risk for dehydration and malnutrition can increase as a result of limiting food and fluids in preparation for diagnostic tests and medications that decrease appetite.

50. The risk for health care–associated infections can increase because of age-related reductions in immune system responses, most commonly urinary catheter–related bacteriuria.

51. Causes of transient urinary incontinence include delirium, untreated UTIs, excessive urine production, medications, depression, restricted mobility, and constipation.

52. Older adults face an increased risk for skin breakdown related to changes in aging and to immobility, incontinence, and malnutrition.

53. Older adults face an increased risk for falls because of intrinsic factors (gait and balance problems, weakness, or cognitive impairment) and extrinsic factors (polypharmacy, poor lighting, cluttered environment).

54. a. The continuation of the recovery from acute illness or surgery that began in the acute care setting

b. The support of chronic conditions that affect day-to-day functioning

55. 4. It potentially is a reversible cognitive impairment that often has physiological causes.

56. 1. Often the result of retinal damage, reduced pupil size, development of opacities in the lens, or loss of lens elasticity

57. 4. It is the stage of life characterized by transitions and role changes.

CHAPTER 15

1. Involves open-mindedness, continual inquiry, and perseverance, combined with a willingness to look at each unique patient situation and determine which identified assumptions are true and relevant

2. Evidence-based knowledge is knowledge based on research or clinical expertise.

3. a. Stop and think about what is going on with your patient.

b. Reflect carefully on critical incidents.

c. Think about your feelings and the painful experiences you sometimes have.

d. Take time to reflect at the end of the day.

e. Keep all written care plans or clinical notes for future resources.

f. Keep a personal journal.

4. a. In basic critical thinking, the learner trusts that experts have the right answers for every problem; thinking is concrete and based on a set of rules or principles.

b. In complex critical thinking, learners begin to separate themselves from experts and analyze and examine choices more independently.

c. In commitment, learners anticipate the need to make choices without assistance from others and accept accountability.

5. c
6. d
7. a
8. g

9. b
10. f
11. e

12. a. Seek the true meaning of a situation.
   b. Be tolerant of different views and one's own prejudices.
   c. Anticipate possible results or consequences.
   d. Be organized.
   e. Trust in your own reasoning processes.
   f. Be eager to acquire new knowledge and value learning.
   g. Reflect on your own judgments.

13. c
14. g
15. j
16. a
17. e
18. h

19. d
20. f
21. b
22. i
23. k

24. a. Diagnostic reasoning: Analytical process for determining a patient's health problems and selecting proper therapies
   b. Inference: The process of drawing conclusions from related pieces of evidence and previous experience with the evidence
25. a. A nurse's understanding of a specific patient
   b. A nurse's subsequent selection of interventions
26. a. Spend more time during initial patient assessment to observe behavior and measure physical findings.
   b. Listen to their accounts of their experiences with illness.
   c. Consistently check on patients to assess and monitor problems.
   d. Ask to have the patient assigned to you over consecutive days.
   e. Social conversation and continuity
27. The five steps are assessment, diagnosis, planning, interventions, and evaluation.
28. a. Intellectual: Clear, precise, specific, accurate, relevant, plausible, consistent, logical, deep, broad, complete, significant, adequate, and fair
   b. Professional: Ethical criteria, criteria for evaluation, professional responsibility
29. Reflective journaling is the process of purposefully thinking back or recalling a situation to discover its purpose or meaning.
30. Concept mapping is a visual representation of patient problems and interventions that shows their relationships to one another.
31. a. Learn to recognize when you are feeling stressed.
   b. Take a time out.
   c. Discuss the difficult and stressful patient care experiences you are having.
   d. Participate in opportunities to make decisions.
   e. Attend a stress management class.
32. 4. Involves recognizing an issue exists, analyzing information, evaluating information, and making conclusions

33. 4. The five steps are assessment, diagnosis, planning, interventions, and evaluation.
34. 3. Identifying a patient's health care needs

CHAPTER 16

1. a. Collection of information from primary and secondary sources
   b. Interpretation and validation of data
2. a. The patient through interviews, observations, and physical exam
   b. Family members or significant others
   c. Other members of the health team
   d. Medical record information
   e. Scientific and medical literature
3. The patient-centered interview during the history and physical exam and periodic assessments during rounding or administering care
4. a. Cue is information that you obtain through your senses.
   b. Inference is your judgment or interpretation of these cues.
5. a. Health perception–health management pattern
   b. Nutritional–metabolic pattern
   c. Elimination pattern
   d. Activity–exercise pattern
   e. Sleep–rest pattern
   f. Cognitive–perceptual pattern
   g. Self-perception–self-concept pattern
   h. Role–relationship pattern
   i. Sexuality–reproductive pattern
   j. Coping–stress tolerance pattern
   k. Value–belief pattern
6. a. Subjective data include patients' verbal descriptions of their health problems.
   b. Objective data include observations or measurements of a patient's health status.
7. Motivational interviewing is a process that addresses a patient's ambivalence to medically indicated behavior change and supports patients in making health care decisions.
8. a. Courtesy
   b. Comfort
   c. Connection
   d. Confirmation
9. a. Orientation and setting an agenda
   b. Working phase: Collecting assessment
   c. Terminating an interview
10. a. Observation: Nonverbal communication
   b. Open ended: Prompts patients to describe a situation (tell their story) in more than one or two words
   c. Leading question: Risky, limits information
   d. Back channeling: Active listening prompts
   e. Probing: Encourages a full description without trying to control the direction of the story
   f. Closed ended: Limit the patient's answers to one or two words

11. f
12. g
13. e

14. h
15. i
16. c

17. j
18. b
19. a
20. d
21. Diagnostic and laboratory data provide further explanation of alterations or problems identified during the history and physical examination.
22. Data validation is the comparison of data with another source to determine data accuracy.
23. Documentation should be timely, thorough, and accurate. Record all observations. Pay attention to facts and be descriptive. Record objective information in accurate terminology. Do not generalize or form judgments.
24. A concept map is a visual representation that allows you to graphically show the connections between a patient's many health problems.
25. 4. Prompts patients to describe a situation in more than one or two words.
26. 1. Some may be focused, and others may be comprehensive.
27. 3. Takes information provided in the patient's story and then more fully describes and identifies specific problem areas
28. 2. Asking questions about the normal functioning of each system and the changes are usually subjective data perceived by the patient.

CHAPTER 17

1. d
2. e
3. b
4. c
5. f
6. a
7. g

8. A data cluster is a set of signs or symptoms gathered during assessment that help you group them together in a logical way.
9. Defining characteristics are clinical criteria that are observable and verifiable.
10. Analyzing clusters of defining characteristics or risk factors
11. A diagnostic label is the name of the diagnosis as approved by NANDA; it describes the essence of the patient's response to health conditions.
12. A related factor is a condition or etiology identified from the patient's assessment data, or actual or potential responses to the health problem.
13. P = problem, E = etiology or related factor, and S = symptoms or defining characteristics
14. a. How has this health problem affected you and your family?
    b. What do you believe will help or fix the problem?
    c. What worries you the most about this problem?
    d. What do you expect from us to help you maintain some of your values or practices?
    e. What cultural practices do you do to keep yourself well?
15. Concept mapping a nursing diagnosis is a way to graphically represent the connections among concepts (nursing diagnosis) and ideas that are related to a central subject (patient's problem).

16. Inaccurate interpretation, failure to consider conflicting cues, insufficient number of cues, invalid cues, failure to consider cultural influences
17. Insufficient cluster of cues, premature or early closure, incorrect clustering
18. Wrong label, evidence exists for another diagnosis, collaborative problem, failure to validate with the patient, failure to seek guidance
19. a. Identify the patient's response, not the medical diagnosis.
    b. Identify a North American Nursing Diagnosis Association (NANDA) diagnostic statement rather than the symptom.
    c. Identify a treatable etiology or risk factor rather than a clinical sign or chronic problem.
    d. Identify the problem caused but the treatment or diagnostic study rather than the treatment or study itself.
    e. Identify the patient's response to the equipment rather than the equipment itself.
    f. Identify the patient's problems rather than your problems with nursing care.
    g. Identify the patient's problem rather than the nursing intervention.
    h. Identify the patient's problem rather than the goal of care.
    i. Make professional rather than prejudicial judgments.
    j. Avoid legally inadvisable statements.
    k. Identify the problem and etiology to avoid a circular statement.
    l. Identify only one patient problem in the diagnostic statement.
20. Enter them either on the written plan of care or in the agency's electronic health information record. List nursing diagnosis chronically, placing the highest priority nursing diagnosis first; date the diagnosis at time of entry; review the list; and reevaluate the priority.
21. 4. Provide the basis for the selection of nursing interventions to achieve outcomes for which the nurse is responsible.
22. 4. It is the diagnostic label that describes the essence of a patient's response to health conditions.
23. 4. It is associated with the patient's actual or potential response to the health problem.
24. 2. It is the patient's actual or potential response to the health problem.

CHAPTER 18

1. Prioritizing the diagnoses, setting patient-centered goals and expected outcomes, prescribing individualized nursing interventions
2. a. If untreated, result in harm to the patient or others
   b. Involve nonemergent, nonthreatening needs of the patient
   c. Are not always directly related to a specific illness or prognosis
3. a. Model for delivering care
   b. Nursing unit's workflow routine

   c. Staffing levels
   d. Interruptions from other care providers
   e. Available resources
   f. Policies and procedures
   g. Supply access
 4. d
 5. b
 6. e
 7. c
 8. f
 9. a
10. Specific, Measurable, Attainable, Realistic, Timed
11. A singular goal or outcome is precise in evaluating a patient response to a nursing action; each goal and outcome should address only one behavior, perception, or physiologic response.
12. Terms describing quality, quantity, frequency, length, or weight allow the nurse to evaluate outcomes precisely.
13. For a patient's health to improve he or she must be able to attain the outcomes of care that are set; mutually set attainable goals and outcomes.
14. A realistic goal or outcome is one that a patient is able to achieve.
15. A time-limited outcome is written so that it indicates when the nurse expects the response to occur.
16. Independent nursing interventions are nurse-initiated interventions that do not require direction or an order from another health care professional.
17. Dependent nursing interventions are physician-initiated interventions that require an order from a physician or other health care professional.
18. Collaborative interventions are interdependent nursing interventions that require the combined knowledge, skill, and expertise of multiple care professionals.
19. a. Desired patient outcomes
     b. Characteristics of the nursing diagnosis
     c. Research base knowledge for the intervention
     d. Feasibility for doing the intervention
     e. Acceptability to the patient
     f. Your own competency
20. The nursing care plan should direct clinical nursing care and decrease the risk of incomplete, incorrect, or inaccurate care. It identifies and coordinates resources for delivering care. It lists the interventions needed to achieve the goals of care.
21. Student care plans are useful for learning problem-solving techniques, nursing process, skills of written communication, and organizational skills needed for nursing care.
22. The interdisciplinary care plan is designed to improve the coordination of all patient therapies and communication among all disciplines.
23. In a "nursing handoff," nurses collaborate and share information that ensures the continuity of care for a patient and prevents errors or delays in providing nursing interventions.
24. Consultation is a process in which the nurse seeks the expertise of a specialist to identify ways to handle problems in patient management or the planning and implementation of therapies.
25. a. Identify the general problem area.
     b. Direct the consultation to the right professional.
     c. Provide the consultant with relevant information about the problem area.
     d. Do not prejudice or influence the consultants.
     e. Be available to discuss the findings and recommendations.
     f. Incorporate the recommendations into the plan of care.
26. 2. An objective behavior or response that you expect a patient to achieve in a short time, usually less than 1 week
27. 4. The measurable change in a patient's condition that you expect to occur in response to the nursing care
28. 3. The nurse sets patient-centered goals and expected outcomes and plans nursing interventions.

CHAPTER 19

 1. Implementation begins after the nurse develops a plan of care based on clear and relevant nursing diagnoses. The interventions are designed to achieve the goals and expected outcomes needed to support or improve the patient's health status.
 2. a. Direct care are treatments performed through interactions with patients.
     b. Indirect care are treatments performed away from the patient but on behalf of the patient.
 3. a. Helping role
     b. Teaching–coaching function
     c. Diagnostic and patient-monitoring function
     d. Effective management of rapidly changing situations
     e. Administering and monitoring therapeutic interventions and regimens
     f. Monitoring and ensuring the quality of health care practices
     g. Organizational and work-role competencies
 4. A clinical practice guideline or protocol is a document that guides decisions and interventions for specific health care problems or conditions.
 5. A standing order is a preprinted document containing orders for the conduct of routine therapies, monitoring guidelines, or diagnostic procedures for patients with identified clinical problems.
 6. Nursing Interventions Classification (NIC) interventions offer a level of standardization to enhance communication of nursing care across settings and to compare outcomes.
 7. a. Review the set of all possible nursing interventions for a patient's problem.
     b. Review all consequences associated with each possible nursing action.
     c. Determine the probability of all possible consequences.
     d. Judge the value of the consequence to the patient.

8. Reassessing the patient is a continuous process that occurs each time you interact with the patient; you collect new data, identify a new patient need, and you modify the care plan.

9. If the patient's status has changed and the nursing diagnosis and related nursing interventions are no longer appropriate, modify the nursing care plan.

10. Time management, equipment, personnel, environment, and the patient

11. Risks to patients come from both the illness and the treatments.

12. Implementation skills include cognitive (application of critical thinking in the nursing process), interpersonal (trusting relationship, level of caring, and communication), and psychomotor skills (integration of cognitive and motor activities).

13. Activities of daily living are activities usually performed in the course of a normal day such as ambulation, eating, dressing, bathing, and grooming.

14. Instrumental activities of daily living include skills such as shopping, preparing meals, writing checks, and taking medications.

15. Physical care techniques involve the safe and competent administration of nursing procedures.

16. Lifesaving measures are physical care techniques that are used when a patient's physiological or psychological state is threatened.

17. Counseling is a direct care method that helps the patient use a problem-solving process to recognize and manage stress and to facilitate interpersonal relationships.

18. The focus of teaching is intellectual growth or the acquisition of new knowledge or psychomotor skills.

19. An adverse reaction is a harmful or unintended effect of a medication, diagnostic test, or therapeutic intervention.

20. Preventive nursing actions promote health and prevent illness to avoid the need for acute or rehabilitative health care.

21. An interdisciplinary care plan represents the contributions of all disciplines caring for the patient.

22. Patient adherence is when patients and families invest time in carrying out required treatments to achieve patient goals.

23. 4. The nurse needs to exercise good judgment and decision making before actually delivering any interventions.

24. 2. Certain nursing situations require you to obtain assistance by seeking additional personnel, knowledge, or nursing skills. You will need assistance with this patient to help turn and position the patient safely.

25. 1. Guides decisions and interventions for specific health care problems or conditions

26. 1. An acquisition of new knowledge or psychomotor skills

CHAPTER 20

1. Evaluation is done after the application of the nursing process and the patient's condition or well-being improves.

2. Are the same as assessment measures, but you perform them at the point of care when you make decisions about a patient's status and progress. The intent is to determine if the known problems have remained the same, improved, worsened, or otherwise changed.

3. a. Being systematic and using criterion-based evaluation
   b. Collaborating with patients and other professionals
   c. Using ongoing assessment data to revise the plan
   d. Communicate results to patients and family

4. The Nursing Outcomes Classification (NOC) identifies, labels, validates, and classifies nurse-sensitive patient outcomes. Its purpose is to field test and validate the classification and to define and test measurement procedures for the outcomes and indicators using clinical data.

5. Expected outcomes are states, behaviors, or perceptions that are measured along a continuum in response to a nursing intervention.

6. a. Examine the outcome criteria to identify the exact desired patient behavior.
   b. Assess the patient's actual behavior or response.
   c. Compare the established outcome criteria with the actual behavior.
   d. Judge the degree of agreement between outcome criteria and the actual behavior.
   e. If there is no agreement between the outcome criteria and the actual behavior, what are the barriers?

7. The nurse's ability to recognize how a patient is responding and then adjusting interventions as a result

8. Each time the nurse evaluates a patient, he or she determines if the plan of care continues or if revisions are necessary. The nurse may have to modify or add nursing diagnoses with appropriate goals, expected outcomes, and interventions.

9. If the nurse and the patient agree that the expected outcomes and goals have been met, then that portion of the care plan is discontinued.

10. Identify the factors that interfere with goal achievement.

11. Being systematic and using criterion-based evaluation, collaborating with patients and health care professionals, using assessment data to revise a plan, and communicating results to patients and families.

12. Interactions in which professionals work together cooperatively with shared responsibility and interdependence toward achieving patient outcomes.

13. The nurse is responsible for consistent, thorough documentation of the patient's progress toward the expected outcomes and use of nursing diagnostic language. When documenting a patient's response to the interventions, the nurse should describe the intervention, the evaluative measures used, the outcomes achieved, and the continued plan of care.

14. 2. Determines whether the patient's condition or well-being has improved after the application of the nursing process

15. 2. Whenever you have contact with a patient, you continually make clinical decisions and redirect nursing care; this is an ongoing process.

16. 2. They are the expected favorable and measurable results of nursing care.
17. 3. If the goals have not been met, you may need to adjust the plan of care by the use of interventions, modify or add nursing diagnoses with appropriate goals and expected outcomes, and redefine priorities.

CHAPTER 21

1. a. Effective communicator
   b. Consistent in managing conflict
   c. Knowledgeable and competent
   d. Role model
   e. Uses participatory approach in decision making
   f. Shows appreciation for a job well done
   g. Delegates appropriately
   h. Sets objectives and guides staff
   i. Displays caring attitude
   j. Motivates others
   k. Proactive and flexible
   l. Focuses on team development
2. a. Focus on change and innovation through team development
   b. Motivate and empower staff to function at a high level of performance
   c. Serve as a role model for the nurses on the unit
3. d   8. f
4. e   9. h
5. b   10. i
6. j   11. g
7. c   12. a
13. a. Assist staff in establishing annual goals for the unit and systems needed
    b. Monitor professional nursing standards of practice
    c. Develop an ongoing staff development plan
    d. Recruit new employees
    e. Conduct routine staff evaluations
    f. Establish self as a role model
    g. Submit staff schedules
    h. Conduct regular patient rounds and problem solve
    i. Establish, monitor, and implement a performance/quality improvement plan
    j. Review and recommend new equipment
    k. Conduct regular staff meetings
    l. Make rounds with health care providers
    m. Establish and support staff and interprofessional committees
14. a. Establishment of nursing practice or problem-solving committees or professional shared governance councils
    b. Interprofessional collaboration
    c. Interprofessional rounding
    d. Staff communication
    e. Staff education
15. A focused and complete assessment of the patient's condition allows for accurate clinical decisions as to the patient's health problems and required nursing therapies.

16. The nurse forms a picture of the patient's total needs and sets priorities by deciding on what patient needs or problems need to be cared for first.
17. Implementing a plan of care requires you to be effective and efficient. Whereas effective use of time means doing the right things, efficient use of time means doing things right.
18. Administration of patient care occurs more smoothly when staff members work together.
19. Learn how, where, and when to use your time. Establish personal goals and time frames. Anticipate interruptions.
20. Evaluation is an ongoing process that compares actual patient outcomes with expected outcomes.
21. A professional environment is one in which staff members respect one another's ideas, share information, and keep one another informed.
22. a. Goal setting
    b. Time analysis
    c. Priority setting
    d. Interruption control
    e. Evaluation
23. a. Right task
    b. Right circumstances
    c. Right person
    d. Right direction or communication
    e. Right supervision
24. a. Assess the knowledge and skills of the delegate.
    b. Match tasks to the delegate's skills.
    c. Communicate clearly.
    d. Listen attentively.
    e. Provide feedback.
25. 4. As a student nurse, you have a responsibility for the care given to your patients, and you assume accountability for that care.

CHAPTER 22

1. d
2. b
3. e
4. c
5. a
6. a. Responsibility
   b. Accountability
   c. Confidentiality
   d. Advocacy
7. A value is a personal belief about the worth of a given idea, attitude, custom, or object that sets standards that influence behavior.
8. Values clarification is the need to distinguish among values, facts, and opinions.
9. Deontology is a system of ethics that defines actions as right or wrong based on their "right-making characteristics such as fidelity to promises, truthfulness, and justice." It does not look at the consequences of actions.
10. Utilitarianism is when the value of something is determined by its usefulness; the main emphasis is on the outcome or consequence of actions.

11. Feminist ethics focus on inequalities between people; they look to the nature of relationships for guidance.
12. An ethic of care focuses on understanding relationships, especially personal narratives.
13. Case-based reasoning turns away from conventional principles of ethics as a way to determine best actions and focuses instead on an intimate understanding of particular situations.
14. a. Gather information relevant to the case.
    b. Clarify values.
    c. Verbalize the problem.
    d. Identify possible causes of action.
    e. Negotiate a plan.
    f. Evaluate the plan over time.
15. The ethics committee provides education, policy recommendations, and case consultation.
16. Quality-of-life measures the value and benefits of certain medical interventions, which is central to discussions in futile care, cancer therapy, and do not resuscitate (DNR).
17. Antidiscrimination laws enhance the economic security of people with physical, mental, or emotional challenges.
18. End-of-life care: Almost any intervention beyond symptom management and comfort measures is seen as futile.
19. 2. Ethical problems come from controversy and conflict.
20. 4. The ethics committee is an additional resource for patients and health care professionals.
21. 4. Incorporate as much information as possible from a variety of sources such as laboratory and test results; the clinical state of the patient; current literature about the condition; and the patient's religious, cultural, and family situation.

CHAPTER 23

1. e	5. c
2. h	6. g
3. f	7. d
4. b	8. a

9. Consumer rights and protection, affordable health care coverage, increase access to care, stronger Medicare
10. It protects the rights of people with disabilities. It also is the most extensive law on how employers must treat health care workers and patients infected with HIV.
11. The EMTALA states that when a patient comes to the emergency department or hospital, an appropriate medical screening occurs within the hospital's capacity. If an emergency exists, the hospital is not to discharge or transfer the patient until the condition stabilizes.
12. Requires compliance with Mental Health Parity and Addiction Equity Act and strengthens mental health services by requiring patients to obtain insurance
13. The Patient Self-Determination Act requires health care institutions to provide written information to patients concerning their rights under state law to

make decisions, including the right to refuse treatment and formulate advance directives.
14. Living wills are written documents that direct treatment in accordance with a patient's wishes in the event of a terminal illness or condition.
15. The Durable Power of Attorney for Health Care is a legal document that designates a person or persons of one's choosing to make health care decisions when the patient is no longer able to make decisions on his or her own behalf.
16. An individual older than the age of 18 years has the right to make an organ donation; the person needs to make the gift in writing with his or her signature.
17. HIPAA provides rights to patients (protects individuals from losing their health insurance when changing jobs by providing portability) and protects employees. It also establishes the basis for privacy and confidentiality.
18. In conjunction with HIPPA and in response to new technology and social media
19. a. Restraints should be used only to ensure the physical safety of the resident or other residents.
    b. Restraints should be used only when less restrictive interventions are not successful.
    c. Restraints should be used only on the written order of a physician, which includes a specific episode with start and end times.
20. The Board of Nursing licenses all RNs in the state in which they practice and can suspend or revoke a license if a nurse's conduct violates provisions in the licensing statute based on administrative law rules that implement and enforce the statute.
21. Good Samaritan laws encourage health care professionals to assist in emergencies, limit liability, and offer legal immunity for nurses who help at the scene of an accident.
22. Public health laws provide protection of the public's health, advocating for the rights of people, regulating health care and health care financing, and ensuring professional accountability for the care provided.
23. Determination of death requires irreversible cessation of circulatory and respiratory functions or that there is irreversible cessation of all functions of the entire brain, including the brainstem.
24. Statute that stated that a competent individual with a terminal disease could make an oral and written request for medication to end his or her life in a humane and dignified manner

25. d	30. c
26. g	31. f
27. e	32. j
28. h	33. b
29. i	34. a

35. a. The nurse (defendant) owed a duty to the patient (plaintiff).
    b. The nurse did not carry out that duty.
    c. The patient was injured.
    d. The nurse's failure to carry out the duty caused the injury.

36. a. Lacks the knowledge or skill needed
    b. Care exceeding the Nurse Practice Act is expected.
    c. Health of the nurse or her unborn child is directly threatened.
    d. Orientation to the unit has not been completed.
    e. Clearly states and documents a conscientious objection based on moral, ethical, or religious grounds
    f. Clinical judgment is impaired due to fatigue.
37. The nurse needs to inform the supervisor of any lack of experience in caring for the type of patients on the unit. The nurse also needs to request an orientation to the unit.
38. Nurses must follow the orders unless they believe the orders are in error or will harm the patients. If there is any controversy with the order, the nurse needs to also inform the supervising nurse or follow the established chain of command.
39. Risk management is a system of ensuring appropriate nursing care that attempts to identify potential hazards and eliminate them before harm occurs.
40. The occurrence (incident) report provides a database for further investigation in an attempt to determine deviations from standards of care; corrective measures are needed to prevent recurrence and to alert risk management to a potential claim situation.
41. 1. Determines the legal boundaries within each state
42. 3. Need to perform only those tasks that appear in the job description for a nurse's aide or assistant
43. 4. Conduct that falls below the standards of care
44. 1. Unintentional touching without consent
45. 4. Need to follow the institution's policies and procedures on how to handle these situations and use the chain of command

CHAPTER 24

1. Communication is a lifelong learning process that is an essential part of patient-centered nursing care.
2. a. Take the initiative in establishing and maintaining communication.
   b. Be authentic (one's self).
   c. Respond appropriately to the other person.
   d. Have a sense of mutuality.
   e. Believe that the nurse–patient relationship is a partnership with equal participants.
3. Perceptual biases are human tendencies that interfere with accurately perceiving and interpreting messages from others.
4. An assessment and communication technique that allows nurses to better understand and perceive the emotions of themselves and others
5. a. Patients who are silent or withdrawn and have difficulty expressing feelings or needs
   b. Patients who are sad and depressed
   c. Patients who require assistance with visual or speech disabilities
   d. Patients who are angry or confrontational and cannot listen to explanations

e. Patients who are uncooperative and resent being asked to help others
f. Patients who are talkative or lonely and want someone else to be with them all the time
g. Patients who are demanding and expect others to meet their requests
h. Patients who are frightened, anxious, and have difficulty coping
i. Patients who are confused and disoriented
j. Patients who speak and/or understand little English
k. Patients who are flirtatious or sexually inappropriate

6. c	16. m
7. d	17. a
8. e	18. h
9. a	19. b
10. b	20. i
11. g	21. k
12. c	22. n
13. f	23. e
14. j	24. d
15. l	

25. a. Voice tone
    b. Eye contact
    c. Body positioning
26. a. Intimate zone (0 to 18 inches)
    b. Personal zone (18 inches to 4 feet)
    c. Socioconsultative zone (9 to 12 feet)
    d. Public zone (12 feet and greater)
27. a. Preinteraction phase
    b. Orientation phase
    c. Working phase
    d. Termination phase
28. A technique for encouraging patients to share their thoughts, beliefs, fears, and concerns with the aim of changing their behaviors.
29. Many nursing situations, especially those in community and home care settings, require the nurse to form helping relationships with entire families.
30. Communication with other members of the health care team affects patient safety and the work environment.
31. Behaviors such as withholding information, backbiting, making snide remarks, nonverbal expressions of disapproval
32. a. Address the behavior when it occurs in a calm manner.
    b. Describe how the behavior affects your functioning.
    c. Ask for the abuse to stop.
    d. Notify the manager to get support for the situation.
    e. Make a plan for taking action in the future.
    f. Document the incidence in detail.
33. a. Courtesy
    b. Use of names
    c. Trustworthiness
    d. Autonomy and responsibility
    e. Assertiveness
34. a. Autonomy is being self-directed and independent in accomplishing goals and advocating for others.
    b. Assertiveness is expressing feelings and ideas without judging or hurting others.

35. a. Physiological status, emotional status, growth and development, unmet needs, attitudes and values, perceptions and personality, self-concept, self-esteem
   b. Social and working relationship, level of trust, level of caring, level of self-disclosure, shared history, balance of power and control
   c. Information exchange, goal achievement, problem resolution, expression of feelings
   d. Privacy level, noise level, comfort and safety level, distraction level
   e. Educational level, language and self-expression, customs and expectations
36. a. Make sure the patient knows that you are talking.
   b. Face the patient with your face/mouth visible and don't chew gum.
   c. Speak clearly, do not shout.
   d. Speak slowly.
   e. Check for hearing aids, etc.
   f. Quiet, well-lit environment with minimal distraction
   g. Allow time for the patient to respond.
   h. Give the patient a chance to ask questions.
   i. Keep communication short and to the point.
37. a. Understand your own cultural values and biases.
   b. Assess the patient's primary language and level of fluency in English.
   c. Provide a professional interpreter, do not use the family.
   d. Speak directly to the patient even if using an interpreter.
   e. Nodding of head or "OK" does not mean the patient understands.
   f. Provide written information in English and primary language.
   g. Learn about cultures that are common in your work area.
   h. Incorporate the patient's communication methods or needs into the plan of care.
38. a. Men tend to use less verbal communication but are more likely to initiate communication and address issues more directly.
   b. Women disclose more personal information and use more active listening.
39. Impaired verbal communication (state in which the individual's experiences are decreased, delayed, or absent or the person has an inability to receive, process, transmit, and use symbols)
40. Defining characteristics are the inability to articulate words, inappropriate verbalization, difficulty forming words, and difficulty in comprehending.
41. Related factors can be physiological, mechanical, anatomical, psychological, cultural, or developmental in nature.
42. a. Patient initiates conversation about the diagnosis.
   b. Patient is able to attend to appropriate stimuli.
   c. Patient conveys clear and understandable messages with health team.
   d. Patient will express increased satisfaction with the communication process.

43. e
44. g
45. m
46. o
47. f
48. a
49. p
50. n
51. l
52. k
53. b
54. j
55. i
56. c
57. d
58. h
59. g
60. k
61. j
62. f
63. h
64. c
65. e
66. d
67. a
68. i
69. b

70. Listen attentively, do not interrupt, ask simple questions, allow time, use visual cues, use communication aids.
71. Use simple sentences, ask one question at a time, allow time for patient to respond, be an attentive listener, include family and friends.
72. Check for hearing aids, reduce environmental noise, get patient's attention, face the patient, do not chew gum, speak in a normal voice, rephrase, provide sign language.
73. Check for glasses, identify yourself, speak in a normal tone, do not rely on gestures or nonverbal communication, use indirect lighting, use 14-point print.
74. Call the patient by name, verbally and by touch; speak to patient as though the patient can hear; explain all procedures; provide orientation.
75. Speak to the patient in normal tone, establish a method to signal the desire to communicate, provide an interpreter, avoid using family members, develop communication aids.
76. a. Determine whether he encourages openness and allow the patient to "tell his story" expressing both thoughts and feelings.
   b. Identify any missed verbal or nonverbal cues or conversational themes.
   c. Examine whether nursing responses blocked or facilitated the patient's efforts to communicate.
   d. Determine whether nursing responses were positive and supportive or superficial and judgmental.
   e. Examine the type and number of questions asked.
   f. Determine the type and number of therapeutic communication techniques used.
   g. Discover any missed opportunities to use humor, silence, or touch.
77. 4. Means of conveying and receiving messages through visual, auditory, and tactile senses
78. 1. Awareness of the tone of verbal response and the nonverbal behavior results in further exploration.
79. 3. The connotative meaning of a word is influenced by the thoughts, feelings, or ideas people have about the word
80. 3. Motivates one person to communicate with the other
81. 4. Personal zone when taking a patient's history

CHAPTER 25

1. The nurse is a visible, competent resource for patients who want to improve their physical and psychological well-being. In the school, home, clinic, or workplace, nurses provide information and skills that allow patients to assume healthier behaviors.

2. As the nurse, you learn to identify patients' willingness to learn and motivate interest in learning. Injured or ill patients need information and skills to help them regain or maintain their levels of health.

3. New knowledge and skills are often necessary for patients to continue ADLs and learn to cope with permanent health alterations.

4. c
5. h
6. f
7. i
8. g
9. e
10. a
11. d
12. b

13. Need to know a patient's level of knowledge and intellectual skills before beginning a teaching plan

14. Learning in children depends on the child's maturation; intellectual growth moves from the concrete to the abstract as the child matures. Information presented to children needs to be understandable and based on the child's developmental stage.

15. Adults tend to be self-directed learners; they often become dependent in new learning situations. The amount of information provided and the amount of time varies depending on the patient's personal situation and readiness to learn.

16. To learn psychomotor skills, the following physical characteristics are necessary: size, strength, coordination, and sensory acuity.

17. a. The nursing process requires assessment of all sources to date to determine a patient's total health care needs.
    b. The teaching process focuses on the patient's learning needs and willingness and capability to learn.

18. a. Information or skills needed by the patient to perform self-care and to understand the implications of a health problem
    b. Patient's experiences that influence the need to learn
    c. Information that the family members require

19. a. Behavior
    b. Health beliefs and sociocultural background
    c. Perception of severity and susceptibility of a health problem and the benefits and barriers to treatment
    d. Perceived ability to perform behaviors
    e. Desire to learn
    f. Attitudes about providers
    g. Learning style preference

20. a. Physical strength, movement, dexterity, and coordination
    b. Sensory deficits

c. Reading level
d. Developmental level
e. Cognitive function
f. Physical symptoms that interfere

21. a. Distractions or persistent noise
    b. Comfort of the room
    c. Room facilities and available equipment

22. a. Willingness to have family members and others involved in the teaching plan
    b. Family members' perceptions and understanding of the illness and its implications
    c. Willingness and ability to participate in care
    d. Financial or material resources
    e. Teaching tools

23. Functional illiteracy is the inability to read above a fifth-grade level.

24. The nurse assesses information related to the patient's ability and need to learn, and interprets data and cluster-defining characteristics to form diagnoses that reflect the patient's specific learning needs. This ensures that teaching will be goal directed and individualized.

25. Identify what a patient needs to achieve to gain a better understanding of the information provided and better manage their illness

26. Priorities should be based on the patient's immediate needs (perception of what is most important, anxiety level, and amount of time available), nursing diagnoses, and the goals and outcomes established for the patient.

27. Time the teaching for when a patient is most attentive, receptive, and alert and organize the activities to provide time for rest and teaching–learning interactions.

28. Organize teaching material into a logical sequence progressing from simple to complex ideas.

29. c
30. e
31. i
32. j
33. h
34. a
35. g
36. d
37. f
38. b

39. The nurse is legally responsible for providing accurate, timely patient information that promotes continuity of care. Documentation of patient teaching supports quality improvement efforts and promotes third-party reimbursement.

40. 2. An internal impulse is a force acting on or within a person that causes the person to behave in a particular way.

41. 4. Psychomotor learning involves acquiring skills that integrate mental and muscular activity.

42. 4. Mr. Jones. A mild level of anxiety motivates learning, but a high level of anxiety prevents learning from occurring.

43. 3. Complicated skills, such as learning to use a syringe, require considerable practice but are developmentally appropriate for school-age children.

44. 4. The objective describes an appropriate and achievable skill that the patient can be expected to master within a realistic time frame.

CHAPTER 26

1. Produces a written account of pertinent patient data, nursing clinical decision and interventions, and patient responses in a health care record
2. c
5. b
3. e
6. d
4. f
7. a
8. a. A positive impact on the quality of patient care through interdisciplinary collaboration with improved data availability
   b. Improve patient safety through the use of clinical decision support
9. a. Providers are required to notify patients of their privacy policy and make a reasonable effort to get written acknowledgment of this notification.
   b. HIPAA requires that disclosure or requests regarding health information are limited to the minimum necessary.
10. The standards of documentation by The Joint Commission require documentation within the context of the nursing process, as well as evidence of patient and family teaching and discharge planning.
11. A factual record contains descriptive, objective information about what a nurse sees, hears, feels, and smells.
12. An accurate record uses exact measurements, contains concise data, contains only approved abbreviations, uses correct spelling, and identifies the date and caregiver.
13. A complete record contains all appropriate and essential information.
14. Current records contain timely entries with immediate documentation of information as it is collected from the patient
15. Organized records communicate information in a logical order.
16. j
24. a
17. c
25. d
18. i
26. d
19. f
27. c
20. h
28. e
21. g
29. b
22. e
30. f
23. b
31. a
32. With telephone reports, the nurse includes when the call was made, who made it, who was called, to whom information was given, what information was given, and what information was received.
33. a. Clearly determine the patient's name, room number, and diagnosis.
   b. Repeat all prescribed orders back to the physician.
   c. Use clarification questions.
   d. Write TO or VO, including the date and time, name of the patient, and the complete order, and sign the physician name and the nurse.
   e. Follow agency policies.
34. An incident or occurrence is any event that is not consistent with the routine operation of a health care unit or routine care of a patient. Examples include patient falls, needle-stick injuries, a visitor with an illness, medication errors, accidental omission of therapies, and any circumstances that lead to patient injury.
35. Health informatics is the application of computer and information science in all biomedical sciences to facilitate acquisition, processing, interpretation, optimal use, and communication.
36. Nursing informatics integrates nursing science, computer science, and information science to manage and communicate data, information, and knowledge in nursing practice.
37. a. Nursing process, NANDA, NIC, and NOC
   b. Protocol or critical pathway
38. a. Better access to information
   b. Enhanced quality of documentation
   c. Reduced errors of omission
   d. Reduced hospital costs
   e. Increased nurse job satisfaction
   f. Compliance with requirements of accrediting agencies
   g. Development of a common clinical database
   h. Enhanced ability to track records
39. 4. The patient's medical record should be the most current and accurate continuous source of information about the patient's health care status.
40. 4. When recording subjective data, document the patient's exact words within quotation marks whenever possible.
41. 2. An effective change-of-shift report describes each patient's health status and lets staff on the next shift know what care the patients will require.
42. 3. An incident is any event that is not consistent with the routine operation of a health care unit or routine care of a patient.
43. 3. Do not erase, apply correction fluid, or scratch out errors made while recording; it may appear as if you were attempting to hide information or deface the record.

CHAPTER 27

1. a. Identify patients correctly
   b. Improve staff communication
   c. Use medicines safely
   d. Use alarms safely
   e. Prevent infection
   f. Prevent mistakes in surgery
2. a. Oxygen
   b. Nutrition
   c. Optimum temperature
3. a. MVAs (leading cause)
   b. Poison
   c. Falls
   d. Fire
   e. Disasters
4. Any microorganism capable of producing an illness with the most common means of transmission by the hands
5. Reduces and in some cases prevents the transmission of disease from person to person

6. A harmful chemical or waste material discharged into the water, soil, or air
7. a. Patient's developmental level
   b. Mobility, sensory, and cognitive status
   c. Lifestyle choices
   d. Knowledge of common safety precautions
8. a. Lifestyle
   b. Impaired mobility
   c. Sensory or communication impairment
   d. Lack of sensory awareness
9. a. Falls
   b. Patient-inherent accidents (seizures, burns, inflicted cuts)
   c. Procedure-related accidents (medication administrations, improper procedures)
   d. Equipment-related accidents (rapid IV infusions, electrical hazards)
10. a. Activity and exercise
    b. Medication history
    c. History of falls
    d. Home maintenance
11. a. Impaired home maintenance
    b. Risk for injury
    c. Deficient knowledge
    d. Risk for poisoning
    e. Risk for suffocation
    f. Risk for trauma
12. a. Demonstrate effective use of technology and standardized practices that support safety and quality.
    b. Demonstrate effective use of strategies to reduce the risk of harm to self or others.
    c. Use appropriate strategies to reduce reliance on memory.
13. Table 27-1, p. 385.
14. Table 27-1, p. 386.
15. Table 27-1, p. 386.
16. Table 27-1, p. 386.
17. Assist them in making lifestyle modifications by referring them to resources
18. Box 27-8, p. 387
19. a. Basic needs related to oxygen, nutrition and temperature
    b. General preventive measures
20. a. On admission
    b. Routinely until discharge
21. A physical restraint is any manual method, physical or mechanical device, material, or equipment that immobilizes or reduces the ability of a patient to move his or her arms, legs, body, or head freely.
22. Medications used to manage a patient's behavior that are not a standard treatment or dosage for the patient's condition
23. a. Reduce the risk of patient injury from falls.
    b. Prevent interruption of therapy.
    c. Prevent a confused or combative patient from removing life support equipment.
    d. Reduce the risk of injury to others by the patient.
24. a. R—Rescue and remove all patients in immediate danger.
    b. A—Activate the alarm.

c. C—Confine the fire by closing doors and windows and turning off oxygen and electrical equipment.
d. E—Extinguish the fire using an extinguisher.
25. Seizure precautions are nursing interventions to protect patients from traumatic injury, positioning for adequate ventilation and drainage of oral secretions, and providing privacy and support after the event.
26. The nurse limits the time spent near the source, makes the distance from the source as great as possible, and uses shielding devices.
27. a. The identification of possible emergency situations and their probable impact
    b. The maintenance of an adequate amount of supplies
    c. A formal response plan for staff and hospital operations to restore essential services and resume normal operations
28. 3. An individual's safety is most threatened when physiological needs are not met, including the need for water, oxygen, basic nutrition, and optimum temperature.
29. 4. Older adulthood is the developmental stage that carries the highest risk of an injury from a fall because of the physiological changes that occur during the aging process, which increase the patient's risk for falls.
30. 3. The nurse should use the RACE to set priorities in case of fire. Rescue and remove all patients in immediate danger first.
31. a. Ms. Cohen states, "I bump into things, and I'm afraid I'm going to fall." Cabinets in her kitchen are disorganized and full of breakable items that could fall out. Throw rugs are on the floors, bathroom lighting is poor (40-watt bulbs), her bathtub lacks safety strips or grab bars; and her home is cluttered with furniture and small objects. Ms. Cohen has kyphosis and has a hesitant, uncoordinated gait. She frequently holds walls for support. Ms. Cohen's left arm and leg are weaker than those on the right. Ms. Cohen has trouble reading and seeing familiar objects at a distance while wearing current glasses.
    b. Basic human needs, potential risks to patient, developmental stage, influence of medication or illness
    c. In the case of safety, the nurse integrates knowledge from previous experiences in caring for patients who had an injury or were at risk.
    d. The American Nurses Association's standards for nursing practice address the nurse's responsibility in maintaining patient safety, agency practice standards, and The Joint Commission's patient safety goals.
    e. Critical thinking attitudes such as perseverance and creativity, collection of unbiased accurate data regarding threats to the patient's safety, and a thorough review of the patient's home environment would be applicable in this case.

CHAPTER 28

1. d
2. c
3. a
4. b

5. Connections between bones—cartilaginous, fibrous, and synovial
6. Aid joint flexibility and support
7. Connect muscle to bone
8. Nonvascular and support connective tissue
9. Contract and relax are the working elements of movement.
10. Regulates movement and posture
11. a. Impaired body alignment, balance, and mobility
    b. Weakness and wasting of muscles, which increase disability and deformity; bruises, contusions, fractures
    c. Impaired body alignment, balance and mobility
12. A person's ability to move about freely
13. The inability to move freely
14. Cells and the tissue reduce in size and function in response to prolonged inactivity resulting from bedrest, trauma, casting, or local nerve damage.
15. Decreases the metabolic rate; alters the metabolism of CHO, fats, and proteins; causes fluid and electrolyte and calcium imbalances; and causes GI disturbances
16. a. Collapse of alveoli
    b. Inflammation of the lung from stasis or pooling of secretions
17. a. A drop in blood pressure greater than 20 mmHg in systolic pressure or 10 mmHg in diastolic pressure
    b. Accumulation of platelets, fibrin, clotting factors, and cellular elements of the blood attached to the interior wall of a vein or artery that occludes the lumen of the vessel
18. a. Loss of endurance, strength, and muscle mass and decreased stability and balance
    b. Impaired calcium metabolism
    c. Impaired joint mobility
    d. Osteoporosis
    e. Joint contractures
    f. Footdrop
19. a. Urinary stasis (renal pelvis fills before urine enters the ureters)
    b. Renal calculi (calcium stones that lodge in the renal pelvis)
20. Pressure ulcers (impairment of the skin as a result of prolonged ischemia in tissues)
21. a. Emotional and behavioral responses
    b. Sensory alterations
    c. Changes in coping
22. Delays the child's gross motor skills, intellectual development, or musculoskeletal development
23. Social isolation
24. Physiological systems are at risk, loss of job
25. Weaker bones, increased risk of falls, increased physical dependence on others
26. a. The maximum amount of movement available at a joint in one of the three planes of the body: sagittal, frontal, or transverse; exercises are active and passive
    b. Particular manner or style of walking; mechanics involve coordination of skeletal, neurological, and muscular systems

c. Physical activity for conditioning the body, improving health, and maintaining fitness
d. Determines normal physiological changes, identifies deviations, learning needs, trauma, and risk factors
27. Inspection (muscle atrophy), anthropometric measurements (decreased amounts of subcutaneous fat), palpation (edema)
28. Inspection (asymmetrical chest wall movement), auscultation (crackles)
29. Auscultation (orthostatic hypotension), palpation (peripheral pulses)
30. Inspection (decreased range of motion), palpation (joint contracture)
31. Inspection (break in skin integrity), palpation (skin)
32. Inspection (decreased urine output), palpation (distended abdomen), auscultation (decreased bowel sounds)
33. a. Ineffective Airway Clearance
    b. Ineffective Coping
    c. Impaired Physical Mobility
    d. Impaired Urinary Elimination
    e. Risk for Impaired Skin Integrity
    f. Risk for Disuse Syndrome
    g. Social Isolation
34. a. Skin color and temperature return to normal baseline within 20 minutes of position change.
    b. Changes position at least every 2 hours
35. a. Prevention of work-related injury
    b. Fall prevention measures
    c. Exercise
    d. Early detection of scoliosis
36. a. A high-protein, high-caloric diet
    b. Vitamin B and C supplements
37. a. Deep breathe and cough every 1 or 2 hours
    b. Chest physiotherapy (CPT)
    c. Ensure intake of 1400 mL/day of fluid
38. a. Reduce orthostatic hypotension; early mobilization
    b. Reduce cardiac workload; avoid Valsalva movements
    c. Prevent thrombus formation; prophylaxis (heparin, SCDs, and TEDs)
39. a. Perform active and passive ROM exercises
    b. CPM machines
40. a. Positioning and skin care
    b. Use of therapeutic devices to relieve pressure
41. a. Well hydrated
    b. Prevent urinary stasis and calculi and infections
42. a. Anticipate change in the patient's status and provide routine and informal socialization
    b. Stimuli to maintain patient's orientation
43. a. Prevents external rotation of the hips when the patient is in supine position
    b. Maintain the thumb in slight adduction and in opposition to the fingers
    c. Allows the patient to pull with the upper extremities to raise the trunk off the bed, assist in transfer, or to perform exercises
44. a. Head of bed (HOB) elevated 45 to 60 degrees and the knees are slightly elevated

b. Rest on their backs; all body parts are in relation to each other

c. Lies face or chest down

d. The patient rests on the side with body weight on the dependent hip and shoulder.

e. Patient places the weight on the anterior ileum humerus and clavicle.

45. Activities beyond ADLs that are necessary to be independent in society

46. Always stand on the patient's affected side and support the patient by using a gait belt.

47. 1. Footdrop. Allowing the foot to be dorsiflexed at the ankles prevents this.

48. 3. Immobility causing decreased lung elastic recoiling and secretions accumulating in portions of the lungs

49. 1. Homan's sign is no longer a reliable indicator in assessing for DVT.

50. 4. This technique produces a forceful, productive cough without excessive fatigue.

CHAPTER 29

1. d	9. a
2. m	10. f
3. o	11. j
4. l	12. b
5. g	13. e
6. n	14. h
7. k	15. c
8. p	16. i

17. a. An infectious agent or pathogen
    b. A reservoir or source
    c. A portal of exit from the reservoir
    d. A mode of transmission
    e. A portal of entry to a host
    f. A susceptible host

18. a. Person-to-person or physical source and susceptible host
    b. Personal contact of a susceptible host with a contaminated inanimate object
    c. Large particles that travel up to 3 feet and come in contact with the host
    d. Droplets that suspend in the air
    e. Contaminated items
    f. Internal and external transmissions

19. a. Incubation period: Interval between entrance of the pathogen into the body and appearance of the first symptoms
    b. Prodromal stage: Onset of nonspecific signs and symptoms to more specific symptoms
    c. Illness stage: Manifests signs and symptoms to type of infection
    d. Convalescence: Acute symptoms of infection disappear

20. a. Patient experiences localized symptoms such as pain, tenderness, warmth, and redness at the wound site
    b. An infection that affects the entire body instead of just a single organ and can become fatal if undetected

21. a. The body contains microorganisms that reside on the surface and deep layers of the skin, in saliva and oral mucosa, and in the intestinal walls and genitourinary tract that maintain health.
    b. The skin, mouth, eyes, respiratory tract, urinary tract, genitourinary tract, and vagina have unique defenses against infection.
    c. Inflammation is the body's response to injury, infection, or irritation. It is a protective vascular reaction that delivers fluid, blood products, and nutrients to an area of injury.

22. a. Acute inflammation: Rapid vasodilatation that causes redness at the site and localized warmth, allowing phagocytosis to occur
    b. Inflammatory exudate is the accumulation of fluid and dead tissue cells; WBCs form at the site. Exudate may be serous, sanguineous, or purulent.
    c. Healing involves the defensive, reconstructive, and maturative stages.

23. a. Exogenous infection comes from microorganisms outside the individual that do not exist in normal floras.
    b. Endogenous infection occurs when part of the patient's flora becomes altered and an overgrowth results.

24. a. Urinary tract
    b. Surgical or traumatic wounds
    c. Respiratory tract
    d. Bloodstream

25. a. Infants have immature defenses, breastfed babies have greater immunity, viruses are common in middle-aged adults, older adult cell-mediated immunity declines
    b. A reduction in the intake of protein, carbohydrates, and fats reduces the body's defenses and impairs wound healing.
    c. Basal metabolic rate increases; increase serum glucose levels and decrease anti-inflammatory responses with elevated cortisone levels
    d. People with diseases of the immune system (leukemia, AIDS) and chronic diseases (AODM) have weakened defenses against infection.

26. a. COPD, heart failure
    b. Communicable/infectious diseases
    c. Health care worker
    d. Invasive radiology
    e. Sickle cell disease
    f. West Nile virus
    g. Fractures
    h. Obesity

27. See Table 29-4, p. 451

28. a. Risk for Infection
    b. Imbalanced Nutrition
    c. Impaired Oral Mucous Membrane
    d. Impaired Skin Integrity
    e. Social Isolation
    f. Impaired Tissue Integrity

29. a. Preventing exposure to infectious organisms
    b. Controlling or reducing the extent of infection

c. Maintaining resistance to infection

d. Verbalizing understanding of infection prevention and control techniques

30. a. Nutrition

b. Rest

c. Maintenance of physiological protective mechanisms

d. Recommended immunizations

e. Eliminate reservoirs of infection

f. Controlling ports of exit and entry

g. Methods to control the spread of microorganisms: Proper use of sterile supplies, barrier precautions, standard precautions, transmission-based precautions, and hand hygiene

31. a. The absence of pathogenic microorganisms; the technique refers to the practices or procedures that assist in reducing the risk for infection.

b. Clean technique: Hand hygiene, using clean gloves, cleaning the environment routinely

32. a. Hand hygiene includes washing hands with soap and water followed by a stream of water.

b. Alcohol-based hand rubs are recommended by Centers for Disease Control and Prevention to improve hand hygiene practices, protect health care workers' hands, and reduce pathogens to patients.

c. Disinfection is a process that eliminates many or all microorganisms with the exception of bacterial spores from inanimate objects.

d. Sterilization is the complete elimination or destruction of all microorganisms, including spores.

33. a. When bathing, use soap and water to remove drainage, dried secretions, and excess perspiration.

b. Change dressings when they are wet or soiled.

c. Place tissues, soiled dressings, or soiled linen in fluid-resistant bags

d. Place all needles, safety needles, and needleless systems into puncture-proof containers.

e. Keep surfaces clean and dry.

f. Do not leave bottle solutions open; date and discard them in 24 hours.

g. Keep drainage tubes and collection bags patent.

h. Wear gloves and protective eyewear and empty all drainage systems at the end of the shift.

34. a. Education of health care facility staff and visitors

b. Posters and written material for agency and visitors

c. Education on how to cover your nose and mouth when you cough, using a tissue, and the prompt disposal of the contaminated tissue

d. Placing a surgical mask on the patient if it will not compromise respiratory function or is applicable

e. Hand hygiene after contact with contaminated respiratory secretions

f. Spatial separation greater than 3 feet from persons with respiratory infections

35. Standard precautions are designed for all patients in all settings regardless of the diagnosis; they apply to contact with blood, body fluid, nonintact skin, and mucous membranes.

36. Isolation precautions are based on the mode of transmission of disease. They are termed airborne; droplet; contact; and a new category, protective environment.

37. Gowns prevent soiling clothing during contact with patients.

38. A full-face protection when you anticipate splashing or spraying of blood or bloody fluid into your face and a mask to satisfy droplet or airborne precautions

39. Protective eyewear should be worn for procedures that generate splashes or splatters.

40. Gloves prevent the transmission of pathogens by direct and indirect contact.

41. a. Wounds

b. Blood

c. Stool

d. Urine

42. a. Provide staff and patient education.

b. Develop and review infection prevention and control policies and procedures.

c. Recommend appropriate isolation procedures.

d. Screen patient records.

e. Consult with health departments.

f. Gather statistics regarding the epidemiology.

g. Notify the public health department of incidences of communicable diseases.

h. Consult with all departments to investigate unusual events or clusters.

i. Monitor antibiotic-resistant organisms.

43. a. During procedures that require intentional perforation of the patient's skin

b. When the skin's integrity is broken

c. During procedures that involve insertion of catheters

44. a. A sterile object remains sterile only when touched by another sterile object.

b. Place only sterile objects on a sterile field.

c. A sterile object or field out of the range of vision or an object held below a person's waist is contaminated.

d. A sterile object or field becomes contaminated by prolonged exposure to air.

e. When a sterile surface comes in contact with a wet, contaminated surface, the sterile object or field becomes contaminated by capillary action.

f. Because fluid flows in the direction of gravity, a sterile object becomes contaminated if gravity causes a contaminated liquid to flow over the object's surface.

g. The edges of a sterile field or container are considered to be contaminated.

45. a. Assemble all equipment.

b. Don caps, masks, and eyewear.

c. Open sterile packages.

d. Open sterile items on a flat surface.

e. Open a sterile item while holding it.

f. Prepare a sterile field.

g. Pour sterile solutions.

h. Surgical scrub.

i. Apply sterile gloves.

j. Don a sterile gown.

46. a. Monitor patients postoperatively, including surgical sites, invasive sites, the respiratory tract, and the urinary tract.
    b. Examine all invasive and surgical sites for swelling, erythema, or purulent drainage.
    c. Monitor breath sounds.
    d. Review laboratory results.
47. 3. Infection occurs in a cycle that depends on the presence of certain elements.
48. 1. The incubation period is the interval between the entrance of the pathogen into the body and appearance of first symptoms.
49. 1. Iatrogenic infections are a type of health care-associated infection (HAI) caused by an invasive diagnostic or therapeutic procedure.
50. 1. If moisture leaks through a sterile package's protective covering, organisms can travel to the sterile object.
51. 1. Patients who are transported outside of their rooms need to wear surgical masks to protect other patients and personnel.

CHAPTER 30

1. a. The nurse may delegate the measurement of vital signs but is responsible for analyzing and interpreting their significance and selecting appropriate interventions.
   b. Equipment needs to be appropriate and functional.
   c. Equipment needs to be based on the patient's condition and characteristics.
   d. Know the patient's usual range of vital signs.
   e. Know the patient's medical history.
   f. Control or minimize environmental factors.
   g. Use a systematic approach.
   h. Collaborate with health care providers to decide on the frequency.
   i. Use measurements to determine the indications for medication administration.
   j. Analyze the results.
   k. Verify and communicate significant changes with the patient's health care provider.
   l. Develop a teaching plan.
2. h   7. g
3. j   8. b
4. f   9. i
5. e   10. c
6. a   11. d
12. Visible perspiration primarily occurring on forehead and upper thorax
13. a. Insulation of the body
    b. Vasoconstriction
    c. Temperature sensation
14. a. The degree of temperature extreme
    b. The person's ability to sense feeling comfortable or uncomfortable
    c. Thought processes or emotions
    d. Person's mobility or ability to remove or add clothes
15. a. Age
    b. Exercise

c. Hormone level
d. Circadian rhythm
e. Stress
f. Environment
g. Temperature alterations (fever, hyperthermia, heat stroke, heat exhaustion, hypothermia)
16. e   20. c
17. h   21. g
18. b   22. d
19. f   23. a
24. Examples of answers can be found in Box 30-4, p. 493.
25. a. Subtract 32 from the Fahrenheit reading and multiply the result by 5/9.
    b. Multiply the Celsius reading by 9/5 and add 32 to the product.
26. a. Risk for Imbalanced Body Temperature
    b. Hyperthermia
    c. Hypothermia
    d. Ineffective Thermoregulation
27. a. Regain normal range of body temperature.
    b. Obtain appropriate clothing to wear in cold weather.
28. Those at risk include the very young and very old; persons debilitated by trauma, stroke, or diabetes; those who are intoxicated by drugs or alcohol; patients with sepsis; and those who have inadequate home heating and shelter. Fatigue, dark skin color, malnutrition, and hypoxemia also increase the risk.
29. a. Children have immature temperature-control mechanisms, so their temperatures can rise rapidly, and they are at risk for fluid-volume deficit.
    b. Drug fevers are often accompanied by other allergy symptoms such as rash or pruritus.
30. a. Pharmacologic therapy includes nonsteroidal drugs and corticosteroids.
    b. Nonpharmacologic therapy includes tepid sponge baths, bathing with alcohol water solutions, applying ice packs to the axillae and groin sites, and cooling fans.
31. Move the patient to a cooler environment; remove excess body clothing; place cool, wet towels over the skin; and use fans.
32. Remove wet clothes; wrap the patient in blankets.
33. Body temperature will return to an acceptable range, other vital signs will stabilize, and the patient will report a sense of comfort.
34. a. Radial
    b. Apical
35. See Table 30-2, p. 498.
36. a. When assessing the radial pulse, consider rate, rhythm, strength, and equality.
    b. When assessing the apical pulse, consider rate and rhythm only.
37. a. 120 to 160
    b. 90 to 140
    c. 80 to 110
    d. 75 to 100
    e. 60 to 90
    f. 60 to 100

38. See answers in Table 30-4, p. 499.
39. Tachycardia is an abnormal elevated heart rate (>100 beats/min in adults).
40. Bradycardia is a slow rate (<60 beats/min in adults).
41. Pulse deficit is an inefficient contraction of the heart that fails to transmit a pulse wave to the peripheral site; it is the difference between the apical and the radial pulse rate.
42. A dysrhythmia is an abnormal rhythm, including early, late, or missed beats.
43. Ventilation is the movement of gases in and out of the lungs.
44. Diffusion is the movement of oxygen and carbon dioxide between the alveoli and the red blood cells.
45. Perfusion is the distribution of red blood cells to and from the pulmonary capillaries.
46. Hypoxemia is low levels of arterial O_2.
47. a. Active
    b. Passive
48. See Box 30-7, p. 501.
49. a. 30 to 60
    b. 30 to 50
    c. 25 to 32
    d. 20 to 30
    e. 16 to 20
    f. 12 to 20
50. Rate of breathing is regular but slow; <12 breaths/min.
51. Rate of breathing is regular but rapid; >20 breaths/min.
52. Respirations are labored and increased in depth, and the rate is >20 breaths/min.
53. Respirations cease for several seconds.
54. Rate and depth of respirations increase.
55. Respiratory rate is abnormally low, and depth of ventilation is depressed.
56. Respiratory rate and depth are irregular; alternating periods of apnea and hyperventilation.
57. Kussmaul respirations are abnormally deep, regular, and increased in rate.
58. Biot respirations are abnormally shallow for two or three breaths followed by an irregular period of apnea.
59. SaO_2 is the percentage of hemoglobin that is bound with oxygen in the arteries and is the percent of saturation of hemoglobin; normal range is usually between 95% and 100%.
60. Blood pressure is the force exerted on the walls of an artery by the pulsing blood under pressure from the heart.
61. Systolic pressure is the peak of maximum pressure when ejection occurs.
62. Diastolic pressure occurs when the ventricles relax; the blood remaining in the arteries exerts a minimum pressure.
63. Pulse pressure is the difference between systolic and diastolic pressure.
64. Cardiac output increases as a result of an increase in heart rate, greater heart muscle contractility, or an increase in blood volume.

65. Peripheral resistance is the resistance to blood flow determined by the tone of vascular musculature and diameter of blood vessels.
66. The volume of blood circulating within the vascular system affects blood pressure, which normally remains constant.
67. Viscosity is the thickness that affects the ease with which blood flows through blood vessels, determined by the hematocrit.
68. With reduced elasticity, there is greater resistance to blood flow, and the systemic pressure rises (systolic pressure).
69. a. Age
    b. Stress
    c. Ethnicity
    d. Gender
    e. Daily variations
    f. Medications
    g. Activity and weight
    h. Smoking
70. a. 40 (mean) mm Hg
    b. 85/54 mm Hg
    c. 95/65 mm Hg
    d. 105/65 mm Hg
    e. 110/65 mm Hg
    f. 119/75 mm Hg
    g. <120/80 mm Hg
71. Family history, obesity, cigarette smoking, heavy alcohol consumption, high sodium, sedentary lifestyle, exposure to continuous stress, diabetics, older, African Americans
72. Dehydrated, anemic, experienced prolonged bed rest, recent blood loss, medications
73. First: Clear, rhythmic tapping corresponding to the pulse rate that gradually increases in intensity (systolic pressure)
    Second: Blowing or swishing sound as the cuff deflates
    Third: A crisper and more intense tapping
    Fourth: Muffled and low-pitched as the cuff is further deflated (diastolic pressure in infants and children)
    Fifth: The disappearance of sound (diastolic pressure in adolescents and adults)
74. See Box 30-13, 511.
75. 4. The skin regulates the temperature through insulation of the body, vasoconstriction, and temperature sensation.
76. 3. The transfer of heat from one object to another with direct contact (solids, liquids, and gases)
77. 3. Victims of heat stroke do not sweat.
78. 2. 156 is the onset of the first Korotkoff sound (systolic pressure), and 88 is the fifth sound that corresponds with the diastolic pressure.

CHAPTER 31

1. a. Gather baseline data about the patient's health status.
   b. Support or refute subjective data obtained in the nursing history.

c. Confirm and identify nursing diagnoses.

d. Make clinical decisions about a patient's changing health status and management.

e. Evaluate the outcomes of care.

2. a. A head-to-toe physical assessment is required daily.

b. Reassessment is performed when the patient's condition changes as it improves or worsens.

c. The environment, equipment, and patient are properly prepared.

d. Safety for confused patients should be a priority.

3. a. Infection control

b. Environment

c. Equipment

d. Physical preparation of the patient

e. Psychological preparation of the patient

4. a. Gather all or part of the histories of infants and children from parents or guardians.

b. Gain a child's trust before doing any type of examination, perform the exam in a nonthreatening area, talk and play first, and do the visual parts of the exam first.

c. Offer support to the parents during the examination and do not pass judgment.

d. Call children by their first names and address the parents as Mr. and Mrs.

e. Treat adolescents as adults, provide confidentiality for adolescents; speak alone with them.

5. a. Do not stereotype about aging patients' level of cognition.

b. Be sensitive to sensory or physical limitations (more time).

c. Adequate space is needed.

d. Use patience, allow for pauses, and observe for details.

e. Certain types of information may be stressful to give.

f. Perform the examination near bathroom facilities.

g. Be alert for signs of increasing fatigue.

6. a. Compare both sides for symmetry.

b. If a patient is ill, first assess the systems of the body part most at risk.

c. Offer rest periods if the patient becomes fatigued.

d. Perform painful procedures near the end of the examination.

e. Record assessments in specific terms in the record.

f. Use common and accepted medical terms and abbreviations.

g. Record quick notes during the examination to avoid delays.

7. Inspection is looking, listening, and smelling to distinguish normal from abnormal findings.

8. a. Adequate lighting is available.

b. Use a direct light source.

c. Inspect each area for size, shape, color, symmetry, position, and abnormality.

d. Position and expose body parts as needed, maintaining privacy.

e. Check for side-to-side symmetry.

f. Validate findings with the patient.

9. Palpation involves using the hands to touch body parts.

10. a. Light palpation involves pressing inward 1 cm (superficial).

b. Deep palpation involves depressing the area 4 cm to assess the conditions of organs.

11. Tapping the skin with the fingertips to vibrate underlying tissues and organs

12. Auscultation is listening to the internal sounds the body makes.

13. a. Frequency indicates the number of sound wave cycles generated per second by a vibrating object.

b. Amplitude describes the loudness, soft to loud.

c. Quality describes sounds of similar frequency and loudness.

d. Duration describes length of time that sound vibrations last.

14. a. Gender and race

b. Age

c. Signs of distress

d. Body type

e. Posture

f. Gait

g. Body movements

h. Hygiene and grooming

i. Dress

j. Body odor

k. Affect and mood

l. Speech

m. Signs of patient abuse

n. Substance abuse

15. Physical injury or neglect are signs of possible abuse (evidence of malnutrition or presence of bruising). Also watch for fear of the spouse or partner, caregiver, or parent.

16. C: Have you ever felt the need to cut down on your use?

A: Have people annoyed you by criticizing your use?

G: Have you ever felt bad or guilty about your use?

E: Have you ever used or had a drink first thing in the morning as an "eye opener" to steady your nerves or feel normal?

17. a. Weigh patients at the same time of day.

b. Weigh patients on the same scale.

c. Weigh patients in the same clothes.

18. a. Oxygenation

b. Circulation

c. Nutrition

d. Local tissue damage

e. Hydration

19. Pigmentation is skin color. It is usually uniform over the body.

20. Answers can be found in Table 31-8 p. 546.

21. a. Diaphoresis

b. Spider angiomas

c. Burns (especially on fingers)

d. Needle marks

e. Contusions, abrasions, cuts, scars

f. "Homemade" tattoos

g. Vasculitis

h. Red, dry skin

22. *Indurated* means hardened.

23. *Turgor* is the skin's elasticity.

24. Occurs in localized pressure areas when patients remain in one position

25. Edema means areas of the skin that are swollen or edematous from a buildup of fluid in the tissues.

26. Unusual findings in the skin—skin tags, senile keratosis, cherry angiomas

27–35. Answers can be found in Box 31-6, p. 549.

36–38. Answers can be found in Box 31-7, p. 550.

39. Asymmetry, Border irregularity, Color, Diameter

40. a. *Pediculus humanus capitis* (head lice)

b. *Pediculus humanus corporis* (body lice)

c. *Pediculus pubis* (crab lice)

41. Clubbing is a change in the angle between the nail and nail base, including softening, flattening, and enlargement of the fingertips.

42. Beau lines are transverse depressions in the nails.

43. Koilonychia are concave curves.

44. Splinter hemorrhages are red or brown linear streaks in nail beds.

45. Paronychia is inflammation of the skin at the base of the nail.

46. Hydrocephalus is the buildup of cerebrospinal fluid in the ventricles.

47. Hyperopia is a refractive error causing farsightedness.

48. Myopia is a refractive error causing nearsightedness.

49. Presbyopia is impaired near vision in middle-age and older adults caused by loss of elasticity of the lens.

50. Retinopathy is a noninflammatory eye disorder resulting from changes in retinal blood vessels.

51. Strabismus is a congenital condition in which both eyes do not focus on an object simultaneously.

52. A cataract is an increased opacity of the lens.

53. Glaucoma is intraocular structural damage resulting from increased intraocular pressure.

54. Macular degeneration is blurred central vision often occurring suddenly caused by progressive degeneration of the center of the retina.

55. a. Visual acuity

b. Visual fields

c. Extraocular movements

d. External eye structures

e. Internal eye structures

56. a. Position and alignment

b. Eyebrows

c. Eyelids

d. Lacrimal apparatus

e. Conjunctivae and sclera

f. Corneas

g. Pupils and irises

57. Exophthalmos is a bulging of the eye.

58. An ectropion is an eyelid margin that turns out.

59. An entropion is an eyelid margins that turns in.

60. Conjunctivitis is the presence of redness, which indicates and allergy or an infection.

61. A ptosis is an abnormal drooping of the eyelid over the pupil.

62. Pupils equal, round, and reactive to light and accommodation

63. a. Retina

b. Choroids

c. Optic nerve disc

d. Macula

e. Fovea centralis

f. Retinal vessels

64. a. External ear (auricle, outer ear canal, and tympanic membrane)

b. Middle ear (three bony ossicles)

c. Inner ear (cochlea, vestibule, and semicircular canals)

65. The normal tympanic membrane appears translucent, shiny, and pearly gray.

66. a. Conduction

b. Sensorineural

c. Mixed

67. Injury to the auditory nerve resulting from high maintenance doses of antibiotics

68. Excoriation is skin breakdown characterized by redness and skin sloughing.

69. Polyps are tumor-like growths.

70. Leukoplakia are thick white patches that are often precancerous lesions seen in heavy smokers and people with alcoholism.

71. Varicosities are swollen, tortuous veins that are common in older adults.

72. Exostosis is extra bony growth between the two palates.

73. a. Neck muscles

b. Lymph nodes of the head and neck

c. Carotid arteries

d. Jugular veins

e. Thyroid gland

f. Trachea

74. 1. Occipital nodes at the base of the skull

2. Postauricular nodes over the mastoid

3. Preauricular nodes at the base of the skull

4. Retropharyngeal nodes at the angle of the mandible

5. Submandibular nodes

6. Submental nodes

75. Malignancy

76. a. Patient's nipples

b. Angle of Louis

c. Suprasternal notch

d. Costal angle

e. Clavicles

f. Vertebrae

77. Symmetrical, separating thumbs 3 to 5 cm; reduced chest excursion may be caused by pain, postural deformity, or fatigue.

78. Vocal or tactile fremitus are vibrations that you can palpate externally caused by sound waves.

79. Vesicular sounds are soft, breezy, and low pitched sounds that are created by air moving through smaller airways.
80. Bronchovesicular sounds are blowing sounds that are medium pitched and of medium intensity that are created by air moving through large airways.
81. Bronchial sounds are loud and high pitched with a hollow quality that are created by air moving through the trachea close to the chest wall.
82. Answers can be found in Table 31-21, p. 571.
83. The point of maximal impulse is where the apex of the heart is touching the anterior chest wall at approximately the fourth to fifth intercostal space just medial to the left midclavicular line.
84. Mitral and tricuspid valve closure causes the first heart sound (S_1).
85. Aortic and pulmonic valve closure causes the second heart sound (S_2).
86. When the heart attempts to fill an already distended ventricle, a third heart sound (S_3) can be heard.
87. When the atria contract to enhance ventricular filling, a fourth sound is heard (S_4).
88. Lies between the sternal body and manubrium and feels the ridge in the sternum approximately 5 cm below the sternal notch
89. Second intercostal space on the right
90. Left second intercostal space
91. Left third intercostal space
92. Fourth or fifth intercostal space along the sternum
93. Fifth intercostal space just to the left of the sternum; left midclavicular line
94. Tip of the sternum
95. A murmur is a sustained swishing or blowing sound heard at the beginning, middle, or end of the systolic or diastolic phase.
96. a. Auscultate all valve areas for placement in the cardiac cycle (timing), where best heard (location), radiation, loudness, pitch, and quality.
    b. Determine if they occur between S_1 and S_2 (systolic), and S_2 and S_1 (diastolic).
    c. The location is not necessarily over the valves.
    d. Listen over areas besides where the murmur is heard best to assess for radiation.
    e. Feel for a thrust or intermittent palpable sensation at the auscultation site in serious murmurs and rate the intensity.
    f. Low-pitched murmur best heard with the bell of the stethoscope; a high-pitched murmur is best heard with the diaphragm.
97. Grade 1 = barely audible in a quiet room
    Grade 2 = clearly audible but quiet
    Grade 3 = moderately loud
    Grade 4 = loud with associated thrill
    Grade 5 = very loud thrill easily palpable
    Grade 6 = louder; heard without stethoscope
98. Syncope is caused by a drop in heart rate and blood pressure.
99. An absent pulse wave (blockage)
100. Narrowing

101. A bruit is the blowing sound caused by turbulence in a narrowed section of a blood vessel.
102. 1. Place the patient in a semi-Fowler position.
     2. Expose the neck; align the head.
     3. Lean the patient back into a supine position; the level of venous pulsations begins to rise as the patient reaches a 45-degree angle.
     4. Use two rulers to measure.
     5. Repeat the same measurement on the other side.
103. See Table 31-25, p. 580.
104. Inspect the calves for localized redness, tenderness, and swelling over vein sites.
105. a. Monthly BSE for women in their 20s and 30s.
     b. Women ages 20 years and older need to report any breast changes.
     c. Women need to have a clinical breast examination every 3 years (ages 20 to 40 years) and yearly after the age of 40 years.
     d. Women with a family history need a yearly examination.
     e. Asymptomatic women need a screening mammogram by age 40 years. Women older than age 40 years need an annual mammogram.
     f. For women with increased risk, additional testing (MRI) should be discussed with the health care provider.
106. a. Clockwise or counterclockwise
     b. Vertical technique
     c. Center of the breast in a radial fashion
107. a. Location in relation to the quadrant
     b. Diameter
     c. Shape
     d. Consistency
     e. Tenderness
     f. Mobility
     g. Discreteness
108. Benign (fibrocystic) breast disease is characterized by bilateral lumpy, painful breast, sometimes with nipple discharge.
109. Striae are stretch marks.
110. A hernia is a protrusion of abdominal organs through the muscle wall.
111. Distention is swelling by intestinal gas, tumor, or fluid in the abdominal cavity.
112. Peristalsis is movement of contents through the intestines, which is a normal function of the small and large intestine.
113. Borborygmi are growling sounds, which are hyperactive bowel sounds.
114. Rebound tenderness is the pain a patient may experience when the nurse quickly lifts his or her hand away after pressing it deeply into the involved area.
115. An aneurysm is a localized dilation of a vessel wall.
116. Chancres are syphilitic lesions, which appear as small, open ulcers that drain serous material.
117. A Papanicolaou specimen is used to test for cervical and vaginal cancer.
118. Common symptoms include a painless enlargement of one testis and the appearance of a palpable, small, hard lump on the side of the testicle.

119. Digital examination is used to detect colorectal cancer in the early stages and prostatic tumors.
120. A kyphosis is a hunchback, an exaggeration of the posterior curvature of the thoracic spine.
121. Lordosis is a swayback, an increased lumbar curvature.
122. Scoliosis is a lateral spinal curvature.
123. Osteoporosis is a metabolic bone disease that causes a decrease in quality and quantity of bone.
124. A goniometer is an instrument that measures the precise degree of motion in a particular joint.
125. Flexion = movement decreasing angle between two adjoining bones
126. Extension = increasing angle between two adjoining bones
127. Hyperextension = beyond its normal resting extended position
128. Pronation = that the frontal or ventral surfaces face downward
129. Supination = front or ventral surface faces upward
130. Abduction = away from the midline
131. Adduction = toward the midline
132. Internal rotation = rotation of the joint inward
133. External rotation = rotation of the joint outward
134. Eversion = turning of the body part away from the midline
135. Inversion = turning the body part toward the midline
136. Dorsiflexion = flexion of toes and foot upward
137. Plantar flexion = bending of toes and foot downward
138. Hypertonicity is increased muscle tone.
139. Hypotonicity is a muscle with little tone.
140. Atrophied muscles are reduced in size; they feel soft and boggy.
141. The Mini-Mental State Examination measures orientation and cognitive function.
142. Delirium is characterized by confusion, disorientation, and restlessness.
143. The Glasgow Coma Scale provides an objective measurement of consciousness on a numerical scale over time.
144. a. A person cannot understand written or verbal speech
    b. A person understands written and verbal speech but cannot write or speak appropriately when attempting to communicate
145. a. Olfactory
    b. Optic
    c. Oculomotor
    d. Trochlear
    e. Trigeminal
    f. Abducens
    g. Facial
    h. Auditory
    i. Glossopharyngeal
    j. Vagus
    k. Spinal accessory
    l. Hypoglossal
146. a. Pain
    b. Temperature
    c. Position
    d. Vibration
    e. Crude and finely localized touch
147. The cerebellum controls muscular activity, maintains balance and equilibrium, and helps to control posture.
148. a. Deep tendon reflexes (biceps, triceps, patellar, Achilles)
    b. Cutaneous reflexes (plantar, gluteal, abdominal)
149. 4. A thorough explanation of the purpose and steps of each assessment lets patients know what to expect and what to do so they can cooperate.
150. 3. Normally, the skin lifts easily and snaps back immediately to its resting position; the back of the hand is not the best place to test for turgor
151. 3. Circumscribed elevation of skin filled with serous fluid, smaller than 1 cm
152. 2. Use a systematic pattern when comparing the right and left sides. You need to compare lung sounds in one region on one side of the body with sounds in the same region on the opposite side of the body.
153. 3. High-velocity airflow through severely narrowed or obstructed airway
154. 4. After the ventricles empty, ventricular pressure falls below that in the aorta and pulmonary artery, allowing the valves to close and causing the second heart sound.

CHAPTER 32

1. a. The federal government protects the health of the people by ensuring that medications are safe and effective. Currently, the Food and Drug Administration ensures that all medications undergo vigorous testing before they are sold.
   b. The state governments conform to federal legislation but also have additional controls such as alcohol and tobacco.
   c. Health care institutions have individual policies to meet federal and state regulations.
   d. The Nurse Practice Act defines the scope of a nurse's professional functions and responsibilities.
2. A chemical name provides an exact description of the medication's composition and molecular structure.
3. A generic name is created by the manufacturer who first develops the medication; this becomes the official name.
4. The trade name is one that the manufacturer has trademarked to identify the particular version they manufacture.
5. A medication classification indicates the effect of the medication on a body system, the symptoms the medication relieves, or the medication's desired effect.
6. The form of the medication determines its route of administration.
7. Pharmacokinetics is the study of how medications enter the body, reach their site of action, metabolize, and exit the body.

8. Absorption refers to the passage of medication molecules into the blood from the site of administration.
9. a. Route of administration
   b. Ability of the medication to dissolve
   c. Blood flow to the site of administration
   d. Body surface area
   e. Lipid solubility
10. a. Circulation
    b. Membrane permeability
    c. Protein binding
    d. Metabolism
    e. Excretion
11. After a medication reaches its site of action, it becomes metabolized into a less active or inactive form that is easier to excrete.
12. The kidneys are the primary organ for drug excretion. When renal function declines, a patient is at risk for medication toxicity.
13. Therapeutic effects are the expected or predictable physiological response to a medication.
14. Side effects are predictable and often unavoidable secondary effects a medication predictably will cause.
15. Adverse effects are unintended, undesirable, and often unpredictable severe responses to medication.
16. Toxic effects develop after prolonged intake of a medication or when a medication accumulates in the blood because of impaired metabolism or excretion.
17. Idiosyncratic reactions are unpredictable effects in which a patient overreacts or underreacts to a medication or has a reaction that is different from normal.
18. Allergic reactions are unpredictable responses to a medication.
19. Anaphylactic reactions are allergic reactions that are life threatening and characterized by sudden constriction of bronchiolar muscles, edema of the pharynx and larynx, and severe wheezing and shortness of breath.
20. Medication interaction occurs when one medication modifies the action of another medication; it may alter the way another medication is absorbed, metabolized, or eliminated from the body.
21. A synergistic effect is when the combined effect of the two medications is greater than the effect of the medications when given separately.
22. The MEC is the plasma level of a medication below which the medication's effect will not occur.
23. The peak concentration is the highest serum level concentration.
24. The trough concentration is the lowest serum level concentration.
25. The biological half-life is the time it takes for excretion processes to lower the serum medication concentration by half.
26. a. Oral
    b. Buccal
    c. Sublingual
27. a. Intradermal
    b. Subcutaneous
    c. Intramuscular
    d. Intravenous

28. Epidural injections are administered in the epidural space via a catheter, usually used for postoperative analgesia.
29. Intrathecal administration is via a catheter that is in the subarachnoid space or one of the ventricles of the brain.
30. Intraosseous infusion of medication is administered directly into the bone marrow; it is commonly used in infants and toddlers.
31. Intraperitoneal medications, such as chemotherapeutic agents, insulin, and antibiotics, are administered into the peritoneal cavity.
32. Intrapleural medications, commonly chemotherapeutics, are administered directly into the pleural space.
33. Intraarterial medications are administered directly into the arteries.
34. Intracardiac medications are injected directly into the cardiac tissue.
35. Intraarticular medications are injected into a joint.
36. a. Directly applying a liquid or ointment
    b. Inserting a medication into a body cavity
    c. Instilling fluid into a body cavity
    d. Irrigating a body cavity
    e. Spraying
37. Inhaled medications are readily absorbed and work rapidly because of the rich vascular alveolar capillary network present in the pulmonary tissue.
38. a. Metric
    b. Household
39. A solution is a given mass of solid substance dissolved in a known volume of fluid or a given volume of liquid dissolved in a known volume of another fluid.
40. Dose ordered/Dose on hand×Amount on hand= Amount to administer
41. If the order is given verbally to the nurse by the provider, it is a verbal order.
42. A standing or routine order is carried out until the prescriber cancels it by another order or until a prescribed number of days elapse.
43. A prn order is a medication that is given only when a patient requires it.
44. A single or one-time dose is given only once at a specified time.
45. A STAT order describes a single dose of a medication to be given immediately and only once.
46. Now is used when a patient needs a medication quickly but not right away; the nurse has up to 90 minutes to administer.
47. a. Unit dose
    b. Automated medication dispensing systems (AMDS)
48. a. Inaccurate prescribing
    b. Administration of the wrong medicine
    c. Giving the medication using the wrong route or time interval
    d. Administering extra doses
    e. Failing to administer a medication
49. a. Obtain, verify, document
    b. Consider and compare

c. Reconcile

d. Communicate

50. a. The right medication

b. The right dose

c. The right patient

d. The right route

e. The right time

f. The right documentation

51. a. Be informed of the medication's name, purpose, action, and potential undesired effects.

b. Refuse a medication regardless of the consequences.

c. Have qualified nurses or physicians assess a medication history.

d. Be properly advised of the experimental nature of medication therapy and give written consent.

e. Receive labeled medications safely without discomfort.

f. Receive appropriate supportive therapy.

g. Not receive unnecessary medications

h. Be informed if medications are a part of a research study.

52. a. History

b. History of allergies

c. Medication data

d. Diet history

e. Patient's perceptual coordination problems

f. Patient's current condition

g. Patient's attitude about medication use

h. Patient's knowledge and understanding of medication therapy

i. Patient's learning needs

53. a. Anxiety

b. Ineffective Health Maintenance

c. Caregiver Role Strain

d. Deficient Knowledge

e. Noncompliance

f. Impaired Memory

g. Impaired Swallowing

54. a. Will verbalize understanding of desired effects and adverse effects of medications

b. Will state signs, symptoms, and treatment of hypoglycemia

c. Will monitor blood sugar to determine if medication is appropriate to take

d. Will prepare a dose of ordered medication

e. Will describe a daily routine that will integrate timing of medication with daily activities

55. a. Health beliefs

b. Personal motivations

c. Socioeconomic factors

d. Habits

56. a. Patient's full name

b. Date and time that the order is written

c. Medication name

d. Dose

e. Route of administration

f. Time and frequency of administration

g. Signature of provider

57. a. The name of the medication

b. Dose

c. Route

d. Exact time of administration

e. Site

58. When patients need to take several medications to treat their illnesses, take two or more medications from the same chemical class, use two or more medications with the same or similar actions or mix nutritional supplements or herbal products with medications, polypharmacy happens.

59. a. Patient responds to therapy.

b. Patient has the ability to assume responsibility for self-care.

60. a. Determine the patient's ability to swallow and cough and check for gag reflex.

b. Prepare oral medications in the form that is easiest to swallow.

c. Allow the patient to self-administer medications if possible.

d. If the patient has unilateral weakness, place the medication in the stronger side of the mouth.

e. Administer pills one at a time, ensuring that each medication is properly swallowed before the next one is introduced.

f. Thicken regular liquids or offer fruit nectars if the patient cannot tolerate thin liquids.

g. Avoid straws because they decrease the control the patient has over volume intake, which increases the risk of aspiration.

h. Have the patient hold the cup and drink from it if possible.

i. Time medications to coincide with meal times or when the patient is well rested and awake if possible.

j. Administer medications using another route if risk of aspiration is severe.

61. a. Medication history and reconciling medications

b. Assess if patient has an existing patch before application.

c. Wear disposable gloves when applying and removing patches.

d. Apply a noticeable label to the patch.

e. Document removal of medication on the MAR.

f. Document the location of the patient's body where the medication was placed on the medication administration record (MAR).

62. Decongestant spray or drops

63. a. Avoid instilling any eye medication directly onto the cornea.

b. Avoid touching the eyelids or other eye structures with eye droppers or ointment tubes.

c. Use medication only for the patient's affected eye.

d. Never allow a patient to use another patient's eye medications.

64. a. Vertigo

b. Dizziness

c. Nausea

65. a. Suppositories

b. Foam

c. Jellies

d. Creams

66. Exerting local effects (promoting defecation) or systemic effects (reducing nausea)
67. a. Delivers a measured dose of medication with each push of a canister often used with a spacer
    b. Releases medication when a patient raises a level and then inhales
    c. Hold dry, powdered medication and create an aerosol when the patient inhales through a reservoir that contains the medication
68. a. Draw medication from ampule quickly; do not allow it to stand open.
    b. Avoid letting the needle touch contaminated surface.
    c. Avoid touching the length of the plunger or inner part of the barrel.
    d. Prepare the skin, use friction and a circular motion while cleaning with an antiseptic swab, and start from the center and move outward.
69. a. The patient's size and weight
    b. Type of tissue into which the medication is to be injected
70. a. Contain single doses of medications in a liquid
    b. A single dose or multidose container with a rubber seal at the top (closed system)
71. a. Do not contaminate one medication with another.
    b. Ensure that the final dose is accurate.
    c. Maintain aseptic technique.
72. Rate of action (rapid, short, intermediate, and long acting); each has a different onset, peak, and duration of action.
73. a. Need to maintain their individual routine when preparing and administering their insulin
    b. Do not mix insulin with any other medication or diluents.
    c. Never mix insulin glargine or insulin detemir with other types of insulin.
    d. Inject rapid-acting insulin mixed with NPH within 15 minutes before a meal.
    e. Verify insulin dosages with another nurse while preparing them.
74. a. Use a sharp beveled needle in the smallest suitable length and gauge.
    b. Position the patient as comfortably as possible to reduce muscle tension.
    c. Select the proper injection site.
    d. Apply a vapocoolant spray or topical anesthetic to the site if possible.
    e. Divert the patient's attention from the injection.
    f. Insert the needle quickly and smoothly.
    g. Hold the syringe while the needle remains in tissues.
    h. Inject the medication slowly and steadily.
75. a. The outer posterior aspect of the upper arms
    b. The abdomen (below the costal margins to the iliac crests)
    c. The anterior aspects of the thighs
76. 0.5 to 1 mL
77. a. 25-gauge, 5/8-inch needle inserted at a 45-degree angle
    b. 1/2-inch needle inserted at a 90-degree angle

78. 90 degrees
79. a. 2 to 5 mL into a large muscle
    b. 2 mL
    c. 1 mL
80. Deep site away from nerves and blood vessels; preferred site for medications for adults; children and infants for large volumes and viscous and irritating solutions
81. For adults and children, muscle is thick and well developed; anterior lateral aspect of the thigh
82. Easily accessible but muscle not well developed; use small amounts; not used in infants or children; potential for injury to radial and ulnar nerves; immunizations for children; recommended site for hepatitis B and rabies injections
83. Minimizes local skin irritation by sealing the medication in muscle tissue
84. Skin testing; injected into the dermis where medication is absorbed slowly
85. a. As mixtures within large volumes of IV fluids
    b. Injection of a bolus or small volume of medication
    c. Piggyback infusion
86. a. Fast-acting medications must be delivered quickly.
    b. It provides constant therapeutic blood levels.
    c. It can be used when medications are highly alkaline and irritating to the muscle and subcutaneous tissue.
87. a. It is the most dangerous method because there is no time to correct errors.
    b. A bolus may cause direct irritation to the lining of blood vessels.
88. a. They reduce risk of rapid infusion by IV push.
    b. They allow for administration of medications that are stable for a limited time in solution.
    c. They allow for control of IV fluid intake.
89. A small (25- to 250-mL) IV bag connected to short tubing lines that connects to the upper Y port of a primary infusion line
90. A small (50- to 150-mL) container that attaches below the primary infusion bag
91. A battery-operated machine that allows medications to be given in very small amounts of fluid (5 to 60 mL)
92. a. Cost saving
    b. Convenience
    c. Increased mobility
    d. Safety
    e. Patient comfort
93. 3. Definition of pharmacokinetics
94. 1. Absorption refers to the passage of medication molecules into the blood from the site of administration.
95. 1. Definition of onset
96. 1. An oral route
97. 2. If mixing rapid- or short-acting insulin with intermediate-acting insulin, take the insulin syringe and aspirate a volume of air equivalent to the dose of insulin to be withdrawn from the intermediate-acting insulin first.

CHAPTER 33

1. Complementary therapies are therapies used in addition to conventional treatment recommended by the patient's provider.

2. Alternative therapies include the same interventions as complementary but frequently become the primary treatment that replaces allopathic medical care.

3–7. See Table 33-1, pp. 689-690.

8. a. Importance of the relationship between practitioner and patient
   b. Focuses on the whole person
   c. Is informed by evidence
   d. Makes use of appropriate therapeutic approaches and health care professionals

9. The stress response is associated with increased heart and respiratory rates, tightened muscles, an increased metabolic rate, a general sense of fear, nervousness, irritability, and a negative mood.

10. The relaxation response is the state of generalized decreased cognitive, physiological, or behavioral arousal.

11. Progressive relaxation training helps to teach the individual how to effectively rest and reduce tension in the body.

12. The goal of passive relaxation is to still the mind and body intentionally without the need to tighten and relax any particular body part.

13. The outcome of relaxation therapy is lowered heart rate and blood pressure, decreased muscle tension, improved sense of well-being, and reduced symptoms of distress.

14. During the first few months when the person is learning to focus on body sensations and tensions, there is increased sensitivity in detecting muscle tension. Occasionally, intensification of symptoms or the development of new symptoms can occur.

15. Meditation is any activity that limits stimulus input by directing attention to a single unchanging or repetitive stimulus.

16. Meditation has been used to successfully reduce hypertensive risks; reduce relapses in alcohol treatment programs; reduce depression, anxiety, and distress in cancer patients; and benefit people with posttraumatic stress disorders and chronic pain.

17. Meditation is contraindicated for people who have a strong fear of losing control or who are hypersensitive; medication use.

18. Imagery is a group of visualization techniques that uses the conscious mind to create mental images to stimulate physical changes in the body, improve perceived well-being, or enhance self-awareness.

19. Creative visualization is one form of self-directed imagery that is based on the principle of mind–body connectivity.

20. Imagery can be helpful in controlling or relieving pain, decreasing nightmares and improving sleep, and treating chronic diseases.

21. Biofeedback is a mind–body technique that uses instruments to teach self-regulation and voluntary self-control over specific physiological responses.

22. Biofeedback can be useful in treating headaches, smoking cessation, strokes, attention deficit hyperactivity, epilepsy, and a variety of gastrointestinal and urinary tract disorders.

23. Repressed emotions or feelings are sometimes uncovered during biofeedback, and the patient may have difficulty coping.

24. Acupuncture can be used for low back pain, myofascial pain, headaches, sciatica, shoulder pain, tennis elbow, osteoarthritis, whiplash, and musculoskeletal sprains.

25. Bleeding disorders and skin infections

26. a. *Qi* is the vital energy of the body.
   b. Meridians are channels of energy that run in regular patterns through the body and over its surface.
   c. Acupoints are holes through which qi can be influenced by the insertion of needles.

27. a. Centering
   b. Assessment
   c. Unruffling
   d. Treatment
   e. Evaluation

28. Therapeutic touch is used in the treatment of pain in adults and children, dementia, trauma, and anxiety.

29. Therapeutic touch is contraindicated in persons who are sensitive to human interaction and touch.

30. The most important concept is yin and yang, which represent opposing yet complementary phenomena that exist in a state of dynamic equilibrium.

31. a. Burning moxa, a cone or stick of dried herbs that have healing properties on or near the skin
   b. Placing a heated cup on the skin to create a slight suction
   c. Martial art—moving meditation
   d. Choreographed movements or gestures

32. Herbal therapy can be used for urinary tract infections, sleep and relaxation, mild gastrointestinal disturbances, and premenstrual symptoms.

33. Problems with herbal therapies include contamination with other chemicals or herbs, toxic agents, a variety of standards used from one company to another.

34. The integrative medicine approach is a multiple-practitioner treatment group; a pluralistic, complementary health care system; it is consistent with the holistic approach nurses learn to practice.

35. 2. The perception that the treatments offered by the medical profession do not provide relief for a variety of common illnesses

36. 3. They have not received approval for use as drugs and are not regulated by the FDA; therefore, they can be sold as food or food supplements only.

37. 2. It is important for the nurse to know the current research being done in this area to provide accurate information not only to patients but also to other health care professionals.

CHAPTER 34

1. Self-concept is an individual's view of him- or herself. It is a complex mixture of unconscious and conscious thoughts, attitudes, and perceptions.

2. a. Sense of competency
   b. Perceived reactions of others to one's body

c. Ongoing perceptions and interpretations of the thoughts and feelings of others

d. Personal and professional relationships

e. Academic and employment-related identity

f. Personality characteristics

g. Perceptions of events

h. Mastery of prior experiences

i. Ethnic, racial, and spiritual identity

3. d

4. a

5. b

6. c

7. A self-concept stressor is any real or perceived change that threatens identity, body image, or role performance.

8. g

9. d

10. f

11. c

12. h

13. b

14. e

15. a

16. a. Thoughts and feelings about lifestyle, health, and illness

b. Awareness of how one's own nonverbal communication affects patients and families

c. Personal values and expectations and how they affect patients

d. Ability to convey a nonjudgmental attitude toward patients

e. Preconceived attitudes toward cultural differences

17. The focus is on identity, body image, and role performance; actual and potential self-concept stressors and coping patterns (nature, number, and intensity of stressors and internal and external resources).

18. See Box 34-5, p. 708.

19. a. Disturbed body image

b. Caregiver role strain

c. Disturbed personal identity

d. Ineffective role performance

e. Readiness for enhanced self-concept

f. Chronic low esteem

g. Situational low self-esteem

h. Risk for situational low self-esteem

20. The patient will discuss a minimum of three areas of her life in which she is functioning well. The patient will be able to voice the recognition that losing her job is not reflective of her worth as a person. The patient will attend a support group for out-of-work professionals.

21. Healthy lifestyle measures include proper nutrition, regular exercise within the patient's capabilities, adequate sleep and rest, and stress-reducing practices.

22. Expected outcomes include nonverbal behaviors indicating positive self-concept, statements of self-acceptance, and acceptance of change in appearance or function.

23. 3. Adolescence is a particularly critical time when many variables affect self-concept and self-esteem.

24. 4. Involves attitudes related to the body, including physical appearance, structure, or function, which is affected by cognitive and physical development as well as cultural and societal attitudes

25. 4. Certain behaviors become common depending on whether they are approved and reinforced.

26. 2. Attitudes toward body image can occur as a result of situational events such as the loss of or change in a body part.

27. a. Observe Mrs. Johnson's behaviors that suggest an alteration in self-concept. Assess Mrs. Johnson's cultural background. Assess Mrs. Johnson's coping skills and resources. Converse with Mrs. Johnson to determine her feelings, perceptions about changes in body image, self-esteem, or role. Assess the quality of Mrs. Johnson's relationships.

b. Self-awareness is critical; nurses derive their self-concepts and professional identify from their public image, work environment, and education as well as their professional, social, and cultural values.

c. Humanities, sciences, nursing research, and clinical practice; components of self-concept (identity, body image, self-esteem, role performance); self-concept stressors related to identity, body image, self-esteem, and role; therapeutic communication principles and nonverbal indicators of distress; cultural and societal issues that influence body image; pharmacologic effects of medicine (pain medication); Erikson's psychosocial theory of development

d. Support Mrs. Johnson's autonomy to make choices and express values that support positive self-concept. Apply intellectual standards of relevance and plausibility for care to be acceptable to Mrs. Johnson. Susan needs to safeguard Mrs. Johnson's right to privacy by judiciously protecting information of a confidential nature.

e. Looking for the range of behaviors suggestive of an altered self-concept; cultural differences, role performance, perception of the stressors and of change; previous coping behaviors

CHAPTER 35

1. f

2. h

3. g

4. i

5. e

6. d

7. j

8. k

9. l

10. b

11. c

12. a

13. a. Contaminated IV needles

b. Anal intercourse

c. Vaginal intercourse

d. Oral–genital sex

e. Transfusion of blood products

14. a. Syphilis

b. Gonorrhea

c. Chlamydia

d. Trichomoniasis

e. HPV

f. Herpes simplex virus

15. a. Impact of pregnancy and menstruation on sexuality

b. Discussing sexual issues

16. a. Contraception
    b. Abortion
    c. STI prevention
17. a. Infertility
    b. Sexual abuse
    c. Personal and emotional conflicts
    d. Sexual dysfunction
18. a. Physical
    b. Functional
    c. Relationship
    d. Lifestyle
    e. Developmental factors
    f. Self-esteem factors
19. Permission, limited information, specific suggestions, intensive therapy
20. a. Anxiety
    b. Ineffective Coping
    c. Interrupted Family Processes
    d. Deficient Knowledge
    e. Sexual Dysfunction
    f. Ineffective Sexuality Pattern
    g. Social Isolation
21. a. Discuss stressors that contribute to sexual dysfunction with partner within 2 weeks.
    b. Identify alternative, satisfying, and acceptable sexual practices for oneself and one's partner within 4 weeks.
22. a. Contraception
    b. Safe sex practices
    c. Prevention of STIs
    d. Women: Regular breast self-examinations, mammograms, Pap smears
    e. Men: Testicular examinations
23. a. Avoid alcohol and tobacco.
    b. Eat well-balanced meals.
    c. Plan sexual activity for times when the couple feels rested.
    d. Take pain medication if needed.
    e. Use pillows and alternate positioning to enhance comfort.
    f. Encourage touch, kissing, hugging, and other tactile stimulation.
    g. Communicate your concerns and fears with your partner.
24. Individuals experience major physical changes, the effects of drugs and treatments, emotional stress of a prognosis, concern about future functioning, and separation from others.
25. a. Ask patients questions about risk factors, sexual concerns, and their level of satisfaction.
    b. Note behavioral cues.
26. 4. The child identifies with the parent of the same sex and develops a complementary relationship with the parent of the opposite sex.
27. 4. Normal sexual changes occur as people age.
28. 1. Methods that are effective for contraception do not always reduce the risk of STIs.
29. a. Assess Mr. Clements' developmental stage in regard to sexuality. Consider self-concept as a factor that will influence sexual satisfaction and

functioning. Provide physical assessment of urogenital area. Determine Mr. Clements' sexual concerns. Assess safe sex practices and the use of contraception. Assess the medical conditions and medications that may be affecting his sexual functioning. Assess the impact of high-risk behaviors on sexual health.
    b. A basic understanding of sexual development, sexual orientation, sociocultural dimensions, the impact of self-concept, STIs, and safe sex practices; ways to phrase questions regarding sexuality and functioning; disease conditions that affect sexual functioning; how interpersonal relationship factors may affect sexual functioning
    c. Explore discomfort by discussing topics related to sexuality and develop a plan for addressing these discomforts. Reflect on personal sexual experiences and how he has responded.
    d. Apply intellectual standards of relevance and plausibility for care to be acceptable to Mr. Clements. Safeguard Mr. Clements' right to privacy by judiciously protecting information of a confidential nature. Apply the principles of ethic of care.
    e. Display curiosity; consider why Mr. Clements might behave or respond in a particular manner. Display integrity; his beliefs and values may differ from Mr. Clements'. Admit to inconsistencies in his and Mr. Clements' values. Risk taking: be willing to explore both personal and Mr. Clements' sexual issues and concerns.

CHAPTER 36

1. Spirituality is an awareness of one's inner self and a sense of connection to a higher being, nature, or to some purpose other than oneself.
2. e   7. c
3. f   8. h
4. d   9. a
5. b   10. i
6. g
11. a. The strength of a patient's spirituality influences how he or she copes with sudden illness and how quickly he or she moves to recovery.
    b. Dependence on others for routine self-care needs often creates feelings of powerlessness; this along with the loss of a sense of purpose in life impairs the ability to cope with alterations in functioning.
    c. Terminal illness creates an uncertainty about what death means and thus makes patients susceptible to spiritual distress.
    d. A near-death experience is a psychological phenomenon of people who either have been close to clinical death or have recovered after being declared dead.
12. Individuals have some source of authority (a supreme being; a code of conduct; a specific religious leader, family or friends, oneself, or a combination) and guidance in their lives that lead them to choose and act on their beliefs.

13. Individuals who accept change in life, make decisions about their lives, and are able to forgive others in times of difficulty have higher levels of spiritual well-being.

14. People who are connected to themselves, others, nature, and God or another supreme being cope with the stress brought on by crisis and chronic illness.

15. When people are satisfied with life, more energy is available to deal with new difficulties and to resolve problems.

16. Remaining connected with their cultural heritage often helps patients define their place in the world and to express their spirituality.

17. Fellowship is a type of relationship that an individual has with other persons.

18. Rituals include participation in worship, prayer, sacraments, fasting, singing, meditating, scripture reading, and making offerings or sacrifices.

19. Expression of spirituality is highly individual and includes showing an appreciation for life in the variety of things that people do, living in the moment and not worrying about tomorrow, appreciating nature, expressing love toward others, and being productive.

20. a. Anxiety
    b. Ineffective Coping
    c. Risk for Impaired Religiosity
    d. Complicated Grieving
    e. Hopelessness
    f. Powerlessness
    g. Readiness for Enhanced Spiritual Well-Being
    h. Spiritual Distress
    i. Risk for Spiritual Distress

21. a. The patient will express an acceptance of his or her illness.
    b. The patient reports the ability to rely on family members for support.
    c. The patient initiates social interactions with family and friends.

22. Giving attention, answering questions, listening, and having a positive and encouraging (but realistic) attitude, being with rather than doing for

23. a. Mobilizing hope for the nurse as well as the patient
    b. Finding an interpretation or understanding of the illness, pain, anxiety, or other stressful emotion that is acceptable to the patient
    c. Assisting the patient in using social, emotional, and spiritual resources

24. Support systems serve as a human link connecting the patient, the nurse, and the patient's lifestyle before an illness. The support system is a source of faith and hope and often is an important resource in conducting meaningful religious rituals.

25. Food and rituals are sometimes important to a person's spirituality.

26. Plan care to allow time for religious readings, spiritual visitations, or attendance at religious services.

27. Prayer offers an opportunity to renew personal faith and belief in a higher being in a specific, focused way that is either highly ritualized and formal or spontaneous and informal.

28. Meditation creates a relaxation that reduces daily stress, lowers blood pressure, slows the aging process, reduces pain, and enhances the function of the immune system.

29. The nurse's ability to enter into a therapeutic and spiritual relationship with the patient will support a patient during times of grief.

30. Reveal the patient's developing an increased or restored sense of connectedness with family; maintaining, renewing, or reforming a sense of purpose in life and for some confidence and trust in a supreme being or power

31. 3. Must be able to practice the five pillars of Islam; health and spirituality are connected

32. 2. Their belief is not to kill any living creature.

33. 3. Muslims wash the body of the dead family member and wrap it in white cloth with the head turned to the right shoulder.

34. 2. The defining characteristics reveal patterns that reflect a person's actual or potential dispiritedness.

35. 3. When patients use meditation in conjunction with their spiritual beliefs, they often report an increased spirituality that they commonly describe as experiencing the presence of power, force or energy, or what was perceived as God.

36. a. Constructs that define spirituality: Self-transcendence, connectedness, faith, and hope
    b. Using the nurse's past experience in selecting interventions that support the patient's well-being, the nurse will exhibit confidence in her skills and develop a trusting relationship with Lisa. Be open to any possible conflict between the patient's opinion and the nurse's; decide how to reach mutually beneficial outcomes
    c. The concepts of faith, hope, spiritual well-being, and religion; caring practices in the individual approach to a patient; available services in the community (health care providers and agencies)
    d. Standards of autonomy and self-determination to support Lisa's decisions about the plan; ANA code of ethics; nurses who are comfortable with their own spirituality often are more likely to care for their patients' spiritual needs
    e. Lisa will express her will to live with family members; Lisa will describe a feeling of peacefulness to her family; Lisa will express a personal sense of spiritual well-being.

CHAPTER 37

1. l	9. i
2. n	10. d
3. m	11. h
4. o	12. c
5. f	13. g
6. k	14. e
7. b	15. a
8. j	

16. a. Human development
    b. Personal relationships

c. Nature of the loss
d. Coping strategies
e. Socioeconomic status
f. Culture and ethnicity
g. Spiritual and religious beliefs
h. Hope
17. It is important to assess the patient's coping style, the nature of the family relationships, personal goals, cultural and spiritual beliefs, sources of hope, and availability of support systems.
18. a. Compromised Family Coping
b. Death Anxiety
c. Grieving
d. Complicated Grieving
e. Risk for Complicated Grieving
f. Hopelessness
g. Pain
h. Spiritual Distress
19. a. Will participate in treatment decisions
b. Will communicate treatment side effects or concerns to the health care team
20. Palliative care is the prevention, relief, reduction, or soothing of symptoms of disease or disorders throughout the entire course of an illness, including care of a dying individual and bereavement follow-up for the family.
21. a. Affirms life and regards dying as a normal process
b. Neither hastens or postpones health
c. Integrates psychological and spiritual aspects of patient care
d. Offers a support system to help
e. Enhances the quality of life
f. Uses a team approach
22. a. Patient and family are the unit.
b. Coordinated home care with access to inpatient and nursing home beds when needed
c. Symptom management
d. Physician-directed services
e. Provision of an interdisciplinary care team
f. Medical and nursing services available at all times
g. Bereavement follow-up
h. Trained volunteers for visitation and respite support
23. a. Use therapeutic communication.
b. Provide psychosocial care.
c. Manage symptoms.
d. Promote dignity and self-esteem.
e. Maintain a comfortable and peaceful environment.
f. Promote spiritual comfort and hope.
g. Protect against abandonment and isolation.
h. Support the grieving family.
i. Assist with end-of-life decision making.
24. a. Help the survivor accept that the loss is real.
b. Support efforts to adjust to the loss using a problem-solving approach.
c. Encourage establishment of new relationships.
d. Allow time to grieve.
e. Interpret normal behavior.
f. Provide continuing support.
g. Be alert for signs of ineffective, harmful coping mechanisms.

25. Organ and tissue donation provides information about who can legally give consent, which organs or tissues can be donated, associated costs, and how donation will affect burial or cremation.
26. Autopsy is the surgical dissection of a body after death to determine the cause and circumstances of death or discover the pathway of a disease.
27. Postmortem care is the care of the body after death, maintaining the integrity of rituals and mourning practices.
28. Short-term goals include talking about the loss without feeling overwhelmed, improved energy level, normalized sleep and dietary patterns, reorganization of life patterns, improved ability to make decisions, and finding it easier to be around people.
29. Long-term goals include the return of a sense of humor and normal life patterns, renewed or new personal relationships, and decrease of inner pain.
30. 1. Life changes are natural and often positive, which are learned as change always involves necessary losses.
31. 3. Care of the terminally ill patient and his or her family
32. 2. Cushions and postpones awareness of the loss by trying to prevent it from happening
33. 3. To help patients and families achieve the best possible quality of life, determine the goals of care, and select the appropriate interventions
34. a. Knowledge related to the characteristics of grief resolution; the clinical symptoms of an improved level of comfort
b. Previous patient responses to planned nursing interventions for symptom management or loss of a significant other
c. Used established expected outcomes to evaluate the patient response to care; evaluated the patient's role in the grieving process
d. Persevere in seeking successful comfort measures for the grieving patient
e. Evaluate signs and symptoms of Mrs. Allison's grief; evaluate family members' ability to provide supportive care; evaluate the patient's level of comfort; ask if the patient's/family's expectations are being met

CHAPTER 38

1. j	11. d
2. c	12. q
3. k	13. s
4. m	14. i
5. g	15. a
6. f	16. e
7. n	17. h
8. o	18. b
9. r	19. l
10. p	20. t

21. a. Uses a systems approach and helps you understand your patients' individual responses to

stressors as well as families' and communities' responses; views a patient, family, or community as constantly changing in response to the environment and stressors

b. People want to live in ways that enable them to be as healthy as possible and capable of assessing their own abilities and assets.

22. Situational factors can arise from job changes (one's own or family) and relocation.

23. Maturational factors vary with life stage: Children (relate to physical appearance), preadolescent (self-esteem issues), adolescent (identity), and adults (major changes in life circumstances).

24. Sociocultural factors include poverty and physical disabilities, loss of parents and caregivers (children), violence, and homelessness.

25. a. Patient safety
    b. Perception of the stressor
    c. Available coping resources
    d. Maladaptive coping used
    e. Adherence to healthy practices

26. a. Grooming and hygiene
    b. Gait
    c. Characteristics of the handshake
    d. Actions while sitting
    e. Quality of speech
    f. Eye contact
    g. The attitude of the patient

27. a. Anxiety
    b. Denial
    c. Fear
    d. Ineffective Coping
    e. Powerlessness
    f. Risk for Posttrauma Syndrome
    g. Situational Low Self-Esteem
    h. Stress Overload

28. a. You direct nursing activities to identify individuals and populations who are possibly at risk for stress
    b. Include actions directed at symptoms
    c. Assist the patient in readapting and can include relaxation training and time management

29. a. Decrease stressful situations
    b. Increase resistance to stress
    c. Learn skills that reduce physiological response to stress

30. Crisis intervention is a specific type of brief psychotherapy with prescribed steps; more directive

31. Reports of feeling better when the stressor is gone; improved sleep patterns and appetite; improved ability to concentrate

32. 1. Stress is an experience a person is exposed to through a stimulus or stressor.

33. 1. Neurophysiological responses to stress function through negative feedback

34. 1. Alarm reaction, resistance stage, and the exhaustion stage

35. 3. The nurse helps the patient make the mental connection between the stressful event and the patient's reaction to it.

36. a. General adaptation syndrome (GAS), communication principles that contribute to assessing a patient's behaviors, factors influencing stress, and coping and sociocultural factors
    b. Experience with previous patients; personal experiences with stress and coping increase your ability to empathize
    c. Practice standards for psychiatric mental health nursing, nursing theories, interprofessional approaches
    d. Maintain ongoing communication with Sandra and John because coping with stress takes time; need to actively involve the patient and his wife in the process of problem identification, prioritizing, and goal setting.
    e. Ask Sandra if her fatigue and stress levels have decreased; ask Sandra and John to describe modifications they have made in their daily routine; any revision in the plan of care includes steps to address patient expectations.

CHAPTER 39

1. k	11. t
2. d	12. f
3. p	13. g
4. n	14. r
5. l	15. b
6. m	16. h
7. e	17. i
8. q	18. j
9. o	19. c
10. s	20. a

21. a. The wider the base of support, the greater the stability of the nurse.
    b. The lower the center of gravity, the greater the stability.
    c. The equilibrium of an object is maintained as long as the line of gravity passes through its base of support.
    d. Facing the direction of movement prevents abnormal twisting of the spine.
    e. Dividing balanced activity between arms and legs reduces the risk of back injury.
    f. Leverage, rolling, turning, or pivoting requires less work than lifting.
    g. When friction is reduced between the object to be moved and the surface on which it is moved, less force is required to move it.

22. a. Congenital defects
    b. Disorders of bones, joints, and muscles
    c. Central nervous system damage
    d. Musculoskeletal trauma

23. The infant's spine is flexed and lacks the anteroposterior curves; as growth and stability increase, the thoracic spine straightens, and the lumbar spinal curve appears, allowing for sitting and standing.

24. Posture is awkward because of slight swayback and protruding abdomen; toward the end of toddlerhood, posture appears less awkward, curves in the cervical

and lumbar vertebrae are accentuated, and foot eversion disappears.

25. Adolescents experience a tremendous growth spurt. In girls, the hips widen, and fat is deposited in upper arms, thighs, and buttocks. In boys, long bone growth and muscle mass are increased.
26. Healthy adults also have the necessary musculoskeletal development and coordination to carry out ADLs.
27. Older adults experience a progressive loss of total bone mass because of physical inactivity, hormonal changes, and increased osteoclastic activity.
28. During standing, the head is erect and midline, body parts are symmetrical, spine is straight with normal curvatures, abdomen is comfortably tucked, knees are in a straight line between the hips and ankles and slightly flexed, and feet are flat on the floor.
29. While sitting, the head is erect and the neck and vertebral column are in straight alignment, body weight is distributed on the buttocks and thighs, thighs are parallel and in a horizontal plane, and feet are supported on the floor.
30. When recumbent, the vertebrae are in straight alignment without observable curves; the head and neck should be aligned without excessive flexion or extension.
31. a. Range of motion
    b. Gait
    c. Exercise
32–34. See Box 39-6, p. 798.
35. a. Activity Intolerance
    b. Ineffective Coping
    c. Impaired Gas Exchange
    d. Risk for Injury
    e. Impaired Physical Mobility
    f. Imbalanced Nutrition
    g. Acute or Chronic Pain
36. a. Participates in prescribed physical activity while maintaining appropriate heart rate, blood pressure, and breathing rate
    b. Verbalizes an understanding of the need to gradually increase activity based on tolerance and symptoms
    c. Expresses understanding of balancing rest and activity
37. Subtract the patient's current age from 220 and obtain the target heart rate by taking 60% to 90% of the maximum.
38. a. Walking, running, bicycling, aerobic dance, jumping rope, and cross-country skiing
    b. Active ROM and stretching all muscle groups and joints
    c. Weight training, raking leaves, shoveling snow, and kneading bread
39. Active: The patient is able to move his or her joints independently.
    Passive: The nurse moves each joint.
40. Walking helps to prevent contractures by increasing joint mobility.

41. a. A single straight-legged cane is used to support and balance a patient with decreased leg strength.
    b. A quad cane provides more support and is used for partial or complete leg paralysis or some hemiplegia.
42. a. Four-point gait: Each leg is moved alternatively with each opposing crutch so three points are on the floor at all times.
    b. Three-point gait: Bears weight on both crutches and then on the uninvolved leg, repeating the sequence.
    c. Two-point gait: There is at least partial weight bearing on each foot.
    d. Swing-through gait: Weight is placed on supportive legs; crutches are one stride in front and then swings through with the crutches, supporting the patient's weight.
43. a. Pulse
    b. Blood pressure
    c. Strength
    d. Endurance
    e. Psychological well-being
44. 4. Ligaments are white, shiny, flexible bands of fibrous tissue that bind joints and connect bones and cartilage.
45. 2. Exercise increases cardiac output.
46. a. Consult and collaborate with members of the health team to increase Mrs. Smith's activity. Involve Mrs. Smith and her family in designing her activity and exercise plan. Consider Mrs. Smith's ability to increase her activity level and follow an exercise program.
    b. The role of physical therapist and exercise trainers in improving Mrs. Smith's activity and exercise program; determine Mrs. Smith's ability to increase her level of activity; impact of medication on Mrs. Smith's activity tolerance
    c. Consider previous patient and personal experiences to therapies designed to improve exercise and activity tolerance. Consider personal experience with exercise regimens.
    d. Therapies need to be individualized to Mrs. Smith's activity tolerance. Apply the goals of the American College of Sports Medicine in the application.
    e. Be responsible and creative in designing interventions to improve Mrs. Smith's activity tolerance.

CHAPTER 40

1. a. The epidermis is the outer layer of the skin.
   b. The dermis is the thicker layer containing bundles of collagen and elastic fibers.
   c. The subcutaneous layer contains blood vessels, nerves, lymph, and loose connective tissue with fat cells.
2. a. Protection
   b. Sensation
   c. Temperature regulation
   d. Excretion and secretion

3. a. Social practices
   b. Personal preferences
   c. Body image
   d. Socioeconomic status
   e. Health beliefs and motivation
   f. Cultural variables
   g. Developmental stage
   h. Physical condition
4. Assessment of the skin includes the color, texture, thickness, turgor, temperature, and hydration.
5. a. Dry skin: Bathe less frequently and rinse the body of all soap because residue left on the skin can cause irritation and breakdown. Add moisture to the air through the use of a humidifier. Increase fluid intake when the skin is dry. Use moisturizing cream to aid healing. (Cream forms a protective barrier and helps maintain fluid within skin.) Use cream such as Eucerin. Use creams to clean skin that is dry or allergic to soaps and detergents.
   b. Acne: Wash hair and skin thoroughly each day with warm water and soap to remove oil. Use cosmetics sparingly because oily cosmetics or creams accumulate in pores and tend to make condition worse. Implement dietary restrictions if necessary. (Eliminate from the diet all foods that aggravate the condition.) Use prescribed topical antibiotics for severe forms of acne.
   c. Skin rashes: Wash the area thoroughly and apply antiseptic spray or lotion to prevent further itching and aid in the healing process. Apply warm or cold soaks to relieve inflammation if indicated.
   d. Contact dermatitis: Avoid causative agents (e.g., cleansers and soaps).
   e. Abrasion: Be careful not to scratch the patient with jewelry or fingernails. Wash abrasions with mild soap and water; dry thoroughly and gently. Observe dressings or bandages for retained moisture because it increases risk of infection.
6. a. Calluses: Thickened portion of epidermis consists of mass of horny, keratotic cells. Calluses are usually flat and painless and are found on undersurface of foot or on palm of hand.
   b. Corns: Friction and pressure from ill-fitting or loose shoes cause keratosis. Corns are seen mainly on or between toes over bony prominences. Corns are usually cone shaped, round, and raised. Soft corns are macerated.
   c. Plantar warts: Fungating lesion appears on sole of foot and is caused by the papilloma virus.
   d. Tinea pedis: Athlete's foot is a fungal infection of the foot; scaliness and cracking of skin occur between the toes and on the soles of the feet. Small blisters containing fluid appear.
   e. Ingrown nails: The toenail or fingernail grows inward into soft tissue around the nail. Ingrown nails often result from improper nail trimming.
   f. Foot odors: Foot odors are the result of excess perspiration that promotes microorganism growth.
7. Halitosis is bad breath.

8. a. Dandruff: Scaling of scalp is accompanied by itching. In severe cases, dandruff is on the eyebrows.
   b. Ticks: Small, gray-brown parasites burrow into the skin and suck blood
   c. Pediculosis: Lice; tiny, grayish-white parasitic insects that infest mammals
   d. Pediculosis capitis: Parasite is on scalp attached to hair strands. Eggs look like oval particles similar to dandruff. Bites or pustules may be observed behind the ears and at the hairline.
   e. Pediculosis corporis: Parasites tend to cling to clothing, so they are not always easy to see. Body lice suck blood and lay eggs on clothing and furniture.
   f. Pediculosis pubis: Parasites are in pubic hair. Crab lice are grayish white with red legs.
   g. Alopecia: Alopecia occurs in all races. Balding patches are in the periphery of the hair line. Hair becomes brittle and broken.
9. a. Oral problems: Patients who are unable to use their upper extremities because of paralysis, weakness, or restriction (e.g., cast or dressing); dehydration; inability to take fluids or food by mouth (NPO); presence of nasogastric or oxygen tubes; mouth breathers; chemotherapeutic drugs; over-the-counter lozenges, cough drops, antacids, and chewable vitamins; radiation therapy to the head and neck; oral surgery, trauma to the mouth, or placement of oral airway; immunosuppression; altered blood clotting; diabetes mellitus
   b. Skin problems: Immobilization; reduced sensation because of stroke, spinal cord injury, diabetes, or local nerve damage; limited protein or caloric intake and reduced hydration (e.g., fever, burns, gastrointestinal alterations, poorly fitting dentures); excessive secretions or excretions on the skin from perspiration, urine, watery fecal material, and wound drainage; presence of external devices (e.g., casts, restraints, bandage, dressing); vascular insufficiency
   c. Foot problems: Patients who are unable to bend over or have reduced visual acuity
   d. Eye care problems: Reduced dexterity and hand coordination
10. a. Activity Intolerance
    b. Bathing Self-Care Deficit
    c. Dressing Self-Care Deficit
    d. Impaired Oral Mucous Membrane
    e. Impaired Physical Mobility
    f. Ineffective Health Maintenance
    g. Risk for Infection
    h. Risk for Impaired Skin Integrity
11. a. Will be able to bathe in front of sink
    b. Will use assist devices
    c. Will dress self, using dressing stick and sock aid
12. a. Make all instructions relevant after assessing knowledge, motivations, and health beliefs.
    b. Adapt instruction of any techniques to the patient's personal bathing facilities.

c. Teach the patient steps to avoid injury.

d. Reinforce infection-control practices.

13. a. Complete bed bath (Skill 40-1): Bath administered to totally dependent patient in bed

b. Partial bed bath (Skill 40-1): Bed bath that consists of bathing only body parts that would cause discomfort if left unbathed, such as the hands, face, axillae, and perineal area. Partial bath also includes washing back and providing a back rub. Dependent patients in need of partial hygiene or self-sufficient bedridden patients who are unable to reach all body parts receive a partial bath.

14. a. Provide privacy

b. Maintain safety

c. Maintain warmth

d. Promote independence

e. Anticipate needs

15. Patients at greatest risk for skin breakdown in the perineal area are male patients who are uncircumcised, patients who have indwelling catheters, and patients recovering from rectal or genital surgery or childbirth.

16. A back rub promotes relaxation, relieves muscular tension, and decreases perception of pain.

17. a. Inspect feet daily

b. Wash feet daily in lukewarm water

c. Wear well-fitting shoes and clean dry socks, never go barefoot

d. Keep skin soft and smooth with emollient lotion

e. Trim toenails straight across and file edges smooth

f. Elevate feet and wiggle toes

g. Protect feet from hot and cold

18. Thorough toothbrushing at least twice a day prevents tooth decay.

19. Flossing removes plaque and tartar between the teeth.

20. Dentures need to be cleaned on a regular basis to avoid gingival infection and irritation.

21. Brushing and combing help keep the hair clean and distribute oil evenly along hair shafts; they also prevent hair from tangling.

22. Shampooing frequency depends on a person's daily routines and the condition of the hair.

23. Mustache and beard require daily grooming because of food particles and mucus that collect on the hair.

24. Shave facial hair after the bath or shampoo; to avoid causing discomfort, gently pull the skin taut and use short, firm razor strokes in the direction the hair grows.

25. Cleansing the eyes involves simply washing with a clean washcloth moistened in water (see Skill 39-1). Never apply direct pressure over the eyeball because it causes serious injury. When cleansing the patient's eyes, obtain a clean washcloth and cleanse from the inner canthus to the outer canthus. Use a different section of the washcloth for each eye.

26. a. To remove an artificial eye, use a small rubber bulb syringe to create a suction effect; place it directly over the eye. Squeezing lifts the eye from the socket.

b. Clean an artificial eye with warm normal saline.

c. To reinsert an artificial eye, retract the upper and lower eyelids and gently slip the eye into the socket.

d. Store an artificial eye in a labeled container filled with tap water or saline.

27. Using a bulb irrigating syringe or a Water Pik set on no. 2 setting, gently wash the ear canal with warm solution (37°C or 98.6°F), being careful not to occlude the canal, which results in pressure on the tympanic membrane. Direct the fluid slowly and gently toward the superior aspect of the ear canal, maintaining the flow in a steady stream.

28. a. An ITC hearing aid is the newest, smallest, and least visible; it fits entirely in the ear canal.

b. An ITE hearing aid fits into the external ear and allows for more fine tuning; it is powerful and easy to adjust.

c. A BTE hearing aid hooks around and behind the ear and is connected to an ear mold; it allows for fine tuning and is useful for patients with progressive hearing loss.

d. A digital hearing aid analyzes sounds to remove background noise; it is beneficial for those with mild to severe hearing loss.

29. a. Fowler: Head of bed raised to angle of 45 degrees or more; semisitting position; the foot of the bed may also be raised at the knees

b. Semi-Fowler: Head of bed raised approximately 30 degrees; inclination less than Fowler position; the foot of the bed may also be raised at the knees

c. Trendelenburg: Entire bed frame tilted with the head of the bed down

d. Reverse Trendelenburg: Entire bed frame tilted with the foot of the bed down

e. Flat: Entire bed frame horizontally parallel with the floor

30. 2. A bath that is administered to a totally dependent patient in bed

31. 1. The condition of the skin depends on the exposure to environmental irritants; with frequent bathing or exposure to low humidity, the skin becomes very dry and flaky.

32. 3. Each patient has individual desires and preferences about when to bathe, shave, and perform hair care.

33. 2. File the toenails straight across and square; do not use scissors or clippers; consult a podiatrist as needed.

34. 3. Use a medicated shampoo for eliminating lice, which are easily able to spread to furniture and other people if not treated.

35. a. Understanding of anatomy and physiology of the skin, pathophysiology of disease states (diabetic, hypertension, body mass index [BMI] of 40), developmental stage

b. Reflection on early clinical experiences

c. Therapeutic communication skills; professional guidelines American Diabetic Association (ADA)

d. Social practices, personal preferences, body image, socioeconomic status for modifications needed at home

e. Current physical conditions, chronic illnesses, limited mobility

CHAPTER 41

1. e	10. c
2. g	11. c
3. i	12. e
4. j	13. h
5. h	14. f
6. d	15. b
7. f	16. g
8. b	17. a
9. a	18. d

19. Conduction through both atria
20. Impulse travel time through the AV node (0.012 to 20 seconds)
21. The impulse traveled through the ventricles (0.06 to 0.12 seconds)
22. Time needed for ventricular depolarization and repolarization (0.12 to 0.42 seconds)
23. a. Physiological
    b. Developmental
    c. Lifestyle
    d. Environmental
24. a. Pregnancy (inspiratory capacity declines)
    b. Obesity (reduced lung volumes)
    c. Musculoskeletal abnormalities (structural configurations, trauma, muscular disease, CNS)
    d. Trauma (flail chest, incisions)
    e. Neuromuscular diseases (decrease the ability to expand and contract the chest wall)
    f. CNS alterations (reduced inspiratory lung volumes)
    g. Chronic diseases (chronic hypoxemia)
25. Hyperventilation is the state of ventilation in which the lungs remove carbon dioxide faster than it is produced by cellular metabolism.
26. Hypoventilation occurs when alveolar ventilation is inadequate to meet the body's oxygen demand.
27. Hypoxia is inadequate tissue oxygenation at the cellular level (decreased hemoglobin levels, high altitudes, poisoning, pneumonia, shock, chest trauma).
28. Cyanosis is blue discoloration of the skin and mucous membranes caused by the presence of desaturated hemoglobin in capillaries.
29. a. Regular rhythm; rate >100 beats/min
    b. Regular rhythm; rate <60 beats/min
    c. Electrical impulse in the atria is chaotic and originates from multiple sites
30. a. Left-sided heart failure is characterized by decreased functioning of the left ventricle (fatigue, breathlessness, dizziness, and confusion).
    b. Right-sided heart failure is characterized by impaired functioning of the right ventricle (weight gain, distended neck veins, hepatomegaly and splenomegaly, and dependent peripheral edema).
31. Myocardial ischemia results when the supply of blood to the myocardium from the coronary arteries is insufficient to meet the myocardial oxygen demand.
32. Angina pectoris is caused by a transient imbalance between myocardial oxygen supply and demand.
33. Myocardial infarction results from a sudden decrease in coronary blood flow or an increase in myocardial oxygen demand without adequate coronary perfusion.
34. Infants and toddlers are at risk for upper respiratory tract infections because of the teething process (develop nasal congestion that encourages bacterial growth), frequent exposures, and secondhand smoke.
35. School-age children and adolescents are at risk from exposure to respiratory infections, secondhand smoke, and smoking.
36. Young and middle-aged adults are at risk from unhealthy diet, lack of exercise, stress, OTC medications, illegal substances, and smoking.
37. Older adults are at risk from aging changes and osteoporosis.
38. a. Smoking cessation
    b. Weight reduction
    c. Low-cholesterol and low-sodium diet
    d. Management of hypertension
    e. Moderate exercise
39. a. Asbestos
    b. Talcum powder
    c. Dust
    d. Airborne fibers
40. a. Cardiac function: Pain, dyspnea, fatigue, peripheral circulation, cardiac risk factors
    b. Respiratory function: Cough, shortness of breath, wheezing, pain, environmental exposure, frequency of infections, risk factors, medication use, smoking use
41. a. Cardiac pain does not occur with respiratory variations.
    b. Pleuritic chest pain is peripheral and radiates to the scapular regions.
    c. Musculoskeletal pain often presents after exercise, trauma, or prolonged coughing episodes.
42. Fatigue is often an early sign of a worsening of the chronic underlying process.
43. Dyspnea is a clinical sign of hypoxia that is usually associated with exercise or excitement associated with many medical and environmental factors.
44. Orthopnea is an abnormal condition in which the patient uses multiple pillows when lying down.
45. Cough is a sudden, audible expulsion of air from the lungs. It is a protective reflex to clear the trachea, bronchi, and lungs of irritants and secretions.
46. Wheezing is a high-pitched musical sound caused by high-velocity movement of air through a narrowed airway.
47. Inspection: Reveals skin and mucous membrane color, general appearance, level of consciousness, adequacy of systemic circulation, breathing patterns, and chest wall movement
48. Palpation: Documents the type and amount of thoracic excursion; areas of tenderness; identifies tactile fremitus, thrills, heaves, and point of maximal impulse (PMI)
49. Percussion: Detects the presence of abnormal fluid or air in the lungs

50. Auscultation: Identifies normal and abnormal heart and lung sounds
51. a. Holter monitor: Portable ECG worn by the patient. The test produces a continuous ECG tracing over a period of time. Patients keep a diary of activity, noting when they experience rapid heartbeats or dizziness. Evaluation of the ECG recording along with the diary provides information about the heart's electrical activity during activities of daily living.
    b. Exercise stress test: ECG is monitored while the patient walks on a treadmill at a specified speed and duration of time. Used to evaluate the cardiac response to physical stress. The test is not a valuable tool for evaluation of cardiac response in women because of an increased false-positive finding.
    c. Thallium stress test: An ECG stress test with the addition of thallium-201 injected IV. Determines coronary blood flow changes with increased activity.
    d. EPS: Invasive measure of intracardiac electrical pathways. Provides more specific information about difficult-to-treat dysrhythmias. Assesses adequacy of antidysrhythmic medication.
    e. Echocardiography: Noninvasive measure of heart structure and heart wall motion. Graphically demonstrates overall cardiac performance.
    f. Scintigraphy: Radionuclide angiography. Used to evaluate cardiac structure, myocardial perfusion, and contractility.
    g. Cardiac catheterization and angiography: Used to visualize cardiac chambers, valves, the great vessels, and coronary arteries. Pressures and volumes within the four chambers of the heart are also measured.
52. a. Pulmonary function tests: Determine the ability of the lungs to efficiently exchange oxygen and carbon dioxide. Used to differentiate pulmonary obstructive disease from restrictive disease.
    b. PEFR: Reflects changes in large airway sizes and is an excellent predictor of overall airway resistance in patients with asthma. Daily measurement is for early detection of asthma exacerbations.
    c. Bronchoscopy: Visual examination of the tracheobronchial tree through a narrow, flexible fiberoptic bronchoscope. Performed to obtain fluid, sputum, or biopsy samples and to remove mucous plugs or foreign bodies.
    d. Lung scan: Used to identify abnormal masses by their size and location. Identification of masses is used in planning therapy and treatments.
    e. Thoracentesis: Specimen of pleural fluid is obtained for cytologic examination. The results may indicate an infection or neoplastic disease. Identification of infection or a type of cancer is important in determining a plan of care.
53. a. Activity Intolerance
    b. Decreased Cardiac Output
    c. Fatigue
    d. Impaired Gas Exchange
    e. Impaired Verbal Communication
    f. Ineffective Airway Clearance
    g. Ineffective Breathing Pattern
    h. Risk for Aspiration
54. a. Lungs are clear to auscultation.
    b. Patient achieves bilateral lung expansion.
    c. Patient coughs productively.
    d. Pulse oximetry is maintained or improved.
55. a. Assess patient's health literacy and determine patient education approaches.
    b. Communicate with patient and family to identify collaborative goals for reducing risk factors.
    c. Explain the link between smoking and respiratory infections.
    d. Hand hygiene techniques
    e. Annual flu vaccine
    f. Signs and symptoms of respiratory infections
56. a. Hydration
    b. Humidification
    c. Nebulization
    d. Coughing and deep breathing
57. a. Patient takes a slow, deep breath and holds for 2 seconds while contracting expiratory muscles, then performs a series of coughs through exhalation.
    b. While exhaling the patient opens the glottis by saying huff.
    c. For patients without abdominal muscle control
58. a. Consists of drainage, positioning, and turning
    b. Chest percussion and vibration
59. a. Bleeding disorders
    b. Osteoporosis
    c. Fractured ribs
60. a. Orotracheal and nasotracheal
    b. Oropharyngeal and nasopharyngeal
    c. Tracheal
61. a. Oral (simplest type, extends from the teeth to oropharynx)
    b. Endotracheal tube (ET) (short term, tube passes the pharynx and into the trachea)
    c. Tracheostomy (long-term assistance, surgical incision into the trachea)
62. Benefits include an increase in general strength and lung expansion.
63. Frequent changes of position are effective for reducing stasis of pulmonary secretions and decreased chest wall expansion (semi-Fowler is the most effective position).
64. Incentive spirometry encourages voluntary deep breathing and prevents atelectasis by using visual feedback.
65. a. Reversing hypoxia and acute respiratory acidosis
    b. Relieving respiratory distress
    c. Preventing or reversing atelectasis and respiratory muscle fatigue
    d. Allowing for sedation and/or other neuromuscular blockage
    e. Decreasing oxygen consumption
    f. Reducing intracranial pressure
    g. Stabilizing the chest wall

66. a. Assist control (AC)
    b. Synchronized intermittent mandatory ventilation (SIMV)
    c. Pressure support ventilation (PSV)
67. Volutrauma (alveolar overdistention), cardiovascular compromise (increased intrathoracic pressure), gastrointestinal disturbances (gastric distention), ventilator associated pneumonia (VAP)
68. a. Continuous positive airway pressure (CPAP)
    b. Bilevel positive airway pressure (BiPAP)
69. Facial and nasal injury, skin breakdown, dry mucus membranes, aspiration
70. a. To remove air and fluids from the pleural space
    b. To prevent air or fluid from reentering the pleural space
    c. To reestablish normal intrapleural and intrapulmonic pressures
71. a. Hemothorax is an accumulation of blood and fluid in the pleural cavity between the parietal and visceral pleurae, usually caused by trauma.
    b. Pneumothorax is a collection of air in the pleural space, caused by loss of negative intrapleural pressure.
72. The goal of oxygen therapy is to prevent or relieve hypoxia.
73. a. Nasal cannula: A nasal cannula is a simple, comfortable device used for oxygen delivery (Skill 41-4). The two cannulas, about 1.5 cm (0.5 inch) long, protrude from the center of a disposable tube, and are inserted into the nares.
    b. Face mask: An oxygen face mask is a device used to administer oxygen, humidity, or heated humidity. It fits snugly over the mouth and nose and is secured in place with a strap. It assists in providing humidified oxygen.
    c. Venturi mask: The Venturi mask delivers oxygen concentrations of 24% to 60% with oxygen flow rates of 4 to 12 L/min, depending on the flow-control meter selected.
74. A PaO_2 of 55 mm Hg or less or an SaO_2 of 88% or less on room air at rest, on exertion, or with exercise is an indication for a patient to receive home oxygen therapy.
75. C = Chest compression
    A = Airway
    B = Breathing
76. a. Physical exercise
    b. Nutrition counseling
    c. Relaxation and stress management techniques
    d. Prescribed medications and oxygen
77. Pursed-lip breathing involves deep inspiration and prolonged expiration through pursed lips to prevent alveolar collapse.
78. Diaphragmatic breathing requires the patient to relax the intercostal and accessory respiratory muscles while taking deep inspirations; it improves efficiency of breathing by decreasing air trapping and reducing the work of breathing.
79. 1. These are the three steps in the process of oxygenation.
80. 1. The heart must work to overcome this resistance to fully eject blood from the left ventricle.
81. 2. Gases move into and out of the lungs through pressure changes (intrapleural and atmospheric).
82. 3. All other answers are related to the subjective sensation of dyspnea.
83. 2. CPT includes postural drainage, percussion, and vibration.
84. a. Identify recurring and present signs and symptoms associated with Mr. Edwards' impaired oxygenation. Determine the presence of risk factors that apply to Mr. Edwards. Ask Mr. Edwards about the use of medication. Determine Mr. Edwards' activity status. Determine Mr. Edwards' tolerance to activity.
    b. Cardiac and respiratory anatomy and physiology; cardiopulmonary pathophysiology; clinical signs and symptoms of altered oxygenation; developmental factors affecting oxygenation; impact on lifestyle; environmental impact
    c. Caring for patients with impaired oxygenation, activity intolerance, and respiratory infections; observations of changes in patient respiratory patterns made during poor air quality days; personal experience with how a change in altitudes or physical conditioning affects respiratory patterns; personal experience with respiratory infections or cardiopulmonary alterations
    d. Apply intellectual standards of clarity, precision, specificity, and accuracy when obtaining a health history for a patient with cardiopulmonary alterations.
    e. Carry out the responsibility of obtaining correct information about Mr. Edwards and explaining risk factors, health promotion and disease prevention activities, and therapies for disease or symptom management. Display confidence in assessing Mr. Edwards' management of illness.

CHAPTER 42

1. a. Extracellular fluid is the fluid outside the cell (interstitial, intravascular, and transcellular fluid).
   b. Intracellular fluid comprises all fluid within the cells of the body (two-thirds of total body water).
2. Cations are positively charged electrolytes (sodium, potassium, and calcium).
3. Anions are negatively charged electrolytes (chloride, bicarbonate, and sulfate).
4. Osmosis is a process by which water moves through a membrane that separates fluids with different particle concentrations.
5. Osmotic pressure is the drawing power of water and depends on the number of molecules in solution.
6. Diffusion is the passive movement of a solute in a solution across a semipermeable membrane from an area of higher concentration to an area of lower concentration.

7. Filtration is the net effect of four forces, two that move fluid out of the capillaries and small venules and two that move fluid back into them.

8. Inward-pulling force caused by blood proteins that helps move fluid from the interstitial area back into the capillaries

9. a. Fluid intake and absorption
   b. Fluid distribution
   c. Fluid output

10. ADH regulates the osmolality of the body fluids by influencing how much water is excreted. The release of ADH decreases if body fluids become too dilute, which allows more water to be excreted in the urine.

11. Renin converts angiotensinogen to angiotensin I, which is then converted to angiotensin II (vasoconstriction). Aldosterone causes reabsorption of sodium and water in isotonic proportion in the distal renal tubules; it also increases urinary excretion of potassium and hydrogen ions.

12. Atrial natriuretic peptide helps regulate extracellular fluid volume by influencing how much sodium and water are excreted.

13. a. Extracellular fluid volume deficit is present when there is insufficient isotonic fluid in the extracellular compartment (hypovolemia).
    b. Extracellular fluid volume excess is too much fluid in the extracellular compartment.

14. a. Water deficit, a hypertonic condition; caused by loss of more water than salt or gain of more salt than water

   b. Water excess, hypotonic condition; caused by more water than salt or a loss of more salt than water

15.

Electrolyte	Values	Function
Potassium	3.5 to 5.0 mEq/L	Maintains resting membrane potential of skeletal, smooth, and cardiac muscle, allowing for normal muscle function
Ionized calcium	4.5 to 5.3 mg/dL	Influences excitability of nerve and muscle cells, necessary for muscle contraction
Magnesium	1.5 to 2.5 mEq/L	Influences function of neuromuscular junctions and is a cofactor for numerous enzymes
Phosphate	2.7 to 4.5 mg/dL	Necessary for production of adenosine triphosphate (ATP), the energy source for cellular metabolism

16.

Imbalance	Laboratory Finding	Signs and Symptoms
Hypokalemia	Serum K$^+$ level <3.5 mEq/L (<3.5 mmol/L); ECG abnormalities may occur	Bilateral muscle weakness that begins in quadriceps and may ascend to respiratory muscles; abdominal distention; decreased bowel sounds; constipation; cardiac dysrhythmias; signs of digoxin toxicity at normal digoxin levels
Hyperkalemia	Serum K$^+$ level >5.0 mEq/L (>5.0 mmol/L); ECG abnormalities may occur	Bilateral muscle weakness in quadriceps, transient abdominal cramps and diarrhea, cardiac dysrhythmias, cardiac arrest
Hypocalcemia	Total serum Ca^{++} <8.4 mg/dL (<2.1 mmol/L) or serum ionized Ca^{++} <4.5 mg/dL (<1.1 mmol/L); ECG abnormalities may occur	Positive Chvostek sign (contraction of facial muscles when facial nerve is tapped), positive Trousseau sign (carpal spasm with hypoxia), numbness and tingling of fingers and circumoral (around mouth) region, hyperactive reflexes, muscle twitching and cramping, tetany, seizures, laryngospasm, cardiac dysrhythmias
Hypercalcemia	Total serum Ca^{++} >10.5 mg/dL (>2.6 mmol/L) or serum ionized Ca^{++} >5.3 mg/dL (>1.3 mmol/L); ECG abnormalities may occur	Anorexia, nausea and vomiting, constipation, fatigue, diminished reflexes, lethargy, decreased level of consciousness, confusion, personality change, cardiac dysrhythmias; possible flank pain from renal calculi; with hypercalcemia caused by shift of calcium from bone: pathological fractures; signs of digoxin toxicity at normal digoxin levels
Hypomagnesemia	Serum Mg^{++} level <1.5 mEq/L (<0.75 mmol/L)	Positive Chvostek and Trousseau signs, hyperactive deep tendon reflexes, insomnia, muscle cramps and twitching, grimacing, dysphagia, tachycardia, hypertension, tetany, seizures, cardiac dysrhythmias; signs of digoxin toxicity at normal digoxin levels
Hypermagnesemia	Serum Mg^{++} level >2.5 mEq/L (>1.25 mmol/L); ECG abnormalities may occur	Lethargy, hypoactive deep tendon reflexes, bradycardia, hypotension; acute elevation in magnesium levels: flushing, sensation of warmth; severe hypermagnesemia: flaccid muscle paralysis, decreased rate and depth of respirations, cardiac dysrhythmias, cardiac arrest

17. a. Acid production—two types: carbonic acid (CO_2) and metabolic acids (lactic acid)
   b. Acid buffering—buffers that work together to maintain normal pH (HCO_3)
   c. Acid excretion—through the lungs (carbonic acid) and kidneys (metabolic acids)

18.

Acid–Base Imbalance	Laboratory Findings	Signs and Symptoms
Respiratory acidosis	pH<7.35 $PaCO_2$>45 mm Hg (6.0 kPa) HCO_3^- level normal if uncompensated or >26 mEq/L (>26 mmol/L) if compensated	Headache, lightheadedness, decreased level of consciousness (confusion, lethargy, coma), cardiac dysrhythmias
Respiratory alkalosis	pH>7.45 $PaCO_2$<35 mm Hg (<4.7 kPa) HCO_3^- level normal if short lived or uncompensated or <22 mEq/L (<22 mmol/L) if compensated K^+ level may be decreased (<3.5 mEq/L) Ionized Ca^{++} level may be decreased (<4.5 mg/dL)	Increased rate and depth of respirations (hyperventilation), lightheadedness, numbness and tingling of extremities and circumoral region (paresthesias), excitement and confusion possibly followed by decreased level of consciousness, cardiac dysrhythmias
Metabolic acidosis	pH<7.35 $PaCO_2$ normal if uncompensated or <35 mm Hg (4.7 kPa) if compensated HCO_3 level <22 mEq/L (<22 mmol/L) Anion gap normal or high, depending on cause K^+ level may be elevated (>5.0 mq/L), depending on cause	Decreased level of consciousness (lethargy, confusion, coma), abdominal pain, cardiac dysrhythmias, increased rate and depth of respirations (compensatory hyperventilation)
Metabolic alkalosis	pH>7.45 $PaCO_2$ normal if uncompensated or >45 mm Hg (>6.0 kPa) if compensated HCO_3^- >26 mEq/L (>26 mmol/L) K^+ level often decreased (<3.5 mEq/L) Ionized Ca^{++} level may be decreased (<4.5 mg/dL)	Lightheadedness, numbness and tingling of fingers, toes, and circumoral region (paresthesias); possible excitement and confusion followed by decreased level of consciousness, cardiac dysrhythmias (may be attributable to hypokalemia)

19. Infants and children have greater water needs and are more vulnerable to fluid volume alterations; fever in children creates an increase in the rate of insensible water loss; adolescents have increased metabolic processes; older adults have decreased thirst sensation that often causes electrolyte imbalances.

20. Respiratory diseases, burns, trauma, GI alterations, and acute oliguric renal disease

21. Second to fifth postoperative day; increased secretion of aldosterone, glucocorticoids, and antidiuretic hormone (ADH) causes increased extracellular fluid volume (ECF); decreased osmolality and increased potassium excretion

22. The greater the body surface burned, the greater the fluid loss.

23. Changes depend on the type and progression of the cancer and its treatment.

24. Decreased cardiac output, which reduces kidney perfusion and activates the RAAS

25. Vomiting and diarrhea can cause ECV deficit; hypernatremia, clinical dehydration and hypokalemia, and nasogastric suctioning can cause metabolic alkalosis.

26. Sweating in a hot environment can lead to ECV deficit, hypernatremia, or clinical dehydration.

27. Recent changes in appetite or the ability to chew and swallow (breakdown of glycogen and fat stores, metabolic acidosis, hypoalbuminemia, edema)

28. History of smoking or alcohol consumption can increase likelihood of respiratory acidosis.

29. a. Diuretics: metabolic alkalosis, hyperkalemia, and hypokalemia
   b. Corticosteroids: metabolic alkalosis, hypokalemia
   c. Hyperkalemia
   d. Hyponatremia
   e. Hypokalemia, hyperkalemia, metabolic alkalosis
   f. Hyperkalemia, mild metabolic alkalosis
   g. Hypermagnesemia
   h. Mild ECV excess, hyponatremia

30. See Table 42-10, p. 950.

31. a. Decreased Cardiac Output
   b. Acute Confusion
   c. Deficient Fluid Volume
   d. Excess Fluid Volume
   e. Impaired Gas Exchange
   f. Risk for Injury
   g. Deficient Knowledge Regarding Disease Management
   h. Risk for Electrolyte Imbalance

32. a. Patient will be free of complications associated with the IV device throughout the duration of IV therapy.
    b. Patient will demonstrate fluid balance as evidenced by moist mucous membranes, balanced I & O, and stable weights within 48 hours.
    c. Patient will have serum electrolytes within the normal range within 48 hours.
33. Enteral replacement of fluids may be appropriate when the patient's GI tract is healthy but the patient cannot ingest fluids.
34. Patients who retain fluids and have fluid volume excess require restriction of fluids.
35. Parenteral replacement of fluids and electrolytes includes total parenteral nutrition (TPN), crystalloids, and colloids.
36. Total parenteral nutrition (TPN) is a nutritionally adequate hypertonic solution consisting of glucose, nutrients, and electrolytes administered centrally or peripherally; it is formulated to meet a patient's needs.
37. IV therapy is used to correct or prevent fluid and electrolyte imbalances.
38. Vascular assist devices (VADs) are catheters, cannulas, or infusion ports designed for repeated access to the vascular system.
39. a. Isotonic: dextrose 5% in water, 0.9% sodium chloride (normal saline), lactated Ringer's solution
    b. Hypotonic: 0.45% sodium chloride (1/2 normal saline), 0.33% sodium chloride (1/3 normal saline), 0.225% sodium chloride (1/4 normal saline)

    c. Hypertonic: dextrose 10% in water, 3% to 5% sodium chloride, dextrose 5% in 0.9% sodium chloride, dextrose 5% in 0.45% sodium chloride, dextrose 5% in lactated Ringer's solution
40. A venipuncture is a technique in which a vein is punctured through the skin by a rigid stylet (butterfly), a stylet covered with a plastic cannula (ONC), or a needle attached to a syringe
41. Electronic infusion pumps deliver an accurate hourly rate.
42. a. Keeping the system sterile and intact
    b. Changing solutions, tubing, and site dressings
    c. Assisting the patient with self-care activities
    d. Monitoring for complications of IV therapy
43. See Table 42-12, p. 960.
44. a. Increase circulating blood volume after surgery, trauma, or hemorrhage.
    b. Increase the number of RBCs and to maintain hemoglobin levels in patients with severe anemia.
    c. Provide selected cellular components as replacement therapy.
45. A, B, O, and AB blood types
46. The universal blood donor is type O.
47. The universal blood recipient is type AB.
48. A transfusion reaction is an antigen–antibody reaction and can range from mild response to severe anaphylactic shock, which can be life threatening.
49. Autotransfusion is the collection and reinfusion of a patient's own blood.
50.

Reaction	Cause	Clinical Manifestations
Acute intravascular hemolytic	Infusion of ABO-incompatible whole blood, RBCs, or components containing ≥10 mL of RBCs Antibodies in recipient's plasma attach to antigens on transfused RBCs, causing RBC destruction	Chills, fever, low back pain, flushing, tachycardia, tachypnea, hypotension, hemoglobinuria, hemoglobinemia, sudden oliguria (acute kidney injury), circulatory shock, cardiac arrest, death
Febrile, nonhemolytic (most common)	Antibodies against donor white blood cells	Sudden shaking chills (rigors), fever (rise in temperature ≥1°C or more), headache, flushing, anxiety, muscle pain
Mild allergic	Antibodies against donor plasma proteins	Flushing, itching, urticaria (hives)
Anaphylactic	Antibodies to donor plasma, especially anti-IgA	Anxiety, urticaria, dyspnea, wheezing progressing to cyanosis, severe hypotension, circulatory shock, possible cardiac arrest
Circulatory overload	Blood administered faster than the circulation can accommodate	Dyspnea, cough, crackles, or rales in dependent portions of lungs, distended neck veins when upright
Sepsis	Bacterial contamination of transfused blood components	Rapid onset of chills, high fever, severe hypotension, and circulatory shock May occur: vomiting, diarrhea, sudden oliguria (acute kidney injury), DIC

51. a. Stop the transfusion immediately.
    b. Keep the IV line open with 0.9% normal saline (NS) by replacing the IV tubing down to the catheter hub.
    c. Notify the health care provider.
    d. Remain with the patient, observing signs and symptoms; monitor vital signs (VS) every 5 minutes.
    e. Prepare to administer emergency drugs per protocol.
    f. Prepare to perform cardiopulmonary resuscitation.
    g. Obtain a urine specimen and send to the laboratory (RBC hemolysis).
    h. Save the blood container, tubing, attached labels, and transfusion record and return them to the laboratory.

52. 4. Extracellular fluid is all the fluid outside of the cell and has three compartments.

53. 3. A combination of increased $PaCO_2$, excess carbonic acid, and an increased hydrogen ion concentration

54. 1. Any condition that results in the loss of GI fluids predisposes the patient to the development of dehydration and a variety of electrolyte disturbances.

55. 3. Is marked by a decreased $PaCO_2$ and an increased pH; anxiety with hyperventilation is a cause

56. a. Knowledge of risk factors for fluid imbalances and physiology of aging; this age group has a high risk for fluid imbalances; specific clinical assessments for signs and symptoms of imbalances; skills and techniques of safe IV therapy
    b. An individualized approach is the foundation of care.
    c. Infusion Nurses Society (INS) standards of practice
    d. Accountability, discipline, and integrity assist you in identifying appropriate nursing diagnoses.
    e. VS return to normal, no postural hypotension, I & O measurements are balanced, daily weight is returned to normal; Mrs. Beck describes effective home management of fluid balance

CHAPTER 43

1. f
2. i
3. h
4. j
5. g
6. k
7. a
8. n
9. b
10. d
11. m
12. l
13. c
14. q
15. p
16. o
17. e

18.

Developmental Stage	Sleep Patterns
Neonates	A neonate up to the age of 3 months averages about 16 hours of sleep a day, sleeping almost constantly during the first week. The sleep cycle is generally 40 to 50 minutes with wakening occurring after one to two sleep cycles. Approximately 50% of this sleep is REM sleep, which stimulates the higher brain centers. This is essential for development because neonates are not awake long enough for significant external stimulation.
Infants	Infants usually develop a nighttime pattern of sleep by 3 months of age. Infants normally take several naps during the day but usually sleep an average of 8 to 10 hours during the night for a total daily sleep time of 15 hours. About 30% of sleep time is in the REM cycle. Awakening commonly occurs early in the morning, although it is not unusual for infants to awaken during the night.
Toddlers	By the age of 2 years, children usually sleep through the night and take daily naps. Total sleep averages 12 hours a day. After 3 years of age, children often give up daytime naps. It is common for toddlers to awaken during the night. The percentage of REM sleep continues to fall. During this period, toddlers may be unwilling to go to bed at night because of a need for autonomy or a fear of separation from their parents.
Preschoolers	On average, preschoolers sleep about 12 hours a night (about 20% is REM). By the age of 5 years, preschoolers rarely take daytime naps except in cultures where a siesta is the custom. Preschoolers usually have difficulty relaxing or quieting down after long, active days and have problems with bedtime fears, waking during the night, or nightmares. Partial wakening followed by normal return to sleep is frequent. In the waking period, children exhibit brief crying, walking around, unintelligible speech, sleepwalking, or bedwetting.
School-age children	The amount of sleep needed varies during the school years. Six-year-old children average 11 to 12 hours of sleep nightly, and 11-year-old children sleep about 9 to 10 hours. Children who are 6 or 7 years old usually go to bed with some encouragement or by doing quiet activities. Older children often resist sleeping because of an unawareness of fatigue or a need to be independent.
Adolescents	On average, teenagers get about 7½ hours of sleep per night. The typical adolescent is subject to a number of changes such as school demands, after-school social activities, and part-time jobs that reduce the time spent sleeping.

Developmental Stage	Sleep Patterns
Young adults	Most young adults average 6 to 8½ hours of sleep a night. Approximately 20% of sleep time is REM sleep, which remains consistent throughout life. It is common for the stresses of jobs, family relationships, and social activities frequently to lead to insomnia and the use of medication for sleep. Daytime sleepiness contributes to an increased number of accidents, decreased productivity, and interpersonal problems in this age group. Pregnancy increases the need for sleep and rest. Insomnia, periodic limb movements, restless leg syndrome, and sleep-disordered breathing are common problems during the third trimester of pregnancy.
Middle adults	During middle adulthood, the total time spent sleeping at night begins to decline. The amount of stage 4 sleep begins to fall, a decline that continues with advancing age. Insomnia is particularly common, probably because of the changes and stresses of middle age. Anxiety, depression, and certain physical illnesses cause sleep disturbances. Women experiencing menopausal symptoms often experience insomnia.
Older adults	Complaints of sleeping difficulties increase with age. More than 50% of adults 65 years or older report problems with sleep. Episodes of REM sleep tend to shorten. There is a progressive decrease in stages 3 and 4 NREM sleep; some older adults have almost no stage 4 sleep, or deep sleep. Older adults awaken more often during the night, and it takes more time for them to fall asleep. The tendency to nap seems to increase progressively with age because of the frequent awakenings experienced at night.
	The presence of chronic illness often results in sleep disturbances for older adults. For example, an older adult with arthritis frequently has difficulty sleeping because of painful joints. Changes in sleep pattern are often attributable to changes in the CNS that affect the regulation of sleep. Sensory impairment reduces an older person's sensitivity to time cues that maintain circadian rhythms.

19. Sleepiness, insomnia, and fatigue often result as a direct effect of commonly prescribed medications, including hypnotics, diuretics, alcohol, caffeine, beta-adrenergic blockers, benzodiazepines, narcotics, anticonvulsants, antidepressants, and stimulants.
20. Rotating shifts cause difficulty adjusting to the altered sleep schedule, performing unaccustomed heavy work, engaging in late-night social activities, and changing evening mealtimes.
21. Most persons are sleep deprived and experience excessive sleepiness during the day, which can become pathological when it occurs at times when individuals need or want to be awake.
22. Personal problems or certain situations (retirement, physical impairment, or the death of a loved one) frequently disrupt sleep.
23. Good ventilation is essential for a restful sleep, as are the size and firmness of the bed; light levels affect the ability to fall asleep.
24. Exercise 2 hours or more before bedtime allows the body to cool down and maintain a state of fatigue that promotes relaxation.
25. Eating a large, heavy, or spicy meal at night often results in indigestion that interferes with sleep; caffeine, alcohol, and nicotine produce insomnia.
26. Patients, bed partners, and parents of children
27. a. Description of sleeping problems
    b. Usual sleep pattern
    c. Physical and psychological illness
    d. Current life events

e. Emotional and mental status
f. Bedtime routines
g. Bedtime environment
h. Behaviors of sleep deprivation
28. a. Anxiety
    b. Ineffective Breathing Pattern
    c. Acute Confusion
    d. Disturbed Sleep Pattern
    e. Ineffective Coping
    f. Fatigue
    g. Insomnia
    h. Readiness for Enhanced Sleep
    i. Sleep Deprivation
29. a. Patient will identify factors in the immediate home environment that disrupt sleep in 2 weeks.
    b. Patient will report having a discussion with family members about environmental barriers to sleep in 2 weeks.
    c. Patient will report changes made in the bedroom to promote sleep within 4 weeks.
    d. Patient will report having fewer than two awakenings per night within 4 weeks.
30. Eliminate distracting noises; promote comfortable room temperature, ventilation, bed, and mattress to provide support and firmness.
31. Sleep when fatigued or sleepy, bedtime routines for children and adults need to avoid excessive mental stimulation before bedtime.
32. Use a small night light and a bell at the bedside to alert family members.

33. Clothing, extra blankets, void before retiring
34. Increasing daytime activity lessens problems with falling asleep.
35. Pursue a relaxing activity for adults; children need comforting and night lights.
36. A dairy product that contains L-tryptophan is often helpful to promote sleep; do not drink caffeine, tea, colas, and alcohol before bedtime.
37. Melatonin (nutritional supplement to aid in sleep), valerian, kava
38. Reduce lights, reduce noise; also refer to Box 43-11 on p. 1008 for other examples
39. Keep beds clean and dry and in a comfortable position; application of dry or moist heat; splints; and proper positioning
40. Plan care to avoid awakening patients for nonessential tasks; allow patients to determine the timing and methods of delivery of basic care.
41. Reduce the risk of postoperative complications for patients with sleep apnea (airway); use of CPAP
42. Giving patients control over their health care minimizes uncertainty and anxiety; back rubs; cautious use of sedatives.
43. a. Patient falls asleep after reducing noise and darkening a room.
    b. Patient describes the number of awakenings during the previous night.
    c. Patient and family demonstrate understanding after receiving instructions on sleep habits.
44. 2. Or another name is the diurnal rhythm
45. 3. A natural protein found in milk, cheeses, and meats
46. 4. See Box 43-3 on p. 997 for other symptoms of sleep deprivation; most physiological symptoms are decreased, not increased.
47. 4. The related factor of the sleep disturbance is physiological for this patient (leg pain).
48. 2. A sleep-promotion plan frequently requires many weeks to accomplish.
49. a. Evaluate the signs and symptoms of Julie's sleep disturbance. Review Julie's sleep pattern. Have her sleep partner report Julie's response to therapies. The expected outcomes developed during the care plan serve as the standards to evaluate its success. Ask the patient if her expectations of care are being met.
    b. The characteristics of a desirable sleep pattern; basis for the expected outcomes in the plan of care
    c. Nursing Scope and Standards of Practice, clinical guidelines for the treatment of primary insomnia as guidelines
    d. Humility may apply if an intervention is unsuccessful; rethink the approach. In the case of chronic sleep problems, perseverance is needed in staying with the plan of care or in trying new approaches.
    e. Use of established expected outcomes to evaluate Julie's plan of care (improved duration of sleep, fewer awakenings, she feels more rested)

CHAPTER 44

1. An unpleasant, subjective sensory and emotional experience associated with actual or potential tissue damage or described in terms of such damage
2. a. Improves quality of life
   b. Reduces physical discomfort
   c. Promotes earlier mobilization and return to previous baseline function
   d. Results in fewer hospital and clinic visits
   e. Decreases length of stay, resulting in lower health care costs
3. a. Transduction: Converts energy produced by stimuli (thermal, chemical, or mechanical) into electrical energy.
   b. Transmission: Excitatory neurotransmitters send electrical impulses across the synaptic cleft between the nerve fibers, enhancing the pain impulse.
   c. Perception: The point the person is aware of the pain; gives awareness and meaning to pain, resulting in a reaction
   d. Modulation: The inhibition of pain impulse is the last phase of the normal pain process, which occurs due to release of inhibitory neurotransmitters.
4. Pain has emotional and cognitive components in addition to physical sensations. Gating mechanisms located along the CNS regulate or block pain impulses. Pain impulses pass through when a gate is open and are blocked when a gate is closed.
5. The point at which a person feels pain; because the amount of circulating substances varies with each individual, the response to pain varies.

6. e	13. b
7. l	14. k
8. f	15. d
9. a	16. g
10. c	17. h
11. j	18. m
12. i	

19. a. Acute pain is protective, has a cause, is of short duration, and has limited tissue damage and emotional response.
    b. Chronic pain lasts longer than anticipated, does not always have a cause, and leads to great personal suffering.
20. a. Chronic episodic pain is pain that occurs sporadically over an extended duration of time.
    b. Idiopathic pain is chronic in the absence of an identifiable physical or psychological cause or pain perceived as excessive for the extent of an organic pathological condition.
21. a. Patients who abuse substances (drugs and alcohol) overreact to discomforts.
    b. Patients with minor illnesses have less pain than those with severe physical alteration.
    c. Administering analgesics regularly leads to drug addiction.
    d. The amount of tissue damage in an injury accurately indicates pain intensity.

e. Health care personnel are the best authorities on the nature of a patient's pain.

f. Psychogenic pain is not real.

g. Chronic pain is psychological.

h. Patients who are hospitalized will experience pain.

i. Patients who cannot speak do not feel pain.

22. a. Age
    b. Fatigue
    c. Genes
    d. Neurologic function

23. a. Attention
    b. Previous experience
    c. Family and social support
    d. Spiritual factors

24. a. Anxiety
    b. Coping styles

25. Individuals learn what is expected and accepted by their culture; different meanings and attitudes are associated with pain across various cultural groups.

26. a. Ask about pain regularly. Assess pain systematically.
    b. Believe the patient and family in their report of pain and what relieves it.
    c. Choose pain-control options appropriate for the patient, family, and setting.
    d. Deliver interventions in a timely, logical, and coordinated fashion.
    e. Empower patients and their families. Enable them to control their course to the greatest extent possible.

27. a. Time, duration, and pattern
    b. Location
    c. Severity
    d. Quality
    e. Aggravating and precipitating factors
    f. Relief measures
    g. Contributing symptoms

28. a. Activity Intolerance
    b. Anxiety
    c. Bathing Self-Care Deficit
    d. Ineffective Coping
    e. Fatigue
    f. Impaired Physical Mobility
    g. Insomnia
    h. Impaired Social Interaction

29. a. Patient reports that pain is a 3 or less on a scale of 0 to 10.
    b. Avoids factors that intensify pain
    c. Uses pain-relief measures safely
    d. Level of discomfort does not interfere with dressing self.

30. a. Change patient's perception of pain, and provide patient with a greater sense of control (distraction, prayer, relaxation, guided imagery, music, and biofeedback).
    b. Aim to provide pain relief, correct physical dysfunction, alter physiological responses, and reduce fears associated with pain-related immobility.

31. a. Tailor the no-pharmacological techniques to the individual.
    b. Cognitive behavioral strategies may not be appropriate for the cognitively impaired.
    c. Physical pain relief strategies focus on promoting comfort and altering physiologic responses to pain and are generally safe and effective.

32. Relaxation is mental and physical freedom from tension or stress that provides individuals with a sense of self-control.

33. Distraction directs a patient's attention to something other than pain and thus reduces the awareness of pain.

34. Music diverts the person's attention away from the pain and creates a relaxation response.

35. Cutaneous stimulation (including massage, warm bath, ice bag, and transcutaneous electrical stimulation [TENS]) reduces pain perception by the release of endorphins, which block the transmission of painful stimuli.

36. Herbals are not sufficiently studied; however, many use herbals such as echinacea, ginseng, gingko biloba, and garlic supplements.

37. One simple way to promote comfort is by removing or preventing painful stimuli; also distraction, prayer, relaxation, guided imagery, music, and biofeedback.

38. a. Nonopioids
    b. Opioids
    c. Adjuvants or coanalgesics

39. Adjuvants or coanalgesics are a variety of medications that enhance analgesics or have analgesic properties that were originally unknown.

40. Refer to Box 44-13, p. 1036.

41. a. Know patient's previous response to analgesics
    b. Select proper medications when more than one is ordered
    c. Know accurate dosage
    d. Assess right time and interval for administration

42. The use of different agents allows for lower than usual doses of each medication, therefore lowering the risk of side effects, while providing pain relief that is good or even better than could be obtained from each of the medications alone.

43. PCA allows patients to self-administer opioids with minimal risk of overdose; the goal is to maintain a constant plasma level of analgesic to avoid the problems of prn dosing.

44. The purpose is to manage pain from a variety of surgical procedures with a pump that is set as a demand or continuous mode and left in place for 48 hours.

45. Local anesthesia is intended for local infiltration of an anesthetic medication to induce loss of sensation to a body part.

46. Regional anesthesia is the injection of a local anesthetic to block a group of sensory nerve fibers.

47. Epidural anesthesia permits control or reduction of severe pain and reduces the patient's overall opioid requirement; can be short or long term.

48. See Table 44-6, p. 1040.

49. a. Incident pain: Pain that is predictable and elicited by specific behaviors such as physical therapy or wound dressing changes

 b. End-of-dose failure pain: Pain that occurs toward the end of the usual dosing interval of a regularly scheduled analgesic

 c. Spontaneous pain: Pain that is unpredictable and not associated with any activity or event

50. a. Patient: Fear of addiction, worry about side effects, fear of tolerance ("won't be there when I need it"), take too many pills already, fear of injections, concern about not being a "good" patient, don't want to worry family and friends, may need more tests, need to suffer to be cured, pain is for past indiscretions, inadequate education, reluctance to discuss pain, pain is inevitable, pain is part of aging, fear of disease progression, primary health care providers and nurses are doing all they can, just forget to take analgesics, fear of distracting primary health care providers from treating illness, primary health care providers have more important or ill patients to see, suffering in silence is noble and expected

 b. Health care provider: Inadequate pain assessment, concern with addiction, opiophobia (fear of opioids), fear of legal repercussions, no visible cause of pain, patients must learn to live with pain, reluctance to deal with side effects of analgesics, fear of giving a dose that will kill the patient, not believing the patient's report of pain, primary health care provider time constraints, inadequate reimbursement, belief that opioids "mask" symptoms, belief that pain is part of aging, overestimation of rates of respiratory depression

 c. Health care system barriers: Concern with creating "addicts," ability to fill prescriptions, absolute dollar restriction on amount reimbursed for prescriptions, mail order pharmacy restrictions, nurse practitioners and physician assistants not used efficiently, extensive documentation requirements, poor pain policies and procedures regarding pain management, lack of money, inadequate access to pain clinics, poor understanding of economic impact of unrelieved pain

51. a. Physical dependence: A state of adaptation that is manifested by a drug class–specific withdrawal syndrome produced by abrupt cessation, rapid dose reduction, decreasing blood level of the drug, or administration of an antagonist

 b. Drug tolerance: A state of adaptation in which exposure to a drug induces changes that result in a diminution of one or more of the drug's effects over time

 c. Addiction: A primary, chronic, neurobiologic disease, with genetic, psychosocial, and environmental factors influencing its development and manifestations. Addictive behaviors include one or more of the following: impaired control over drug use, compulsive use, continued use despite harm, and craving.

52. A placebo is a medication or procedure that produces positive or negative effects in patients that are not related to the placebo's specific physical or chemical properties.

53. Pain clinics treat persons on an inpatient or outpatient basis; multidisciplinary approach to find the most effective pain-relief measures.

54. Palliative care is care provided where the goal is to live life fully with an incurable condition.

55. Hospice care is provided at the end of life; it emphasizes quality of life over quantity.

56. Evaluate the patient for the effectiveness of the pain management after an appropriate period of time; entertain new approaches if no relief; evaluate the patient's perception of pain.

57. 2. Only the patient knows whether pain is present and what the experience is like.

58. 1. When the brain perceives pain, there is a release of inhibitory neurotransmitters such as endogenous opioids (e.g., endorphins) that hinder the transmission of pain and help produce an analgesic effect.

59. 2. A patient's self-report of pain is the single most reliable indicator of the existence and intensity of pain.

60. 2. The reticular activating system inhibits painful stimuli if a person receives sufficient or excessive sensory input; with sufficient sensory stimulation, a person is able to ignore or become unaware of pain.

61. a. Determine Mrs. Mays' perspective of pain, including history of pain; its meaning; and its physical, emotional, and social effects. Objectively measure the characteristics of Mrs. Mays' pain. Review potential factors affecting Mrs. Mays' pain.

 b. Physiology of pain. Factors that potentially increase or decrease responses to pain; pathophysiology of conditions causing pain; awareness of biases affecting pain assessment and treatment; cultural variations in how pain is expressed; knowledge of nonverbal communication

 c. Caring for patients with acute, chronic, and cancer pain; caring for patients who experienced pain as a result of a health care therapy; personal experience with pain

 d. Refer to practice guidelines for acute and chronic pain management. Apply intellectual standards (clarity, specificity, accuracy, and completeness) with gathering assessment. Apply relevance when letting Mrs. Mays explore the pain experience.

 e. Persevere in exploring causes and possible solutions for chronic pain. Display confidence when assessing pain to relieve Mrs. Mays' anxiety. Display integrity and fairness to prevent prejudice from affecting assessment.

CHAPTER 45

1. c
2. h
3. i
4. n
5. o
6. j
7. k
8. v

9. d
10. s
11. p
12. f
13. m
14. e
15. r
16. q
17. w
18. g
19. l
20. u
21. t
22. a

23. b
24. f
25. h
26. b
27. g
28. l
29. k
30. j
31. m
32. d
33. e
34. c
35. a
36. i

37. a. The EAR is the recommended amount of nutrition that appears sufficient to maintain a specific body function for 50% of the population based on age and gender.
   b. The RDA is the average needs of 98% of the population, not the individual.
   c. The AI is the suggested intake for individuals based on observed or experimentally determined estimates of nutrient intakes and used when there is not enough evidence to set the RDA.
   d. The UL is the highest level that likely poses no risk of adverse health events.

38. a. Stage of development
   b. Body composition
   c. Activity levels
   d. Pregnancy and lactation
   e. Presence of disease

39. a. Breastfeeding reduces food allergies and intolerances.
   b. Breastfed infants have fewer infections.
   c. Breast milk is easier for an infant to digest.
   d. Breast milk is convenient, available, and fresh.
   e. Breast milk is the correct temperature.
   f. Breastfeeding is economical.
   g. Breastfeeding increases the time for mother and infant interaction.

40. Cow's milk causes GI bleeding, is too concentrated for infants' kidneys to manage, increases the risk of mild product allergies, and is a poor source of iron and vitamins C and E.

41. Honey and corn syrup are potential sources of botulism toxin and should not be used in the infant's diet.

42. a. Nutritional needs
   b. Physical readiness to handle different forms of foods
   c. The need to detect and control allergic reactions

43. a. Diet rich in high-calorie foods
   b. Food advertising targeting children
   c. Inactivity
   d. Genetic predisposition
   e. Use of food for coping mechanism for stress or boredom
   f. Family and social factors

44. a. Body image and appearance
   b. Desire for independence
   c. Eating at fast-food restaurants
   d. Fad diets
   e. Peer pressure

45. a. Anorexia nervosa: Refusal to maintain body weight over a minimal normal weight for age and height such as weight loss leading to maintenance of body weight less than 85% of ideal body weight (IBW) or failure to make expected weight gain during period of growth, leading to body weight less than 85% of that expected; intense fear of gaining weight or becoming fat, although underweight; disturbance in the way in which one's body weight, size, or shape is experienced (e.g., the person claims to "feel fat" even when emaciated, believes that one area of the body is "too fat" even when obviously underweight); in women, absence of at least three consecutive menstrual cycles when otherwise expected to occur (primary or secondary amenorrhea). (A woman is considered to have amenorrhea if her periods occur only after hormone, e.g., estrogen, administration.)
   b. Bulimia nervosa: Recurrent episodes of binge eating (rapid consumption of a large amount of food in a discrete period of time); a feeling of lack of control over eating behavior during the eating binges; the person regularly engages in either self-induced vomiting, use of laxatives or diuretics, strict dieting or fasting, or vigorous exercise to prevent weight gain; a minimum average of two binge eating episodes a week for at least 3 months.

46. Folic acid is important for DNA synthesis and the growth of RBCs; inadequate intake will lead to possible neural tube defects, anencephaly, or maternal megaloblastic anemia.

47. a. Age-related gastrointestinal changes that affect digestion of food and maintenance of nutrition include changes in the teeth and gums, reduced saliva production, atrophy of oral mucosal epithelial cells, increased taste threshold, decreased thirst sensation, reduced gag reflex, and decreased esophageal and colonic peristalsis.
   b. The presence of chronic illnesses (e.g., diabetes mellitus, end-stage renal disease, cancer) often affects nutrition intake.
   c. Adequate nutrition in older adults is affected by multiple causes, such as lifelong eating habits, ethnicity, socialization, income, educational level, physical functional level to meet activities of daily living, loss, dentition, and transportation.
   d. Adverse effects of medications cause problems such as anorexia, xerostomia, early satiety, and impaired smell and taste perception.
   e. Cognitive impairments such as delirium, dementia, and depression affect the ability to obtain, prepare, and eat healthy foods.

48. Ovolactovegetarians avoid meat, fish, and poultry but eat eggs and milk.

49. Lactovegetarians drink milk but avoid eggs, meat, fish, and poultry.

50. Vegans consume only plant foods.

51. Fruitarians eat only fruits, nuts, honey, and olive oil.

52. a. Screening for malnutrition for risk factors (unintentional weight loss, presence of a modified diet, presence of nutrition impact symptoms)
    b. Anthropometry (size and makeup of the body) including IBW and BMI
    c. Laboratory and biochemical tests (albumin, transferrin, prealbumin, retinal binding protein, total iron-binding capacity, and hemoglobin)
    d. Dietary history and health history (see Box 45-6)
    e. Physical exam: Carefully assessing dysphagia (difficulty swallowing)
53. Dysphagia is difficulty swallowing (neurogenic, myogenic, and obstructive causes).
54. a. General appearance: Listless, apathetic, cachectic
    b. Weight: Obesity (usually 10% above IBW) or underweight (special concern for underweight)
    c. Posture: Sagging shoulders, sunken chest, humped back
    d. Muscles: Flaccid, poor tone, underdeveloped tone; "wasted" appearance; impaired ability to walk properly
    e. Nervous system: Inattention, irritability, confusion, burning and tingling of the hands and feet (paresthesia), loss of position and vibratory sense, weakness and tenderness of the muscles (may result in inability to walk), decrease or loss of ankle and knee reflexes, absent vibratory sense
    f. Gastrointestinal: Anorexia, indigestion, constipation or diarrhea, liver or spleen enlargement
    g. Cardiovascular: Rapid heart rate (>100 beats/min), enlarged heart, abnormal rhythm, elevated blood pressure
    h. General vitality: Easily fatigued, no energy, falls asleep easily, tired and apathetic
    i. Hair: Stringy, dull, brittle, dry, thin, sparse, depigmented; easily plucked
    j. Skin: Rough, dry, scaly, pale, pigmented, irritated; bruises; petechiae; subcutaneous fat loss
    k. Face and neck: Greasy, discolored, scaly, swollen; dark skin over cheeks and under eyes; lumpiness or flakiness of skin around nose and mouth
    l. Lips: Dry, scaly, swollen; redness and swelling (cheilosis); angular lesions at corners of mouth; fissures or scars (stomatitis)
    m. Mouth, oral membranes: Swollen, boggy oral mucous membranes
    n. Gums: Spongy gums that bleed easily; marginal redness, inflammation; receding
    o. Tongue: Swelling, scarlet and raw; magenta, beefiness (glossitis); hyperemic and hypertrophic papillae; atrophic papillae
    p. Teeth: Unfilled caries; missing teeth; worn surfaces; mottled (fluorosis) or malpositioned
    q. Eyes: Eye membranes pale (pale conjunctivas), redness of membrane (conjunctival injection), dryness, signs of infection, Bitot spots, redness and fissuring of eyelid corners (angular palpebritis), dryness of eye membrane (conjunctival xerosis), dull appearance of cornea (corneal xerosis), soft cornea (keratomalacia)
    r. Neck (glands): Thyroid or lymph node enlargement
    s. Nails: Spoon shape (koilonychia), brittleness, ridges
    t. Legs, feet: Edema, tender calf, tingling, weakness
    u. Skeleton: Bowlegs, knock-knees, chest deformity at diaphragm, prominent scapulae and ribs
55. a. Risk for Aspiration
    b. Diarrhea
    c. Deficient Knowledge
    d. Imbalanced Nutrition: Less Than Body Requirements
    e. Readiness for Enhanced Nutrition
    f. Feeding Self-Care Deficit
    g. Impaired Swallowing
56. a. Nutritional intake meets the minimal DRIs
    b. Fat nutritional intake is less than 30%
    c. Removes sugared beverages from the diet
    d. Refrains from eating unhealthy foods between meals and after dinner
    e. Loses at least 0.5 to 1 lb per week
57. a. Botulism: Improperly home-canned foods, smoked and salted fish, ham, sausage, shellfish
    b. *Escherichia coli*: Undercooked meat (ground beef)
    c. Listeriosis: Soft cheese, meat (hot dogs, pate, lunch meats), unpasteurized milk, poultry, seafood
    d. Perfringens enteritis: Cooked meats, meat dishes held at room or warm temperature
    e. Salmonellosis: Milk, custards, egg dishes, salad dressings, sandwich fillings, polluted shellfish
    f. Shigellosis: Milk, milk products, seafood, salads
    g. *Staphylococcus*: Custards, cream fillings, processed meats, ham, cheese, ice cream, potato salad, sauces, casseroles
58. a. Keep patient's environment free of odors.
    b. Provide oral hygiene as needed.
    c. Maintain patient comfort.
59. a. Dysphagia puree
    b. Dysphagia mechanically altered
    c. Dysphagia advanced
    d. Regular
60. a. Thin liquids (low viscosity)
    b. Nectar-like liquids (medium viscosity)
    c. Honey-like liquids
    d. Spoon-thick liquids (pudding)
61. a. 1.0 to 2.0 kcal/mL: Milk-based blenderized foods
    b. 3.8 to 4.0 kcal/mL: Single macronutrient preparations; not nutritionally complete
    c. 1.0 to 3.0 kcal/mL: Predigested nutrients that are easier for a partially dysfunctional GI tract to absorb
    d. 1.0 to 2.0 kcal/mL: Designed to meet specific nutritional needs in certain illnesses
62. a. Pulmonary aspiration: Regurgitation of formula, feeding tube displaced, deficient gag reflex, delayed gastric emptying
    b. Diarrhea: Hyperosmolar formula or medications, antibiotic therapy, bacterial contamination, malabsorption
    c. Constipation: Lack of fiber, lack of free water, inactivity

d. Tube occlusion: Pulverized medications given per tube, sedimentation of formula, reaction of incompatible medications or formula

e. Tube displacement: Coughing, vomiting, not taped securely

f. Abdominal cramping, nausea, or vomiting: High osmolality of formula, rapid increase in rate or volume, lactose intolerance, intestinal obstruction, high-fat formula used, cold formula used

g. Delayed gastric emptying: Diabetic gastroparesis, serious illnesses, inactivity

h. Serum electrolyte imbalance: Excess GI losses, dehydration, presence of disease states such as cirrhosis, renal insufficiency, heart failure, or diabetes mellitus

i. Fluid overload: Refeeding syndrome in malnutrition, excess free water or diluted (hypotonic) formula

j. Hyperosmolar dehydration: Hypertonic formula with insufficient free water

63. a. Appropriate assessment of nutrition needs
    b. Meticulous management of the central venous catheter (CVC) line
    c. Careful monitoring to prevent or treat metabolic complications

64. Intravenous fat emulsions provide supplemental kcal, prevent fatty acid deficiencies, and control hyperglycemia.

65. When the patient meets one-third to half of his or her caloric needs per day, PN is usually decreased to half the original volume; increase the EN to meet needs (75%).

66. Medical nutrition therapy is the use of nutritional therapies to treat an illness, injury, or condition.

67. *Helicobacter pylori* is a bacteria that causes peptic ulcers and is confirmed by laboratory tests. Infection is treated with antibiotics.

68. Crohn disease and ulcerative colitis are treated with elemental diets or PN, supplemental vitamins, and iron. Manage by increasing fiber, reducing fat, avoiding large meals, and avoiding lactose.

69. Celiac disease is treated with a gluten-free diet.

70. Diverticulitis is treated with moderate-to low-residue and high-fiber diet.

71. Diabetes mellitus is managed with a diet of 45% to 75% carbohydrates; limit fat to less than 7% and cholesterol to less than 200 mg/day.

72. Cardiovascular disease is managed by balancing caloric intake with exercise; a diet high in fruits, vegetables, and whole-grain fiber; fish at least twice per week; limit food high in added sugar and salt.

73. The goal with patients who have cancer is to meet the increased metabolic needs of the patient by maximizing intake of nutrients and fluids.

74. The diets of patients who have HIV should include small, frequent, nutrient-dense meals that limit fatty foods and overly sweet foods.

75. Ongoing comparisons need to be made with baseline measures of weight, serum albumin, and protein and calorie intake and changes in condition.

76. 4. Each gram of CHO produces 4 kcal and serves as the main source of fuel (glucose) for the brain, skeletal muscles during exercise, erythrocyte and leukocyte production, and cell function of the renal medulla.

77. 3. When the intake of nitrogen is greater than the output, which is used for building, repairing, and replacing body tissues

78. 4. The growth rate slows during the toddler years (1 to 3 years) and therefore needs fewer kcal but an increased amount of protein in relation to body weight; appetite often decreases at 18 months of age.

79. 1. All of the other patients are at risk for a nutritional imbalance.

80. 2. The measurement of pH of secretions withdrawn from the feeding tubes helps to differentiate the location of the tube.

81. 1. The recommended diet from the AHA to reduce risk factors for the development of hypertension and coronary heart disease

82. a. Select nursing interventions to promote optimal nutrition. Select nursing interventions consistent with therapeutic diets. Consult with other health care professionals (dietitians, nutritionists, physicians, pharmacists, and physical and occupational therapists) to adopt interventions that reflect Mrs. Cooper's needs. Involve the family when designing interventions.

    b. Persevere in exploring causes and possible solutions for imbalanced nutrition; display integrity and fairness to prevent prejudice from affecting assessment.

    c. Apply intellectual standards (clarity, specificity, accuracy, and completeness) when gathering assessment. Previous patient responses to nursing interventions for altered nutrition; personal experiences with dietary change strategies (what worked and what did not)

    d. Integrate knowledge from other disciplines and Healthy People 2020

    e. Inquire about her food intake during the last few days; social interaction; weigh patient and assess posture; signs of poor nutrition

CHAPTER 46

1. d
2. c
3. g
4. f
5. b
6. e
7. a

8. a. Growth and development
   b. Sociocultural factors
   c. Psychological factors
   d. Personal habits
   e. Fluid intake
   f. Pathological conditions
   g. Surgical procedures
   h. Medications
   i. Diagnostic exams

9. Medical conditions that in many cases are reversible

10. Causes outside the urinary tract, usually related to functional deficits

11. Involuntary loss of urine caused by an overdistended bladder often related to obstruction of weak contractions

12. Leakage of small volumes usually related to urethral hypermobility of incompetent sphincter

13. Involuntary passage of urine associated with a strong sense of urgency usually related to neurological or infectious processes

14. Involuntary loss usually at predictable intervals with specific bladder volumes

15. Urinary retention is an accumulation of urine resulting from an inability of the bladder to empty properly.

16. Hospital-acquired UTIs result from catheterization or surgical manipulation. *Escherichia coli* is the most common pathogen.

17. a. Dysuria
    b. Cystitis
    c. Urgency
    d. Frequency
    e. Incontinence
    f. Suprapubic tenderness
    g. Foul-smelling cloudy urine

18. Created from a distal portion of the ileum and proximal portion of the colon; a catheter needs to be inserted through the stoma to empty the urine 4 to 6 times a day.

19. Ileal pouch to replace the bladder; able to void using a Valsalva technique

20. Permanent diversion created by transplanting the ureters into closed-off position of the ileum and then creating a stoma with continuous flow of urine collected in a pouch

21. Small tubes into the renal pelvis to relieve obstruction

22. a. Self-care ability
    b. Cultural considerations
    c. Health literacy

23. j   29. l
24. e   30. b
25. g   31. d
26. i   32. f
27. h   33. a
28. k   34. c

35. Pale, straw-colored to amber-colored depending on its concentration

36. Appears transparent at voiding; becomes more cloudy on standing in a container

37. Has a characteristic ammonia odor; the more concentrated the urine, the stronger the odor

38. a. Random: Collect during normal voiding from an indwelling catheter or urinary diversion collection bag. Use a clean specimen cup.
    b. Clean-voided or midstream: Use a sterile specimen cup. For girls and women: After donning sterile gloves, spread the labia with thumb and forefinger of the nondominant hand. Cleanse the area with a cotton ball or gauze, moving from front (above urethral orifice) to back (toward anus). Using a fresh swab each time, repeat the front-to-back motion three times (begin with the center, then left side, then right side). If agency policy indicates, rinse the area with sterile water and dry with dry cotton ball or gauze. While continuing to hold the labia apart, have the patient initiate the urine stream. After the patient achieves a stream, pass the container into the stream and collect 30 to 60 mL. Remove the specimen container before the flow of urine stops and before releasing the labia. The patient finishes voiding in a bedpan or toilet. For boys and men: After donning sterile gloves, hold the penis with one hand, and using circular motion and antiseptic swab, cleanse the end of the penis, moving from the center to the outside. In uncircumcised men, retract the foreskin before cleansing. If agency procedure indicates, rinse the area with sterile water and dry with cotton or gauze. After the patient has initiated the urine stream, pass the specimen collection container into the stream and collect 30 to 60 mL. Remove the specimen container before the flow of urine stops and before releasing the penis. The patient finishes voiding in a bedpan or toilet.
    c. Sterile: If the patient has an indwelling catheter, collect a sterile specimen by using aseptic technique through the special sampling port (Figure 46-12, p. 1121) found on the side of the catheter. Clamp the tubing below the port, allowing fresh, uncontaminated urine to collect in the tube. After the nurse wipes the port with an antimicrobial swab, insert a sterile syringe hub and withdraw at least 3 to 5 mL of urine (check agency policy). Using sterile aseptic technique, transfer the urine to a sterile container.
    d. Timed urine: Time required may be 2-, 12-, or 24-hour collections. The timed period begins after the patient urinates and ends with a final voiding at the end of the time period. The patient voids into a clean receptacle, and the urine is transferred to the special collection container, which often contains special preservatives. Each specimen must be free of feces and toilet tissue. Missed specimens make the whole collection inaccurate. Check with agency policy and the laboratory for specific instructions.

39. A urinalysis will analyze values of pH (4.6 to 8.0), protein (none or ≤8 mg/100 mL), glucose (none), ketones (none), blood, specific gravity (1.0053 to 1.030) and microscopic values for RBCs (up to 2), WBCs (0 to 4 per low-power field), bacteria (none), casts (none), and crystals (none).

40. Specific gravity measures concentration particles in the urine. High specific gravity in the urine reflects concentrated and low reflects diluted urine.

41. A urine culture is performed on a sterile or clean voided sample of urine and can report bacterial growth in 24 to 48 hours.

42. a. Abdominal radiography: Determines the size, shape, symmetry, and location of the kidneys.

b. IVP: Views the collecting ducts and renal pelvis and outlines the ureters, bladder, and urethra. A special intravenous injection (iodine based) that converts to a dye in urine is injected intravenously.

c. Direct visualization, specimen collection, and treatment

d. CT scan: Obtains detailed images of structures within a selected plane of the body. The computer reconstructs cross-sectional images and thus allows the health care provider to view pathologic conditions such as tumors and obstructions.

e. Ultrasonography: Renal ultrasonography identifies gross renal structures and structural abnormalities in the kidney using high-frequency, inaudible sound waves. Bladder ultrasonography identifies structural abnormalities of bladder or lower urinary tract. It can also be used to estimate the volume of urine in the bladder.

43. a. Urinary Incontinence (Functional, Stress, Urge)
   b. Pain (Acute, Chronic)
   c. Risk for Infection
   d. Self-Care Deficit, Toileting
   e. Impaired Skin Integrity
   f. Impaired Urinary Elimination
   g. Urinary Retention

44. a. Normal elimination
   b. Patient will be able to independently use the toilet
   c. Decrease the number of pads by one to two within 8 weeks

45. a. Maintain elimination habits
   b. Maintain adequate fluid intake
   c. Promote complete bladder emptying
   d. Prevent infection

46. a. Intermittent: Used to measure post void residual (PVR) when a bladder scanner is not available or as a way to manage chronic urinary retention
   b. Short- or long-term indwelling: Used for accurate monitoring of urinary output, perioperative or postoperative after urologic or GYN procedures, and when the bladder inadequately empties due to obstruction or neurological condition.

47. The nurse should perform personal hygiene at least three times a day for a patient with an indwelling catheter with soap and water.

48. Catheter care requires special care three times a day and after defecation.

49. Fluid intake should be 2000 to 2500 mL if permitted.

50. To maintain the patency of indwelling catheters, it may be necessary to irrigate or flush with sterile normal saline (NS). Blood, pus, or sediment can collect within the tubing, resulting in the need to change the catheter.

51. For a suprapubic catheter, a catheter is surgically placed through the abdominal wall above the symphysis pubis and into the urinary bladder.

52. A external catheter is suitable for incontinent or comatose men who still have complete and spontaneous bladder emptying.

53. Improve the strength of pelvic muscles and consist of repetitive contractions of muscle groups. They are effective in treating stress incontinence, overactive bladders, and mixed causes of urinary incontinence.

54. Bladder retraining is used to reduce the voiding frequency and to increase the bladder capacity, specifically for patients with urge incontinence related to overactive bladder.

55. Benefits patients with functional incontinence by improving voluntary control over urination.

56. A nurse would evaluate for change in the patient's voiding pattern and continued presence of urinary tract alterations.

57. 2. Involuntary leakage of urine during increased abdominal pressure in the absence of bladder muscle contraction

58. 1. Pain or burning (dysuria) as well as fever, chills, nausea or vomiting, and malaise

59. 3. Symptoms of an allergic response

60. 4. Antibiotics help the situation; the other choices are interventions to teach the patient to prevent UTIs.

61. a. Gather nursing history of the urination pattern, symptoms, and factors affecting urination. Conduct a physical assessment of body systems potentially affected by urinary change. Assess the characteristics of urine. Assess perceptions of urinary problems as they affect self-concept and sexuality.
   b. Physiology of fluid balance; anatomy and physiology of normal urine production and urination; pathophysiology of selected urinary alterations; factors affecting urination; principles of communication used to address issues related to self-concept and sexuality
   c. Caring for patients with alterations in urinary elimination; caring for patients at risk for UTI; personal experience with changes in urinary elimination
   d. Maintain privacy and dignity. Apply intellectual standards to ensure history and assessment are complete and in depth. Apply professional standards of care from professional organizations such as ANA and AHCPR.
   e. Display humility in recognizing limitations in knowledge.

CHAPTER 47

1. The teeth masticate food, breaking it down to swallow, and saliva is produced to dilute and soften the food for easier swallowing.

2. The bolus of food travels down and is pushed along by peristalsis, which propels the food through the length of the GI tract.

3. The stomach stores swallowed food and liquid; mixing of food, liquid, and digestive juices and empties its contents into the small intestine; produces HCl, mucus, pepsin, and intrinsic factor, which is essential for the absorption of vitamin B_{12}.

4. Segmentation and peristaltic movement facilitate both digestion and absorption; chyme mixes with digestive juices.

5. The lower GI tract (colon) is divided into the cecum, colon, and rectum. It is the primary organ of elimination.

6. Contraction and relaxation of the internal and external sphincters, innervated by sympathetic and parasympathetic stimuli, aid in control of defecation.
7. a. Normal GI tract function
   b. Sensory awareness of rectal distention and rectal contents
   c. Voluntary sphincter control
   d. Adequate rectal capacity and compliance
8. a. Age
   b. Diet
   c. Fluid intake
   d. Physical activity
   e. Psychological factors
   f. Personal habits
   g. Position during defecation
   h. Pain
   i. Pregnancy
   j. Surgery and anesthesia
   k. Medications
   l. Diagnostic tests
9. Fiber is a nondigestible residue in the diet that provides the bulk of fecal material. Good sources include whole grains, fresh fruits, and vegetables.
10. Fluid liquefies the intestinal contents, easing its passage through the colon; reduced fluid intake slows the passage of food through the intestine and results in hardening of stool contents.
11. Physical activity promotes peristalsis; weakened abdominal and pelvic floor muscles impair the ability to increase intraabdominal pressure and to control the external sphincter.
12. Stress is associated with ulcerative colitis, irritable bowel syndrome, certain gastric and duodenal ulcers, and Crohn disease.
13. Squatting
14. a. Hemorrhoids
   b. Rectal surgery
   c. Rectal fistulas
   d. Abdominal surgery
15. General anesthetic agents used during surgery cause temporary cessation of peristalsis; direct manipulation of the bowel temporarily stops peristalsis (paralytic ileus).
16. a. Improper diet
   b. Reduced fluid intake
   c. Lack of exercise
   d. Certain medications
17. a. Infrequent bowel movements <3 days
   b. Hard, dry stools that are difficult to pass
18. Fecal impaction occurs when a collection of hardened feces that a person cannot expel (as a result of unrelieved constipation) becomes wedged in the rectum.
19. a. Oozing of diarrhea
   b. Loss of appetite (anorexia)
   c. Nausea or vomiting
   d. Abdominal distention and cramping
   e. Rectal pain
20. Diarrhea is an increased number of stools and the passage of liquid, unformed feces associated with disorders affecting digestion, absorption, and secretion.

21. a. Contamination and risk of skin ulceration
   b. Fluid and electrolyte or acid–base imbalances
22. *C. difficile* is a causative agent of mild diarrhea to severe colitis acquired by the use of antibiotics, chemotherapy, invasive bowel procedures, or a health care worker's hands or direct contact with environmental surfaces.
23. a. Fecal incontinence is the inability to control passage of feces and gas from the anus caused by physical conditions that impair anal sphincter function or control.
   b. Flatulence is a gas accumulation in the lumen of the intestine; stretches and distends (a common cause of abdominal fullness, pain, and cramping).
24. Dilated, engorged veins in the lining of the rectum; either internal or external
25. A stoma is an artificial opening in the abdominal wall.
26. An ileostomy is a surgical opening in the ileum.
27. A colostomy is a surgical opening in the colon.
28. a. Determination of the usual elimination pattern
   b. Patient's description of usual stool characteristics
   c. Identification of routines followed to promote normal elimination
   d. Presence and status of bowel diversions
   e. Changes in appetite
   f. Diet history
   g. Description of daily fluid intake
   h. History of surgery or illness
   i. Medication history
   j. Emotional state
   k. History of exercise
   l. History of pain or discomfort
   m. Social history
   n. Mobility and dexterity
29. Inspect all four quadrants for contour, shape, symmetry, and skin color.
30. Assess bowel sounds in all four quadrants.
31. Palpate for masses or areas of tenderness.
32. Use percussion to detect lesions, fluid, or gas.
33. Fecal occult blood testing, or guaiac test, measures microscopic amounts of blood in feces; useful as a screening tool for colon cancer.
34. a. Color: Infants: yellow; adults: brown
   b. Odor: Malodorous; affected by food type
   c. Consistency: Soft, formed
   d. Frequency: Varies: infants, four to six times daily (breastfed) or one to three times daily (bottle fed); adults, daily or two to three times a week
   e. Amount: 150 g/day (adult)
   f. Shape: Resembles diameter of rectum
   g. Constituents: Undigested food, dead bacteria, fat, bile pigment, cells lining intestinal mucosa, water
35. a. Endoscopy
   b. Anorectal manometry
   c. Plain film of abdomen/kidneys, ureter and bladder (KUB)
   d. Barium enema
   e. Ultrasonography
   f. Computed tomography
   g. Colonic transit study
   h. Magnetic resonance imaging

36. a. Bowel Incontinence
    b. Constipation
    c. Risk for Constipation
    d. Perceived Constipation
    e. Diarrhea
    f. Self-Care Deficit: Toileting
    g. Disturbed Body Image
    h. Nausea
    i. Deficient Knowledge (Nutrition)
    j. Acute Pain
37. a. Patient establishes a regular defecation schedule.
    b. Patient is able to list proper fluid and food intake needed to achieve elimination.
    c. Patient implements a regular exercise program.
    d. Patient reports daily passage of soft, formed brown stool.
    e. Patient does not report any discomfort associated with defecation.
38. a. Sitting position
    b. Positioning on bedpan
39. Cathartics and laxatives (bulk forming, emollient or wetting, saline, stimulant, lubricant) have the short-term action of emptying the bowel.
40. Antidiarrheal opiate agents decrease intestinal muscle tone to slow passage of feces.
41. Enemas provide temporary relief of constipation, emptying the bowel before diagnostic tests, and bowel training.
42. Cleansing enemas include tap water, normal saline, soapsuds solution, and low-volume hypertonic saline. Cleansing enemas promote the complete evacuation of feces from the colon.
43. A tap water enema is hypotonic and exerts a lower osmotic pressure than fluid in interstitial spaces.
44. Normal saline enema is the safest enema solution; it exerts the same osmotic pressure as fluids in interstitial spaces surrounding the bowel.
45. Hypertonic solutions exert osmotic pressure that pulls out of interstitial spaces; they are contraindicated in patients who are dehydrated and in young infants.
46. Soapsuds create the effect of interstitial irritation to stimulate peristalsis.
47. Oil retention enemas lubricate the rectum and the colon and make the feces softer and easier to pass.
48. A carminative enema provides relief from gaseous distention; it improves the ability to pass flatus.
49. a. Can cause irritation to the mucosa
    b. Can cause bleeding
    c. Can cause stimulation of the vagus nerve, which results in a reflex slowing of the heart rate
50. a. Decompression
    b. Enteral feeding
    c. Compression
    d. Lavage
51. The nurse should assess the condition of the nares and mucosa for inflammation and excoriation, frequent changing of the tape and lubrication of the nares, and frequent mouth care.
52. a. Assessing the normal elimination pattern and recording times when the patient is incontinent

b. Incorporating principles of gerontologic nursing when providing bowel training programs for older adults
c. Choosing a time in the patient's pattern to initiate defection-control measures
d. Offering a hot drink or fruit juice before the defecation time
e. Assisting the patient to the toilet at the designated time
f. Providing privacy and setting a time limit for defecation
g. Instructing the patient to lean forward at the hips when on the toilet, apply manual pressure with the hands over the abdomen, and bear down but not strain to stimulate colon emptying
h. Unhurried environment and a nonjudgmental caregiver
i. Maintaining normal exercise within the patient's physical ability
53. Patient is able to have regular, pain-free defecation of soft, formed stool.
54. 4. Reabsorption in the small intestine is very efficient.
55. 1. See Box 47-5, p. 1158 for rationale.
56. 1. An infant's stool is yellow, and an adult's stool is brown.
57. 2. In a supine position, it is impossible to contract the muscles used during defecation; raising the HOB assists the patient to a more normal sitting position, enhancing the ability to defecate.
58. 3. Correct volume for a school-aged child
59. a. Javier needs to select nursing interventions to promote normal bowel elimination. Consult with nutritionists and enteral stoma therapists. Involve Mr. Johnson and his family in designing nursing interventions.
    b. Role of the other health care professionals in returning the patient's bowel elimination pattern to normal; impact of specific therapeutic diets and medication on bowel elimination patterns; expected results of cathartics, laxatives, and enemas on bowel elimination
    c. Previous patient response to planned nursing therapies for improving bowel elimination (what worked and what did not)
    d. Individualize therapies to Mr. Johnson's bowel elimination needs. Select therapies consistent within wound and ostomy professional practice standards.
    e. Javier needs to be creative when planning interventions for Mr. Johnson to achieve normal elimination patterns. Display independence when integrating interventions from other disciplines in Mr. Johnson's plan of care. Act responsibly by ensuring that interventions are consistent within standards.

CHAPTER 48

1. e
2. f
3. a
4. b

5. d
6. c
7. a. Pressure intensity
   b. Pressure duration
   c. Tissue tolerance
8. a. Impaired sensory perception
   b. Impaired mobility
   c. Alteration in level of consciousness
   d. Shear
   e. Friction
   f. Moisture
9. I.   Intact skin with nonblanchable redness of a localized area over a bony prominence
   II. Partial-thickness skin loss involving epidermis, dermis, or both
   III. Full-thickness with tissue loss
   IV. Full-thickness tissue loss with exposed bone, tendon, or muscle
10. Red, moist tissue composed of new blood vessels, which indicates wound healing
11. Stringy substance attached to wound bed that is soft, yellow, or white tissue
12. Black or brown necrotic tissue
13. Describes the amount, color, consistency, and odor of wound drainage
14. Wound that is closed by epithelialization with minimal scar formation
15. Wound is left open until it becomes filled by scar tissue; chance of infection is greater.
16. a. Inflammatory response
    b. Epithelial proliferation (reproduction)
    c. Migration with reestablishment of the epidermal layers
17. a. Injured blood vessels constrict, and platelets gather to stop bleeding; clots form a fibrin matrix for cellular repair.
    b. Damaged tissues and mast cells secrete histamine (vasodilates) with exudation of serum and WBC into damaged tissues.
    c. With the appearance of new blood vessels as reconstruction progresses, the proliferative phase begins and lasts from 3 to 24 days. The main activities during this phase are the filling of the wound with granulation tissue, contraction of the wound, and resurfacing of the wound by epithelialization.
    d. Maturation, the final stage, may take up to 1 year; the collagen scar continues to reorganize and gain strength for several months.
18. a. Bleeding from a wound site that occurs after hemostasis indicates a slipped surgical suture, a dislodged clot, infection, or erosion of a blood vessel by a foreign object (internal or external).
    b. Localized collection of blood underneath the tissue
    c. Second most common nosocomial infection; purulent material drains from the wound (yellow, green, or brown, depending on the organism).
    d. A partial or total separation of wound layers; risks are poor nutritional status, infection, or obesity.

   e. Total separation of wound layers with protrusion of visceral organs through a wound opening requiring surgical repair
19. a. Sensory perception
    b. Moisture
    c. Activity
    d. Mobility
    e. Nutrition
    f. Friction or shear
20. a. Nutrition
    b. Tissue perfusion
    c. Infection
    d. Age
    e. Psychosocial impact of wounds
21. a. Potential effects of impaired mobility; muscle tone and strength
    b. Malnutrition is a major risk factor; a loss of 5% of usual weight, weight less than 90% of ideal body weight, or a decrease of 10 lb in a brief period
    c. Continuous exposure of the skin to body fluids, especially gastric and pancreatic drainage, increases the risk for breakdown.
    d. Adequate pain control and patient comfort will increase mobility, which in turn reduces risk.
22. a. Is superficial with little bleeding and is considered a partial-thickness wound
    b. Sometimes bleeds more profusely depending on depth and location (>5 cm or 2.5 cm in depth)
    c. Bleeds in relation to the depth and size, with a high risk of internal bleeding and infection
23. Whether the wound edges are closed, the condition of tissue at the wound base; look for complications and skin coloration
24. Amount, color, odor, and consistency of drainage, which depends on the location and the extent of the wound
25. See Table 48-2, p. 1192
26. Observe the security of the drain and its location with respect to the wound and the character of the drainage; measure the amount.
27. Surgical wounds are closed with staples, sutures, or wound closures. Look for irritation around staple or suture sites and note whether the closures are intact.
28. a. Risk for Infection
    b. Imbalanced Nutrition: Less Than Body Requirements
    c. Acute or Chronic Pain
    d. Impaired Skin Integrity
    e. Impaired Physical Mobility
    f. Risk for Impaired Skin Integrity
    g. Ineffective Tissue Perfusion
    h. Impaired Tissue Integrity
29. a. Higher percentage of granulation tissue in the wound base
    b. No further skin breakdown in any body location
    c. An increase in the caloric intake by 10%
30. a. Skin care and management of incontinence
    b. Mechanical loading and support devices
    c. Education

31. a. Prevent and manage infection.
    b. Cleanse the wound.
    c. Remove nonviable tissue.
    d. Maintain the wound in moist environment.
    e. Eliminate dead space.
    f. Control odor.
    g. Eliminate or minimize pain.
    h. Protect the wound.
32. Remove nonviable necrotic tissue to rid the ulcer of a source of infection, enable visualization of the wound bed, and provide a clean base necessary for healing.
33. a. Mechanical
    b. Autolytic
    c. Chemical
    d. Sharp or surgical
34. Control bleeding by applying direct pressure in the wound site with a sterile or clean dressing, usually after trauma, for 24 to 48 hours.
35. Gentle cleansing rather than vigorous cleansing with NS (physiological and will not harm tissue)
36. Applying sterile or clean dressings and immobilizing the body part
37. a. Protects a wound from microorganism contamination
    b. Aids in hemostasis
    c. Promotes healing by absorbing drainage and debriding a wound
    d. Supports or splints the wound site
    e. Promotes thermal insulation of the wound surface
    f. Provides a moist environment
38. See Box 48-9, p. 1209.
39. a. Adheres to undamaged skin
    b. Serves as a barrier to external fluids and bacteria but allows the wound surface to breathe
    c. Promotes a moist environment
    d. Can be removed without damaging underlying tissues
    e. Permits viewing
    f. Does not require a secondary dressing
40. a. Absorbs drainage through the use of exudate absorbers
    b. Maintains wound moisture
    c. Slowly liquefies necrotic debris
    d. Impermeable to bacteria
    e. Self-adhesive and molds well
    f. Acts as a preventive dressing for high-risk friction areas
    g. May be left in place for 3 to 5 days, minimizing skin trauma and disruption of healing
41. a. Soothing and reduces pain
    b. Provides a moist environment
    c. Debrides the wound
    d. Does not adhere to the wound base and is easy to remove
42. a. Assessment of the skin beneath the tape
    b. Performing thorough hand hygiene before and after wound care
    c. Wear sterile gloves

    d. Removing or changing dressings over closed wounds when they become wet or if the patient has signs and symptoms of infection
43. Assess the size, depth, and shape of the wound; dressing (moist) needs to be flexible and in contact with all of the wound surface; do not pack tightly (overpacking causes pressure); do not overlap the wound edges (maceration of the tissue).
44. Applies localized negative pressure to draw the edges of a wound together by evacuating wound fluids and stimulating granulation tissue formation, reduces the bacterial burden of a wound, and maintains a moist environment
45. a. Cleanse in a direction from the least contaminated area to the surrounding skin.
    b. Use gentle friction when applying solutions locally to the skin.
    c. When irrigating, allow the solution to flow from the least to the most contaminated area.
46. Use of an irrigating syringe to flush the area with a constant low-pressure flow of solution of exudates and debris. Never occlude a wound opening with a syringe.
47. Portable units that connect tubular drains lying within a wound bed and exert a safe, constant low-pressure vacuum to remove and collect drainage
48. a. Creating pressure over a body part
    b. Immobilizing a body part
    c. Supporting a wound
    d. Reducing or preventing edema
    e. Securing a splint
    f. Securing dressings
49. a. Inspecting the skin for abrasions, edema, discoloration, or exposed wound edges
    b. Covering exposed wounds or open abrasions with a sterile dressing
    c. Assessing the condition of underlying dressings and changing if soiled
    d. Assessing the skin for underlying areas that will be distal to the bandage for signs of circulatory impairment
50. a. Improves blood flow to an injured part; if applied for more than 1 hour, the body reduces blood flow by reflex vasoconstriction to control heat loss from the area
    b. Diminishes swelling and pain, prolonged results in reflex vasodilation
51. a. A person is better able to tolerate short exposure to temperature extremes.
    b. More sensitive to temperature variations: neck, inner aspect of the wrist and forearm, and perineal region
    c. The body responds best to minor temperature adjustments.
    d. A person has less tolerance to temperature changes to which a large area of the body is exposed.
    e. Tolerance to temperature variations changes with age.
    f. Physical conditions that reduce the reception or perception of sensory stimuli.

g. Uneven temperature distribution suggests that the equipment is functioning improperly.

52. Improve circulation, relieve edema, and promote consolidation of pus and drainage.

53. Promotes circulation, lessens edema, increases muscle relaxation, and provides a means to debride wounds and apply medicated solutions

54. The pelvic area is immersed in warm fluid, causing wide vasodilation.

55. Disposable hot packs that apply warm, dry heat to an area

56. Relieves inflammation and swelling

57. Immersing a body part for 20 minutes

58. Used for muscle sprain, localized hemorrhage, or hematoma

59. a. Was the etiology of the skin impairment addressed?
    b. Was wound healing supported by providing the wound base with a moist, protected environment?
    c. Were issues such as nutrition assessed and a plan of care developed?

60. 3. The force exerted parallel to the skin resulting from both gravity pushing down on the body and resistance between the patient and the surface

61. 1. Age is not a subscale. Perception, moisture, activity, mobility, nutrition, friction, and shear are the subscales.

62. 3. The recommended protein intake for adults is 0.8 g/kg; a higher intake of up to 1.8 g/kg/day is necessary for healing.

63. 2. See Table 48-8, p. 1211, for choice and rationale for dressings for ulcer stages.

64. a. Identify the risk for developing impaired skin integrity. Identify signs and symptoms associated with impaired skin integrity or poor wound healing. Examine Mrs. Stein's skin for actual impairment in skin integrity.
    b. Pathogenesis of pressure ulcers; factors contributing to pressure ulcer formation or poor wound healing; factors contributing to wound healing; impact of underlying disease process on skin integrity; impact of medication on skin integrity and wound healing

c. Caring for patients with impaired skin integrity or wounds; observation of normal wound healing.

d. Apply intellectual standards of accuracy, relevance, completeness, and precision when obtaining health history regarding skin integrity and wound management; knowledge of AHCPR standards for prevention of pressure ulcers.

e. Use discipline to obtain complete and correct assessment data regarding Mrs. Stein's skin and wound integrity. Demonstrate responsibility for collecting appropriate specimens for diagnostic and laboratory tests related to wound management.

CHAPTER 49

1. c	10. j
2. f	11. l
3. d	12. d
4. b	13. i
5. a	14. k
6. e	15. b
7. c	16. g
8. f	17. a
9. h	18. e

19. The patient's thoughts to race; attention scatters in many directions and anxiety and restlessness occur

20. a. Age
    b. Meaningful stimuli
    c. Amount of stimuli
    d. Social interaction
    e. Environmental factors
    f. Cultural factors

21. Older adults because of normal physiological changes, individuals who live in confined environments, acutely ill patients

22. a. Has your family member shown any recent mood swings?
    b. Have you noticed the family member avoiding social activities?

23.

Sense	Assessment Technique	Child Behavior	Adult Behavior
Vision	Ask patient to read newspaper, magazine, or lettering on menu. Ask patient to identify colors on color chart or crayons. Observe patient performing ADLs.	Self-stimulation, including eye rubbing, body rocking, sniffing or smelling, arm twirling; hitching (using legs to propel while in sitting position) instead of crawling	Poor coordination, squinting, underreaching or overreaching for objects, persistent repositioning of objects, impaired night vision, accidental falls
Hearing	Assess patient's hearing acuity and history of tinnitus. Observe patient conversing with others. Inspect ear canal for hardened cerumen. Observe patient behaviors in a group.	Frightened when unfamiliar people approach, no reflex or purposeful response to sounds, failure to be awakened by loud noise, slow or absent development of speech, greater response to movement than to sound, avoidance of social interaction with other children	Blank looks, decreased attention span, lack of reaction to loud noises, increased volume of speech, positioning of head toward sound, smiling and nodding of head in approval when someone speaks, use of other means of communication such as lip-reading or writing, complaints of ringing in ears
Touch	Check patient's ability to discriminate between sharp and dull stimuli. Assess whether patient is able to distinguish objects (coin or safety pin) in the hand with eyes closed. Ask whether patient feels unusual sensations.	Inability to perform developmental tasks related to grasping objects or drawing, repeated injury from handling of harmful objects (e.g., hot stove, sharp knife)	Clumsiness, overreaction or underreaction to painful stimulus, failure to respond when touched, avoidance of touch, sensation of pins and needles, numbness Unable to identify object placed in hand
Smell	Have patient close eyes and identify several nonirritating odors (e.g., coffee, vanilla).	Difficult to assess until child is 6 or 7 years old, difficulty discriminating noxious odors	Failure to react to noxious or strong odor, increased body odor, increased sensitivity to odors
Taste	Ask patient to sample and distinguish different tastes (e.g., lemon, sugar, salt). (Have patient drink or sip water and wait 1 minute between each taste.)	Inability to tell whether food is salty or sweet, possible ingestion of strange-tasting things	Change in appetite, excessive use of seasoning and sugar, complaints about taste of food, weight change

24. a. Uneven, cracked walkways leading to doors
  b. Doormats with slippery backing
  c. Extension and phone cords in walkways
  d. Loose area rugs and runners
  e. Bathrooms without shower or tub grab bars
  f. Unmarked water faucets
  g. Unlit stairways, lack of railings
25. a. Expressive aphasia, a motor type, is the inability to name common objects or to express simple ideas in words or writing.
  b. Receptive aphasia, a sensory type, is the inability to understand written or spoken language.
26. a. Risk-Prone Health Behavior
  b. Impaired Verbal Communication
  c. Risk for Injury
  d. Impaired Physical Mobility
  e. Bathing Self-Care Deficit
  f. Situational Low Self-Esteem
  g. Social Isolation
  h. Risk for Falls
27. a. Use communication techniques to send and receive messages.

  b. Demonstrate technique for cleansing hearing aid within 1 week.
  c. Self-report improved hearing acuity.
28. a. Screening for rubella or syphilis in women who are considering pregnancy
  b. Advocate adequate prenatal care to prevent premature birth.
  c. Administer eye prophylaxis in the form of erythromycin ointment approximately 1 hour after an infant's birth.
  d. Periodic screening of children, especially newborns through preschoolers, for congenital blindness and visual impairment caused by refractive error and strabismus
29. Refractive error such as nearsightedness
30. a. Family history
  b. Prenatal infection
  c. Low birth weight
  d. Chronic ear infection
  e. Down syndrome

31.

Sense	Common Sensory Deficits	Interventions to Minimize Loss
Vision	Presbyopia: A gradual decline in the ability of the lens to accommodate or to focus on close objects. Individual is unable to see near objects clearly.	Wearing sunglasses
	Cataract: Cloudy or opaque areas in part of the lens or the entire lens that interfere with passage of light through the lens, causing problems with glare and blurred vision. Cataracts usually develop gradually without pain, redness, or tearing in the eye.	Use of yellow or amber lenses and shades or blinds on windows to minimize the glare
	Dry eyes: Result when tear glands produce too few tears, resulting in itching, burning, or even reduced vision.	Warm incandescent lighting
	Glaucoma: A slowly progressive increase in intraocular pressure that causes progressive pressure against the optic nerve, resulting in peripheral visual loss, decreased visual acuity with difficulty adapting to darkness, and a halo effect around lights if left untreated.	Use glasses
	Diabetic retinopathy: Pathological changes occur in the blood vessels of the retina, resulting in decreased vision or vision loss caused by hemorrhage and macular edema.	A pocket magnifier
	Macular degeneration: Condition in which the macula (specialized portion of the retina responsible for central vision) loses its ability to function efficiently. First signs include blurring of reading matter, distortion or loss of central vision, and distortion of vertical lines.	Larger print in books
Hearing	Presbycusis: A common progressive hearing disorder in older adults.	Amplify the sound of telephones and TVs
	Cerumen accumulation: Buildup of earwax in the external auditory canal. Cerumen becomes hard, collects in the canal, and causes a conduction deafness.	Ensure that the problem is not cercumen
Taste and smell	Xerostomia: Decrease in salivary production that leads to thicker mucus and a dry mouth. Often interferes with the ability to eat and leads to appetite and nutritional problems.	Good oral hygiene keeps the taste buds well hydrated. Well-seasoned, differently textured food eaten separately heightens taste perception. Flavored vinegar or lemon juice adds tartness to food. Always ask the patient what foods are most appealing. Improvement in taste perception improves food intake and appetite as well.
		Stimulation of the sense of smell with aromas such as brewed coffee, cooked garlic, and baked bread heightens taste sensation. The patient needs to avoid blending or mixing foods because these actions make it difficult to identify tastes. Older persons need to chew food thoroughly to allow more food to contact remaining taste buds.

Sense	Common Sensory Deficits	Interventions to Minimize Loss
		You improve smell by strengthening pleasant olfactory stimulation. Make the patient's environment more pleasant with smells such as cologne, mild room deodorizers, fragrant flowers, and sachets. The removal of unpleasant odors (e.g., bedpans, soiled dressings) will also improve the quality of a patient's environment.
Touch	With aging, there are decreased skin receptors. Patients with reduced tactile sensation usually have the impairment over a limited portion of their bodies.	Providing touch therapy stimulates existing function. If the patient is willing to be touched, hair brushing and combing, a back rub, and touching of the arms or shoulders are ways of increasing tactile contact. When sensation is reduced, firm pressure is often necessary for the patient to feel the nurse's hand. Turning and repositioning will also improve the quality of tactile sensation. When performing invasive procedures, it is important to use touch by holding the patient's hands and keeping them warm and dry.
		If a patient is overly sensitive to tactile stimuli (hyperesthesia), minimize irritating stimuli. Keeping bed linens loose to minimize direct contact with the patient and protecting the skin from exposure to irritants are helpful measures.

32. a. Listen to the patient and wait for the patient to communicate. Do not shout or speak loudly (hearing loss is not the problem). If the patient has problems with comprehension, use simple, short questions and facial gestures to give additional clues. Speak of things familiar and of interest to the patient. If the patient has problems speaking, ask questions that require simple yes or no answers or blinking of the eyes. Offer pictures or a communication board so the patient can point. Give the patient time to understand; be calm and patient; do not pressure or tire the patient. Avoid patronizing and childish phrases.

b. Use pictures, objects, or word cards so that the patient can point. Offer a pad and pencil or Magic Slate for the patient to write messages. Do not shout or speak loudly. Give the patient time to write messages because these patients become easily fatigued. Provide an artificial voice box (vibrator) for the patient with a laryngectomy to use to speak.

c. Get the patient's attention. Do not startle the patient when entering the room. Do not approach a patient from behind. Be sure the patient knows that you wish to speak. Face the patient and stand or sit on the same level. Be sure your face and lips are illuminated to promote lip-reading. Keep your hands away from your mouth. Be sure that patients keep eyeglasses clean so they are able to see your gestures and face. If the patient wears a hearing aid, make sure it is in place and working. Speak slowly and articulate clearly. Older adults often take longer to process verbal messages. Use a normal tone of voice and inflections of speech. Do not

speak with something in your mouth. When you are not understood, rephrase rather than repeat the conversation. Use visible expressions. Speak with your hands, your face, and your eyes. Do not shout. Loud sounds are usually higher pitched and often impede hearing by accentuating vowel sounds and concealing consonants. If you need to raise your voice, speak in lower tones. Talk toward the patient's best or normal ear. Use written information to enhance the spoken word. Do not restrict a deaf patient's hands. Never have IV lines in both of the patient's hands if the preferred method of communication is sign language. Avoid eating, chewing, or smoking while speaking. Avoid speaking from another room or while walking away.

33. a. Orientation to the environment: name tags are visible, address the patient by name, explain to the patient any transfers, note physical boundaries

b. Communication: Depends on the type of aphasia (Box 49-8, p. 1255).

c. Control sensory stimuli: Prevent overload by organizing patient's care with periods of rest; control extraneous noise.

d. Safety measures: Help with ambulation, sighted guide, frequent repositioning.

34. a. Spend time with a person in silence or conversation.

b. Use physical contact (holding a hand, embracing a shoulder) to convey caring.

c. Help recommend alterations in living arrangements if physical isolation is a factor.

d. Assist older adults in keeping in contact with people important to them.

e. Help obtain information about mutual help groups.

f. Arrange for security escort services as needed.

g. Bring a pet that is easy to care for into the home.

h. Link a person with religious organizations attuned to the social needs of older adults.

35. The nature of a patient's alterations influences how the nurse would evaluate the outcome of care. If the expected outcomes have not been achieved, there needs to be a change in the interventions or an alteration in the patient's environment. The nurse also needs to evaluate the integrity of the sensory organs and the patient's ability to perceive stimuli.

36. 1. Caused by sensory deprivation related to restrictive environment of the hospital

37. 4. The presence or absence of meaningful stimuli (i.e., constant TV) influences alertness and the ability to participate in care.

38. 3. Priorities need to be set in regard to the type and extent of the sensory alteration, and safety is always a top priority.

39. 4. Motor type of aphasia

40. a. Understanding of how a sensory deficit can affect the patient's functional status; knowledge of therapies that promote or restore sensory function; the role of other health care professionals that might provide sensory function management; services of community resources; adult learning principles to apply when educating the patient and the family

b. Previous patient responses to planned nursing interventions to promote sensory function

c. Individualized therapies that allow the patient to adapt to sensory loss in any setting; standards of safety

d. Using creativity to find interventions that help the patient adapt to the home environment

e. Ms. Long will maintain independence in a safe home environment by selecting strategies to assist the patient in remaining functional at home, adapting therapies for any sensory deficit, involving the family in helping the patient; refer to appropriate health care professional agencies.

CHAPTER 50

1. a. Preoperative (before)
   b. Intraoperative (during)
   c. Postoperative (after surgery)

2. d   8. b
3. h   9. l
4. j   10. f
5. c   11. k
6. g   12. a
7. i   13. e

14. See Table 50-2, p. 1263.

15. a. Smoking
    b. Age: Very young and older adult
    c. Nutrition: Poor tolerance to anesthesia, negative nitrogen balance
    d. Obesity: Atelectasis and pneumonia
    e. Obstructive sleep apnea: Oxygen desaturation
    f. Immunosuppression: Infection
    g. Fluid and electrolyte imbalance

h. Post op nausea and vomiting

i. Venous thromboembolism

16. See Table 50-3, pp. 1264-1265.

17. Identify a patient's normal preoperative function and the presence of any risks to recognize, prevent, and minimize possible postoperative complications.

18. See Table 50-4, p. 1268.

19. See Table 50-5, p. 1270.

20. a. Smoking places the patient at greater risk for pulmonary complication because of an increased amount and thickness of mucous secretions in the lungs.

b. Alcohol and substance use predisposes the patient to adverse reactions to anesthetic agents and cross-tolerance to anesthetic agents; malnourishment also leads to delayed wound healing.

21. a. The patient and family's expectations for pain management after surgery

b. The patient's perceived tolerance to pain

c. Exploring past experiences and prior successful interventions used

22. Have the patient identify personal strengths and weaknesses; poor self-concept hinders the ability to adapt to the stress of surgery and aggravates feelings of guilt or inadequacy.

23. Assess for body image alterations that patients perceive will result, taking into consideration culture, age, self-concept, and self-esteem; removal of body parts often leaves permanent disfigurement, alteration in body function, or concern over mutilation, loss of body function.

24. Discussion of feelings and self-concept reveals whether the patient is able to cope with the stress of surgery, past stress management and behaviors used, and coping resources.

25. a. General survey
    b. Head and neck
    c. Integument
    d. Thorax and lungs
    e. Heart and vascular system
    f. Abdomen
    g. Neurologic status

26. See Table 50-6, p. 1274.

27. a. Ineffective Airway Clearance
    b. Anxiety
    c. Ineffective Coping
    d. Impaired Skin Integrity
    e. Risk for Aspiration
    f. Risk for Perioperative Positioning Injury
    g. Risk for Infection
    h. Deficient Knowledge
    i. Impaired Physical Mobility
    j. Ineffective Thermoregulation
    k. Nausea
    l. Acute Pain
    m. Delayed Surgical Recovery

28. a. Performs deep breathing and coughing exercises upon awakening from anesthesia

b. Performs postoperative leg exercises and ambulation

c. Performs incentive spirometry upon return to patient care

d. Patient verbalizes rationale for early ambulation 24 hours postoperatively.

29. Informed consent for surgery (surgeon's responsibility) involves the patient's understanding of the need for a procedure, steps involved, risks, expected results, and alternative treatments.

30. a. Improves the ability and willingness to deep breathe and cough effectively
   b. Improves understanding and willingness to ambulate and resume activities of ADL
   c. Have less anxiety
   d. Reduces stay by preventing or minimizing complications
   e. Less anxious about pain; ask what they need and require less after surgery

31. a. Patient understands reasons for preoperative instructions and exercises.
   b. Preoperative routines
   c. Surgical procedure
   d. Time of surgery
   e. Postoperative unit and location of family during surgery and recovery
   f. Anticipated postoperative monitoring and therapies
   g. Sensory preparation
   h. Postoperative activity resumption
   i. Pain-relief measures

32. a. Reduction of risk of surgical wound infection—skin asepsis
   b. Maintain normal fluid and electrolyte balance
   c. Prevention of bowel and bladder incontinence

33. a. Hygiene
   b. Hair and cosmetics
   c. Removal of prostheses
   d. Safeguarding valuables
   e. Preparing the bowel and bladder
   f. Vital signs
   g. Prevention of deep vein thrombosis (DVT)
   h. Administering preoperative medications
   i. Documentation and handoff
   j. Eliminating the wrong site and wrong procedure surgery

34. a. The circulating nurse reviews the preoperative assessment, establishes and implements the intraoperative plan of care, evaluates the care, and provides for continuity of care postoperatively.
   b. The scrub nurse maintains a sterile field during the surgical procedure and assists with supplies.

35. a. Ineffective Airway Clearance
   b. Risk for Deficient Fluid Volume
   c. Risk for Perioperative Positioning Injury
   d. Risk for Impaired Skin Integrity
   e. Risk for Thermal Injury
   f. Risk for Injury

36. General anesthesia is given by IV and inhalation routes through three phases (induction, maintenance, and emergence), resulting in an immobile, quiet patient who does not recall the surgical procedure.

37. Regional anesthesia results in loss of sensation in an area of the body via spinal, epidural, or a peripheral nerve block with no loss of consciousness.

38. Local anesthesia involves the loss of sensation at the desired site; common for minor procedures.

39. Conscious sedation is routinely used for procedures that do not require complete anesthesia but rather a depressed level of consciousness.

40. a. Immediate postoperative recovery (phase I)
   b. Recovery in ambulatory surgery (phase II)

41. Responsibilities include maintaining the patient's airway, respiratory, circulatory, and neurologic status and managing pain.

42. The patient will show vital sign stability, temperature control, good ventilatory function and oxygenation status, orientation to surroundings, absence of complications, minimal pain and nausea, controlled wound drainage, adequate output, and fluid and electrolyte balance.

43. Every 15 minutes twice, every 30 minutes twice, and then hourly for 2 hours and then every 4 hours or per orders

44. a. History of obstructive sleep apnea (OSA)
   b. Weak pharyngeal or laryngeal muscle tone from anesthetics
   c. Secretions in the pharynx, bronchial tree, or trachea
   d. Laryngeal or subglottic edema

45. Careful assessment of heart rate and rhythm, along with blood pressure, reveals the patient's cardiovascular status; capillary perfusion—note refill, pulses, and the color and temperature of the nail beds.

46. Hypercarbia, tachypnea, tachycardia, premature ventricular contractions (PVC), unstable blood pressure, cyanosis, skin mottling, and muscular rigidity

47. a. Assess the hydration status and monitor cardiac and neurological function.
   b. Monitor and compare laboratory values.
   c. Maintain patency of IV lines.
   d. Record accurately the I & O, daily weights.
   e. Assess daily weight for the first several days after surgery and compare with the preoperative weight.

48. a. Orientation to self and the hospital
   b. Pupil and gag reflexes, hand grips, and movement of all extremities
   c. Neurologic assessment
   d. Extremity strength

49. a. A rash can indicate a drug sensitivity or allergy.
   b. Abrasions or petechiae result from inappropriate positioning or restraining that injures skin layers or from a clotting disorder.
   c. Burns may indicate that an electrical cautery grounding pad was incorrectly placed.

50. a. Accumulation of gas
   b. Development of a paralytic ileus

51. a. Ineffective Airway Clearance
   b. Anxiety
   c. Fear
   d. Risk for Infection

e. Deficient Knowledge
f. Impaired Physical Mobility
g. Nausea
h. Acute Pain
i. Delayed Surgical Recovery
j. Impaired Skin Integrity

52. a. Frequency of VS assessments
    b. Types of IV fluids and rates
    c. Postoperative medications
    d. Resumption of preoperative medications
    e. Fluid and food allowed
    f. Level of activity
    g. Positions
    h. Intake and output
    i. Laboratory tests and radiography studies
    j. Special directions related to drains, irrigations, and dressings

53. a. Patient's incision remains closed and intact.
    b. Patient's incision remains free of infectious drainage.
    c. Patient remains afebrile.

54. a. Encourage diaphragmatic breathing exercises every hour.
    b. Administer CPAP or NIPPV to patients who use this modality at home.
    c. Use incentive spirometer for maximum inspiration.
    d. Early ambulation.
    e. Turn the patient on his or her sides every 1 to 2 hours and have the patient sit when possible.
    f. Keep the patient comfortable.
    g. Encourage coughing exercises every 1 to 2 hours and maintain pain control.
    h. Provide oral hygiene.
    i. Initiate orotracheal or nasotracheal suction for inability to cough.
    j. Administer oxygen and monitor saturation.

55. See Table 50-8, pp. 1291-1292.

56. a. Encourage the patient to perform leg exercises at least every 4 hours while awake.
    b. Apply graded compression stockings or pneumatic compression stockings.
    c. Encourage early ambulation.
    d. Avoid positioning the patient in a manner that interrupts blood flow to the extremities.
    e. Administer anticoagulant drugs as ordered.
    f. Provide adequate fluid intake orally or IV.

57. Incision area, drainage tubes, tight dressing or casts, muscular strains caused by positioning

58. a. Maintain a gradual progression in dietary intake (clear liquids, full liquids, light diet, usual diet).
    b. Promote ambulation and exercise.
    c. Maintain an adequate fluid intake.
    d. Stimulate the patient's appetite (remove noxious odors, positioning, desired foods, oral hygiene).
    e. Fiber supplements, stool softeners
    f. Provide meals when patient is rested and free from pain.

59. a. Assume normal position.
    b. Check frequently for the need to void.
    c. Assess for bladder distention.
    d. Monitor I & O.

60. a. Provide privacy with dressing changes or inspection of the wound.
    b. Maintain patient's hygiene.
    c. Prevent drainage devices from overflowing.
    d. Provide a pleasant environment.
    e. Offer opportunities for the patient to discuss fears or concerns.
    f. Provide the families with opportunities to discuss ways to promote self-concept.

61. 1. Increases susceptibility to infection and impairs wound healing from altered glucose metabolism and associated circulatory impairment

62. 1. That is a medical decision and the responsibility of the provider.

63. 3. All of the other patients are predisposed to an imbalance either to existing losses, fluid overload, or the inability to obtain oral fluids.

64. 2. Promotes normal venous return and circulatory blood flow

65. 2. Not always a sign of hypothermia but rather a side effect of certain anesthetic agents

66. a. Evaluate Mrs. Campana's knowledge of surgical procedure and planned postoperative care. Have Mrs. Campana demonstrate postoperative exercises. Observe behaviors or nonverbal expressions of anxiety or fear. Ask if patient's expectations are being met.
    b. Behaviors that demonstrate learning; characteristics of anxiety or fear; signs and symptoms or conditions that contraindicate surgery
    c. Previous patient responses to planned preoperative care; any personal experience with surgery
    d. Use established expected outcomes to evaluate Mrs. Campana's plan of care (ability to perform postoperative exercises).
    e. Demonstrate perseverance when Mrs. Campana has difficulty performing postoperative exercises.